PATHOGENESIS OF ENCEPHALITIS

Edited by **Daisuke Hayasaka**

Pathogenesis of Encephalitis
Edited by Daisuke Hayasaka

Published by InTech

Janeza Trdine 9, 51000 Rijeka, Croatia

Publishing Process Manager Masa Vidovic

Technical Editor Teodora Smiljanic

Cover Designer InTech Design Team

Additional hard copies can be obtained from orders@intechopen.com

Pathogenesis of Encephalitis, Edited by Daisuke Hayasaka
p. cm.
ISBN 978-953-307-741-3

For EU product safety concerns:
IN TECH d.o.o., Prolaz Marije Krucifikse Kozulić 3, 51000 Rijeka, Croatia,
info@intechopen.com or visit our website at intechopen.com.

Meet the editor

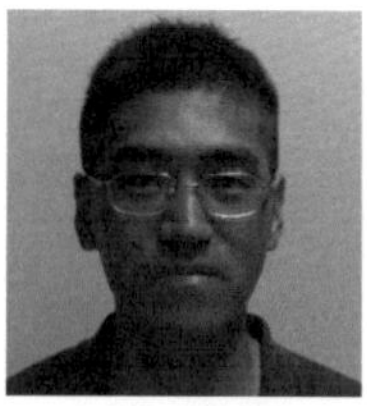

Dr. Daisuke Hayasaka is a research scientist at the Institute of Tropical Medicine (Nekken) at Nagasaki University in Japan. He received his PhD in Veterinary Medicine at the Graduate school of Veterinary Medicine at Hokkaido University. He had a postdoctoral training at the Center for Infectious Disease and Vaccine Research at the University of Massachusetts Medical School in the USA. His research interest is on the pathogenesis of neurotropic viruses, especially encephalitic viruses that include Japanese encephalitis virus and tick-borne encephalitis virus.

Contents

Preface

Many infectious agents, including viruses, bacteria, and parasites, can cause central nervous system (CNS) inflammation. Encephalitis is an inflammation of the brain parenchyma, and those cases with more serious and advanced symptoms usually result in meningoencephalitis. In order to overcome encephalitis, it is a priority to elucidate the mechanism of pathogenesis, to establish accurate diagnosis, and develop effective vaccines and drugs. This book provides comprehensive commentaries on encephalitis. The first section covers diagnoses and clinical symptoms: the topics on biomarkers, diagnosis, childhood and elderly population, limbic encephalitis, language and cognitive impairment, and standardized case. The second section reviews some virus infections concerning SSPE, HSV, and HIV, while providing outlines of inflammatory and chemokine responses. The third section addresses the other agents of encephalitis, such as angiostrongyliasis, cryptococcal meningitis, and clostridium, and describes superantigen-mediated encephalitis, Rasmussen's encephaliti, anti-NMDA receptor encephalitis, and non-herpetic acute limbic encephalitis. The last section discusses the experimental model of encephalitis, including topics on the mechanism of ADEM and AHLE, autoimmune encephalitis in a non-human primate, antibody phage display, and alternative medicines for encephalitis. These chapters provide valuable and important information not only to researchers, but also to physician and health care workers.

I am deeply grateful to all of the authors for preparing the chapter assigned to them, and for doing a great job. Also, I would like to thank Masa Vidovic and Ana Nikolic, from InTech Open Access, for kind and helpful support during the completion of this book.

Daisuke Hayasaka
Department of Virology, Institute of Tropical Medicine,
Nagasaki University,
Japan

Part 1

Diagnosis and Clinical Symptoms of Encephalitis

1

Biomarkers of Encephalitis

Dafna Bonneh-Barkay
Department of Pathology, University of Pittsburgh, USA

1. Introduction

The development of encephalitis presents a dilemma to the clinician as during the early stages, when treatment would be most effective, the symptoms can be nonspecific with a broad differential. Imaging tests (e.g. magnetic resonance imaging and computed axial tomography scan), blood and urine tests as well as lumbar puncture are used to isolate and identify viruses, and together with careful and continuous neurological assessment provide data that may be suggestive of viral encephalitis. In the case of post-infectious or autoimmune encephalitis, a more intense investigation is needed to generate an accurate diagnosis. In addition to imaging tests and electroencephalography, blood and cerebrospinal fluid (CSF) need to be analyzed for evidence of inflammation and the presence of antibodies against cellular antigens. In recent years clinicians and investigators have pursued biomarkers that can aid in the diagnosis as well as prognosis and monitoring of patients with encephalitis. These biomarkers are increasingly important in the recognition and treatment of inflammatory and autoimmune central nervous system (CNS) disorders. This chapter will review the current literature of emerging biomarkers in the different types of encephalitis.

2. Infectious encephalitis

2.1 HIV encephalitis

HIV encephalitis (HIVE) is characterized by the presence of microglial nodules, multinucleated giants cells, glial activation and neuronal loss (Budka 1991). About 25% of immunosuppressed patients infected with HIV develop neurological deficits ranging from cognitive impairments, motor abnormalities, behavioral symptoms to HIV-associated dementia (HAD) (Dore et al 1999; Nath & Sacktor 2006). In HIVE macrophages/microglia are productively infected with HIV and are hypothesized to play a pivotal role in the neurodegenerative process leading to HAD (Ellis et al 2007; Navia et al 1986). The need to diagnose the pathogenic process of HIVE and HAD led to the pursuit for plasma and CSF biomarkers that might provide insight into pathogenesis and also facilitate the diagnosis and disease staging in addition to clinical signs and symptoms.

Historically, HIV-1 RNA load was measured in the brain and CSF of HIV-infected patients to verify whether it could be a marker of HIV-induced neuropathology (Achim et al 1994; Cinque et al 1998). Cinque et al. examined HIV-infected patients with neurological symptoms for the presence of HIV-1 p24 antigen by immunohistochemistry as well as CSF HIV-1 RNA by quantitative polymerase chain reaction (PCR). Their results showed that CSF

HIV-1 RNA copy numbers were significantly higher in patients with HIV encephalitis than in patients without encephalitis. From this study they concluded that CSF HIV-1 RNA levels were associated with HIVE and the associated neuropathology (Cinque et al 1998). Although there were studies that did not show significant difference in CSF levels of HIV-1 RNA between patients with or without HIVE (Bossi et al 1998) many studies in non-human primates infected with simian immunodeficiency virus (SIV) confirmed a correlation between SIV viral load and encephalitis (Bissel et al 2008; Bonneh-Barkay et al 2008; Zink et al 1999; Zink et al 2005).

Because macrophages are the predominant immune cell and the predominant infected cell in the brains of patients with HIVE, it was assumed that immune activation-associated factors in the CSF could serve as a surrogate biomarker for the disease. One of those factors is neopterin, an intermediate of pteridine metabolism, that is produced by activated macrophages in response to cytokines (Anderson et al 2002; Williams & Hickey 2002) that was also found to predict systemic disease progression (Fuchs et al 1989b) . Several studies showed that neopterin was elevated in the CSF of HIV-infected patients, particularly patients with HAD (Brew et al 1990; Fuchs et al 1989a; Sonnerborg et al 1989). However Wiley et al. did not find a strong correlation between CSF neopterin and severity of encephalitis in autopsied patients with HIVE (Wiley et al 1992). A recent study by Hagberg at al. showed that in untreated HIV-infected patients CSF neopterin concentrations were almost always elevated and increased progressively as immunosuppression worsens and blood CD4 cell counts fell. Patients with HAD exhibit particularly high CSF neopterin concentrations, above those of patients without neurological disease suggesting that this might be a useful CNS disease marker (Hagberg et al 2010).

Additional factors that suggest immune activation are of course cytokines and chemokines. Previous studies showed that some HIV patients exhibited elevated CSF levels of interleukin-1β (IL-1β) and interleukin-6 (IL-6) but no tumor necrosis factor-α (TNFα) or interleukin-2 (IL-2) were detected (Gallo et al 1989). In contrast other studies reported high levels of CSF TNFα in HIV-1 sero-positive patients who had neurologic involvement (Sharief et al 1992). The profile of cytokines may differ according to the level of macrophage/microglia infection or activation or the presence of opportunistic infections. Previous studies have also tried to establish correlations between CSF chemokines and CSF HIV viral load. Increased CSF levels of chemokines like CCL2 (also known as MCP-1), were reported in patients with HIVE and HAD (Kelder et al 1998). Moreover, recent reports showed a possible association between CSF CCL2 levels and the development of HAD, suggesting that this chemokine could be used as a biomarker of disease progression (Cinque et al 2005; Sevigny et al 2004; Sevigny et al 2007). Furthermore Almeida et al. obtained similar results and also suggested that CCL2 expression was associated with leukocyte transmigration into the CNS (Monteiro de Almeida et al 2006; Monteiro de Almeida et al 2005). In addition, CXCL10 was found to be positively correlated with CSF HIV viral load (Christo et al 2009; Gisolf et al 2000) and CSF pleocytosis (Cinque et al 2005; Kolb et al 1999) suggesting that this chemokine may contribute to HAD pathogenesis (Christo et al 2005).

Activation of the plasminogen system has been reported in different neurological disorders such as stroke and other forms of acute brain injury (Bonneh-Barkay & Wiley 2008). Expression of the urokinase plasminogen activator (uPA) and its receptor (uPAR) was also found in HIV-1-associated CNS disease (Sidenius et al 2004). CSF soluble uPAR levels were significantly higher in HIV-infected patients than in HIV-negative controls. Moreover CSF soluble uPAR levels correlated with CSF HIV-1 RNA, but not with plasma soluble uPAR concentrations. In addition, highly active antiretroviral therapy (HAART) was associated with a significant decrease of CSF soluble uPAR in parallel to reduction in viral load (Cinque et al 2004).

A recently identified biomarker for HIVE is YKL-40 (chitinase 3-like protein 1, HC-gp39). YKL-40 is up-regulated in inflammatory conditions (e.g. Crohn's disease and rheumatoid arthritis) as well as in cancers (e.g. melanoma, glioblastoma, and myeloid leukemia) (Kirkpatrick et al 1997; Rehli et al 2003). In addition it was found to be induced in astrocytes in acute and chronic neurological conditions (Bonneh-Barkay et al 2010a).

Unbiased proteomics approach was used to identify proteins that are differentially expressed in the CSF of SIV-infected macaques that develop encephalitis. Among the proteins that showed differential up-regulation was YKL-40. Longitudinal analysis of CSF from SIV-infected pigtailed macaques showed an increase in YKL-40 concentration 2 to 8 weeks before death from encephalitis. This increase in YKL-40 correlated with an increase in CSF viral load (Bonneh-Barkay et al 2008). Similar results were obtained in CSF from HIV patients. YKL-40 was higher in patients with HIV viral load higher than 10,000 copies/ml (Figure 1A) and there was a significant elevation in CSF YKL-40 in HIV patients with HIVE

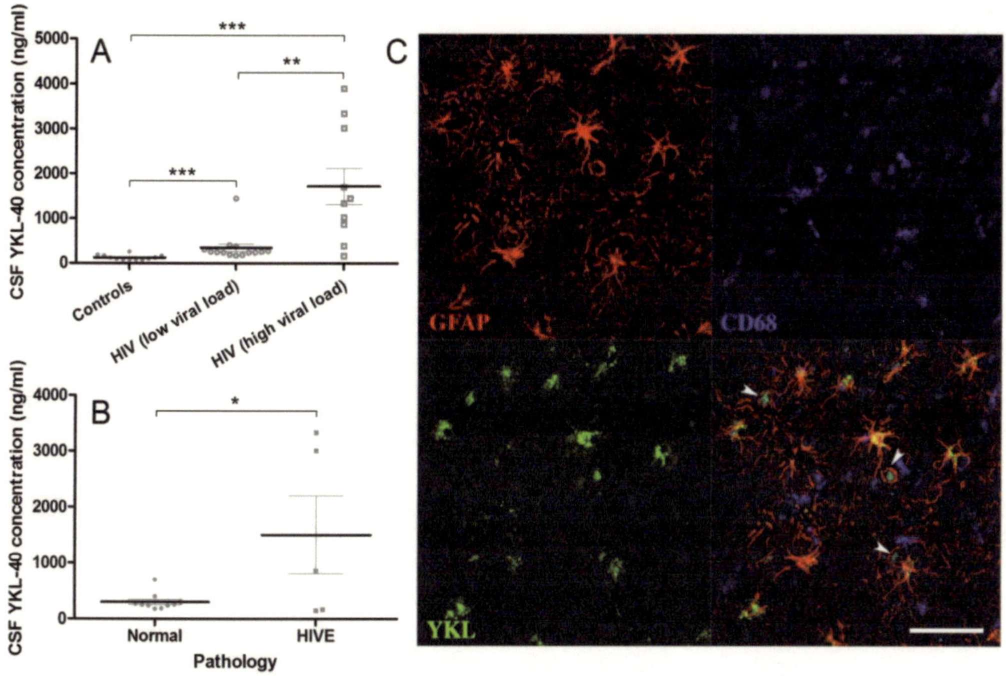

Fig. 1. (A) CSF from HIV-infected patients categorized on the basis of CSF HIV RNA copies (Low viral load=<10,000 HIV copies; High viral load=>10,000 HIV copies) was analyzed for YKL-40. (B) CSF YKL-40 correlation with HIVE pathology. (C) YKL-40 localized in astrocytes and occasional CNS activated macrophage/microglia in HIVE. Triple-label immunofluorescence for YKL-40 (green) and CD68 (blue) or glial fibrillary acidic protein (GFAP) (red). Co-localization of YKL-40 and astrocytes appears as yellow and co-localization of YKL-40 and CD68 positive macrophages is evident as aqua signal (arrowheads); scale bar=50μm (Bonneh-Barkay et al 2008).

versus patients without encephalitis (Figure 1B). Previous studies have shown that high viral load in the CSF correlates with the severity of SIV encephalitis (SIVE) (Bissel et al 2006; Zink et al 1999) and HIVE (Cinque et al 1998; Wiley et al 1998). The correlation between YKL-40 levels and CSF viral load in SIVE and HIVE further support its potential use as a biomarker of HIVE. Immunohistochemistry showed that YKL-40 is expressed in astrocytes in the vicinity of microglial nodules in HIVE (Figure 1C).

It seems that YKL-40 can serve as a biomarker for Neuroinflammation in general as our recent study also showed that CSF YKL-40 levels are elevated in patients with severe traumatic brain injury (TBI), and that they correspond to levels of inflammatory cytokines (Bonneh-Barkay et al 2010b). In addition our previous study showed more pronounced YKL-40 expression in patients with acute infarcts and diminished expression in subacute or older infarcts (Bonneh-Barkay et al 2010a). In that previous study, combined ISH and GFAP staining showed induced YKL-40 expression in astrocytes that was restricted to the penumbra of the infarct. While the precise biological functions of YKL- 40 are speculative, its expression is related to inflammation in a variety of disease states. Further work is required to further evaluate the utility of YKL-40 as a biomarker and its role in Neuroinflammation.

2.2 Herpes simplex encephalitis

Herpes simplex encephalitis (HSE) is an acute or subacute illness, causing both general and focal signs of cerebral dysfunction induced by Herpes simplex virus type 1 (HSV–1) (Kennard & Swash 1981; Koskiniemi et al 1996; Miller & Ross 1968; Sivertsen & Christensen 1996; Whitley et al 1989). HSV invades the CNS and is capable of replicating in neurons and glial cells which produce acute focal, necrotizing encephalitis localized in the temporal and subfrontal regions of the brain, often with a progressive course (Booss & Kim 1984). Early treatment with acyclovir is important to decrease mortality and limit CNS injury in HSE (Skoldenberg 1991). In addition corticosteroids may be given as therapy during the acute phase of HSE in order to reduce inflammation and edema in the CNS (Skoldenberg et al 1984). Despite adequate treatment almost all surviving patients suffer from neurological sequelae. The most common long-term symptoms after HSE are memory impairment, personality and behavioral abnormalities and epilepsy (McGrath et al 1997).

Confirmation of the diagnosis depends on the identification of HSV in the CSF by means of PCR although in some cases the PCR can be negative. In these cases detection of intrathecal synthesis of specific immunoglobulins could be useful (Denes et al 2010; Felgenhauer et al 1982; Felgenhauer & Reiber 1992; Reiber & Lange 1991). Widespread viral replication has not generally been found beyond the acute stage of HSE. Histopathologic studies of autopsy specimens showed that HSV antigen was detected in the brains of 21 out of 29 who died within 3 weeks after the onset of neurologic disease but not in the 8 who died thereafter (Booss & Kim 1984). HSV DNA seems to be cleared from the CSF in about the same period (Aurelius et al 1991), but PCR has shown HSV DNA at autopsy in a few cases of late-stage HSE. Despite lack of firm evidence, it seems that a low-grade continuous or recurrent viral replication may occur in certain foci resulting in continued antigen stimulation. Thus in general PCR is more useful in diagnosing acute HSE.

In HSE there is evidence of a vigorous intrathecal immune response during the acute phase, as shown by increased levels of β2-microglobulin and neopterin in CSF, followed by a chronic phase of low-grade intrathecal inflammation (Aurelius et al 1993). In addition the levels of a variety of CSF cytokines and their receptors are elevated like IL-6, IFNγ, soluble IL-2 receptor (sIL-2R) and soluble CD8 (Asaoka et al 2004; Aurelius et al 1994; Ichiyama et al 2008; Linde et al 1992; Rosler et al 1998). IFNγ and IL-6 levels increased during the first week of HSE while TNFα, IL-2, and soluble CD8 became elevated at 2–6 weeks (Aurelius et al 1994). A more recent study tried to assess whether there is a correlation between cytokines levels and outcomes. Kamei et al. showed that initial IFNγ and maximum IL-6 levels in patients with a poor outcome were higher than those with a good outcome and thus could serve as prognostic biomarkers in HSE (Kamei et al 2009).

Patients with viral CNS infections have previously been studied with regard to neuronal and astroglial markers in CSF (Rosengren et al 1994; Sindic et al 1985). The concentrations and kinetics of these markers in HSE imply that they may be used as brain damage markers to follow individual patients longitudinally or to evaluate therapeutics. Studahl et al. followed neuronal and astroglial marker proteins for up to 6 months in patients with HSE and found markedly higher CSF levels of neuron specific enolase (NSE), neurofilament protein, GFAP and S100 in the acute stage of HSE that was decreased within 45 days after acute infection (Studahl et al 2000). Although high levels of these markers were associated with neurological damage in other acute CNS damaging disorders, such as cerebral infarction (S100 and GFAP) (Aurell et al 1991), neonatal asphyxia (Blennow et al 1995), and after cardiac arrest (NSE) (Karkela et al 1993) Studahl et al. were not able to evaluate the prognostic use of these CSF markers in HSE. It seems that other factors (e.g. duration of disease before start of treatment, age, localization of the infected area and size of hemorrhagic necrosis) can influence the clinical outcome. Bigger cohorts may be needed to determine whether concentrations are correlated with clinical outcome (Studahl et al 2000).

Additional biomarker that might indicate the severity and progression of cerebral injury in HSE is soluble Fas (sFas) which is involved in apoptosis through the Fas/Fas Ligand pathway (Sabri et al 2006). Elevated levels of sFas have been reported in a variety of neurological diseases like HIVE, TBI and multiple sclerosis (De Milito et al 2000; Felderhoff-Mueser et al 2001; Lenzlinger et al 2002; Mogi et al 1996; Sabri et al 2001; Towfighi et al 2004; Zipp et al 1998). Sabri et al. found high levels of sFas in CSF samples collected after neurological onset in 84% of HSE patients. In addition they observed that HSE patients with severe neurological sequels had an increase in changes of CSF sFas as compared to patients with mild or moderate neurological outcome.

In summary, markers of immune activation (e.g. IL-6, IFNγ, neopterin and β2-microglobulin) are found early during the course of HSE and high levels are found to correlate with severe clinical outcome as well as with mortality (Aurelius et al 1993). Additionally there are markers that are indicative of persistent immune activation like soluble IL-2R and CD68 (Aurelius et al 1994).

2.3 Influenza-associated encephalopathy

Influenza-associated encephalopathy (IAE) is a CNS complication with high mortality and neurological sequelae with estimated mortality rate of 27% to 44% (Morishima et al 2002). The clinical symptoms of IAE include symptoms of both flu and CNS dysfunction. CNS neurological manifestations including seizure, altered or loss of consciousness, decreased cognitive performance, motor paralysis or sensory loss, abnormal or delirious behavior, and change in mental status. The neurological complications usually appear within several days of the first symptoms of flu (Wang et al 2010).

The influenza-virus usually can not be detected in the CNS of IAE patients and thus the pathophysiology of IAE remains unclear. The early studies reported that thrombocytopenia and severely elevated serum aspartate aminotransaminase levels were associated with a poor prognosis (Morishima et al 2002). High concentration levels of various cytokine such as IL-6 and TNFα have been reported (Aiba et al 2001; Hosoya et al 2005; Ichiyama et al 1998; Togashi et al 2004). Ichiyama et al. reported significantly higher levels of serum and CSF IL-6 in the IAE group with a poor prognosis relative to the group without sequelae. In addition serum levels of soluble TNFR1 and IL-10 levels were higher (Hasegawa et al 2011; Ichiyama et al 2004). Hosoya et al. reported significantly elevated levels of TNFα and cytochrome c concentrations in patients with poor prognosis as compared to good outcome (Hosoya et al 2005). The authors suggested that apoptosis of the CNS parenchyma contributes to the cerebral atrophy observed in patients with sequelae.

Recently, a new test for the evaluation of oxidative status, the Diacron-Reactive Oxygen Metabolites (d-ROM) test, has become available (Cesarone et al 1999). Yamanaka et al. assessed the prognostic value of serum and CSF d-ROM levels of patients with IAE in the initial stage (Yamanaka et al 2008; Yamanaka et al 2006). CSF d-ROM levels showed that the oxidative trend status corresponds to the therapeutic response and thus oxidative stress may be related to the pathogenesis of IAE. Similar results by Kawashima et al. showed high concentrations of NOx levels in the serum and CSF of the patients with IAE during the initial stage (Kawashima et al 2002; Kawashima et al 2003).

Another approach to discovering specific biomarkers of patients with IAE was to analyze all metabolites in CSF by using metabolome analysis. Two metabolites (molecular weights: 246.0092 and 204.0611) were significantly higher than those in other diseases including influenza without convulsion. These results indicate that the metabolites detected in CSF could serve as primary markers for the diagnosis of IAE (Kawashima et al 2006).

2.4 West Nile Virus encephalitis

West Nile virus (WNV) is a mosquito-borne, neurotropic , single-stranded sense RNA flavivirus (Brehin et al 2008). The classical symptoms of WNV infection range from fever (Hayes & Gubler 2006; Leis & Stokic 2005; Leis et al 2002; Leis et al 2003; Nash et al 2001; Sejvar et al 2003; Tilley et al 2007) to CNS disease of severe meningoencephalitis (Petersen & Marfin 2002). Clinical symptoms of CNS disease include persistent weakness, flaccid paralysis, myelitis, ataxia, seizures, or change in mental status. Neurological signs in WNV infection have been reported in about 42% of the cases.

One of the main diagnostic criteria for neurologic involvement in WNV infection is the presence of WNV IgM in CSF though it can be detected in the CSF for more than 6 months (Kapoor et al 2004). Therefore a more specific marker is necessary in order to distinguish WNV from other infections with neurological symptoms. Nixon et al. evaluated CSF WNV IgA as a marker of WNV neuroinvasive infection but found that it had equivalent value to IgM (Nixon & Prince 2006).

In addition to specific antibodies, protein biomarkers are an attractive tool for assessing neuronal death and glial pathology. Petzold et al. showed a significant elevation of those CSF proteins like GFAP, S100B, and neurofilament-SMI35 in patients suffering from WNV CNS disease (Petzold et al 2010). However, CSF GFAP and S100B were also increased in all of patients with WNV fever only thus decreasing their usefulness as a biomarker for CNS disease. Interestingly, in patients that died from the disease high CSF S100B levels were related to a shorter time to death.

In summary, most of the studies aiming to discover biomarkers of viral encephalitides were targeted towards studying known pathways believed to be involved in immune activation or cell damage. These studies, however, have achieved limited success. Over the last few years, unbiased proteomic techniques have been utilized to discover novel biomarkers in different diseases without the a priori selection of specific proteins (Romeo et al 2005). In recent years there are more and more studies using those techniques to discover biomarkers in neurological conditions and neurodegenerative diseases (e.g. multiple sclerosis and Alzheimer's disease) (Craig-Schapiro et al 2010; Ottervald et al 2010; Perrin et al 2011). Unbiased proteomics profiling is very complex and requires a multi-discipline approach from sample preparation and protein identification to data processing and validation. These analyses most likely will result a combination of candidate biomarkers that will need to be tested in larger cohorts.

3. Autoimmune encephalitis

Autoimmune encephalitis encompasses a variety of disorders resulting from an immune reaction against antigens expressed in neurons. As a result there is rapidly progressive cognitive decline and behavioral abnormalities. The antibodies against those antigens are important markers for these disorders (Vitaliani et al 2008).

3.1 Limbic encephalitis

Paraneoplastic neurologic disorders are immunologic complications induced by malignancies that express proteins that are usually restricted to the CNS (Vernino et al 2007). They are characterized by memory impairment, temporal lobe seizures and psychiatric symptoms. The most common tumors associated with paraneoplastic neurological disorders are small-cell lung carcinoma (SCLC), testicular cancer, thymoma and breast cancer (Ahern et al 1994; Gultekin et al 2000; Vernino & Lennon 2004).

A variety of autoantibody markers are associated with limbic encephalitis like anti-Hu and anti-CV2/CRMP5 (Gultekin et al 2000; Voltz 2002). In recent years different subtypes of this disorder have been discovered as well as new antigens. Anti-N-Methyl-D-aspartate receptor (NMDAR) encephalitis was identified as a subtype of limbic encephalitis. This disease usually starts with an episode of fever, headache, or malaise, followed by mood and behavioral changes, psychiatric symptoms and decline of consciousness that could deteriorate to death. It usually affects young women and is associated with ovarian teratoma. These patients demonstrate serum and CSF presence of antibodies against NMDA receptor subunit 1 (NR1) and NMDA receptor subunit 2 (NR2) (Iizuka et al 2008). Additional subtype of limbic encephalitis is characterized by antibodies against voltage gated potassium channels (VGKC) (Buckley et al 2001; Thieben et al 2004; Vincent et al 2004). VGKC limbic encephalitis is mostly non-paraneoplastic, although VGKC antibodies have been found in a small number of patients with tumors (Pozo-Rosich et al 2003). Jarius et al. showed that even patients without CSF pathological findings or inflammatory changes can be positive for VGKC antibodies (Jarius et al 2008).

Non-herpetic acute limbic encephalitis (NHALE) has been identified as a new subgroup of limbic encephalitis with a clinical presentation which is similar to HSE (Asaoka et al 2004; Ichiyama et al 2009; Kusuhara et al 1994; Shoji et al 2004). Autopsy cases showed neuronal loss and severe gliosis with inflammatory cell infiltrations in the hippocampus and amygdala. Examination of the CSF revealed occasional mild pleocytosis, and increased IL-6 levels (Ichiyama et al 2008; Shoji 2010). Recent reports associate the disease with the presence of anti-glutamate receptor epsilon 2 antibodies (Shoji 2010). Takahashi et al. reported the presence of those antibodies in the serum and CSF of patients in acute and chronic stages (Takahashi et al 2010).

3.2 Hashimoto's encephalopathy

Hashimoto's encephalopathy (HE) is a rare autoimmune disease affecting mostly women that is associated with elevated titers of antithyroid antibodies in serum and CSF (Brain et al 1966; Chong et al 2003). HE is characterized by various neuropsychological symptoms, including personality changes, cognition deterioration, seizures, myoclonus and loss consciousness (Ghika-Schmid et al 1996; Henchey et al 1995; Kothbauer-Margreiter et al 1996; Mijajlovic et al 2010; Peschen-Rosin et al 1999; Shaw et al 1991). HE patients show high CSF protein levels (oligoclonal bands or an increased total protein concentration) without pleocytosis and high titer of antithyroid antibodies (Archambeaud et al 2001; Ferracci & Carnevale 2006; Hartmann et al 2000; Shaw et al 1991). The etiology of the disease is not entirely clear but there are some reports claiming an inflammatory response to antineuronal antibodies (Oide et al 2004; Takahashi et al 1994).

3.3 Rasmussen's encephalitis

Rasmussen's encephalitis is an acquired progressive inflammatory encephalopathy characterized by seizures and cognitive deterioration resulting from an atrophy of a single brain hemisphere. Rasmussen's encephalitis is divided into two clinical subtypes by the existence of epilepsia partialis continua (EPC). EPC is characterized by continuous myoclonic jerks of the extremities and/or the face, usually without impairment of consciousness (Takahashi et al 1997). The etiology of the disease has been hypothesized to be associated with an autoimmune process mediated through antibodies against the glutamate receptor subunit 3, (Mastrangelo et al 2010). Takahashi et al. reported that antibodies against NMDA type GluRε2 were detected in Rasmussen's encephalitis patients with and without EPC (Pleasure 2008; Takahashi et al 2003; Takahashi et al 2005). This suggests that autoantibodies against GluRε2 are important for the diagnosis of both subtypes of Rasmussen's encephalitis, independent of EPC.

4. Conclusion

Viral and autoimmune disorders of the CNS are a heterogeneous group of disorders. Many viruses are known to cause acute viral encephalitis in humans which can cause a variable degree of meningeal as well as parenchymal inflammation. CSF abnormalities typically consists lymphocytic pleocytosis and protein elevation. Identification of viral antigens, viral nucleic acid or antibody analysis may provide an important diagnostic help in addition to imaging (e.g. CT scan and MRI) (Debiasi & Tyler 2004). The clinical and laboratory findings in many of those viral and autoimmune disorders are largely similar and thus more specific biomarkers for diagnostic and prognostic purposes are warranted. These biomarkers are increasingly important in the recognition and treatment of viral and autoimmune CNS disorders (Dale & Brilot 2010).

Many of the viral encephalitides are accompanied by CSF markers for immune activation like β_2 microglobulin and neopterin or elevated levels of cytokines and chemokines in addition to the presence of the virus or viral antigens. Many studies also tried to predict the progression of the disease and response to therapeutics base on those biomarkers. Despite the plethora of surrogate markers of immune activation and neuronal and glial destruction, their clinical use is still obscure in that there are no clinical trials that showed a correlation with clinical status and that they respond to a therapeutic intervention. There is a great need for validation of these studies in larger trials before surrogate marker measurements would be accepted universally as clinical end-points. In conclusion, although more and more studies were aimed to identify specific biomarkers for each type of encephalitis there is still need for more studies to validate their use in larger trials.

5. References

Achim CL, Wang R, Miners DK, Wiley CA. 1994. Brain viral burden in HIV infection. *J Neuropathol Exp Neurol* 53:284-94

Ahern GL, O'Connor M, Dalmau J, Coleman A, Posner JB, et al. 1994. Paraneoplastic temporal lobe epilepsy with testicular neoplasm and atypical amnesia. *Neurology* 44:1270-4

Aiba H, Mochizuki M, Kimura M, Hojo H. 2001. Predictive value of serum interleukin-6 level in influenza virus-associated encephalopathy. *Neurology* 57:295-9

Anderson E, Zink W, Xiong H, Gendelman HE. 2002. HIV-1-associated dementia: a metabolic encephalopathy perpetrated by virus-infected and immune-competent mononuclear phagocytes. *J Acquir Immune Defic Syndr* 31 Suppl 2:S43-54

Archambeaud F, Galinat S, Regouby Y, Magy L, Rebeyrotte I, et al. 2001. [Hashimoto encephalopathy. Analysis of four case reports]. *Rev Med Interne* 22:653-9

Asaoka K, Shoji H, Nishizaka S, Ayabe M, Abe T, et al. 2004. Non-herpetic acute limbic encephalitis: cerebrospinal fluid cytokines and magnetic resonance imaging findings. *Intern Med* 43:42-8

Aurelius E, Andersson B, Forsgren M, Skoldenberg B, Strannegard O. 1994. Cytokines and other markers of intrathecal immune response in patients with herpes simplex encephalitis. *J Infect Dis* 170:678-81

Aurelius E, Forsgren M, Skoldenberg B, Strannegard O. 1993. Persistent intrathecal immune activation in patients with herpes simplex encephalitis. *J Infect Dis* 168:1248-52

Aurelius E, Johansson B, Skoldenberg B, Staland A, Forsgren M. 1991. Rapid diagnosis of herpes simplex encephalitis by nested polymerase chain reaction assay of cerebrospinal fluid. *Lancet* 337:189-92

Aurell A, Rosengren LE, Karlsson B, Olsson JE, Zbornikova V, Haglid KG. 1991. Determination of S-100 and glial fibrillary acidic protein concentrations in cerebrospinal fluid after brain infarction. *Stroke* 22:1254-8

Bissel SJ, Wang G, Bonneh-Barkay D, Starkey A, Trichel AM, et al. 2008. Systemic and brain macrophage infections in relation to the development of simian immunodeficiency virus encephalitis. *J Virol* 82:5031-42

Bissel SJ, Wang G, Trichel AM, Murphey-Corb M, Wiley CA. 2006. Longitudinal analysis of activation markers on monocyte subsets during the development of simian immunodeficiency virus encephalitis. *J Neuroimmunol* 177:85-98

Blennow M, Hagberg H, Rosengren L. 1995. Glial fibrillary acidic protein in the cerebrospinal fluid: a possible indicator of prognosis in full-term asphyxiated newborn infants? *Pediatr Res* 37:260-4

Bonneh-Barkay D, Bissel SJ, Wang G, Fish KN, Nicholl GC, et al. 2008. YKL-40, a marker of simian immunodeficiency virus encephalitis, modulates the biological activity of basic fibroblast growth factor. *Am J Pathol* 173:130-43

Bonneh-Barkay D, Wang G, Starkey A, Hamilton RL, Wiley CA. 2010a. In vivo CHI3L1 (YKL-40) expression in astrocytes in acute and chronic neurological diseases. *J Neuroinflammation* 7:34

Bonneh-Barkay D, Wiley CA. 2008. Brain Extracellular Matrix in Neurodegeneration. *Brain Pathol*

Bonneh-Barkay D, Zagadailov P, Zou H, Niyonkuru C, Figley M, et al. 2010b. YKL-40 expression in traumatic brain injury - an initial analysis. *J Neurotrauma*

Booss J, Kim JH. 1984. Biopsy histopathology in herpes simplex encephalitis and in encephalitis of undefined etiology. *Yale J Biol Med* 57:751-5

Bossi P, Dupin N, Coutellier A, Bricaire F, Lubetzki C, et al. 1998. The level of human immunodeficiency virus (HIV) type 1 RNA in cerebrospinal fluid as a marker of HIV encephalitis. *Clin Infect Dis* 26:1072-3

Brain L, Jellinek EH, Ball K. 1966. Hashimoto's disease and encephalopathy. *Lancet* 2:512-4

Brehin AC, Mouries J, Frenkiel MP, Dadaglio G, Despres P, et al. 2008. Dynamics of immune cell recruitment during West Nile encephalitis and identification of a new CD19+B220-BST-2+ leukocyte population. *J Immunol* 180:6760-7

Brew BJ, Bhalla RB, Paul M, Gallardo H, McArthur JC, et al. 1990. Cerebrospinal fluid neopterin in human immunodeficiency virus type 1 infection. *Ann Neurol* 28:556-60

Buckley C, Oger J, Clover L, Tuzun E, Carpenter K, et al. 2001. Potassium channel antibodies in two patients with reversible limbic encephalitis. *Ann Neurol* 50:73-8

Budka H. 1991. Neuropathology of human immunodeficiency virus infection. *Brain Pathol* 1:163-75

Cesarone MR, Belcaro G, Carratelli M, Cornelli U, De Sanctis MT, et al. 1999. A simple test to monitor oxidative stress. *Int Angiol* 18:127-30

Chong JY, Rowland LP, Utiger RD. 2003. Hashimoto encephalopathy: syndrome or myth? *Arch Neurol* 60:164-71

Christo PP, Greco DB, Aleixo AW, Livramento JA. 2005. HIV-1 RNA levels in cerebrospinal fluid and plasma and their correlation with opportunistic neurological diseases in a Brazilian AIDS reference hospital. *Arq Neuropsiquiatr* 63:907-13

Christo PP, Vilela Mde C, Bretas TL, Domingues RB, Greco DB, et al. 2009. Cerebrospinal fluid levels of chemokines in HIV infected patients with and without opportunistic infection of the central nervous system. *J Neurol Sci* 287:79-83

Cinque P, Bestetti A, Marenzi R, Sala S, Gisslen M, et al. 2005. Cerebrospinal fluid interferon-gamma-inducible protein 10 (IP-10, CXCL10) in HIV-1 infection. *J Neuroimmunol* 168:154-63

Cinque P, Nebuloni M, Santovito ML, Price RW, Gisslen M, et al. 2004. The urokinase receptor is overexpressed in the AIDS dementia complex and other neurological manifestations. *Ann Neurol* 55:687-94

Cinque P, Vago L, Ceresa D, Mainini F, Terreni MR, et al. 1998. Cerebrospinal fluid HIV-1 RNA levels: correlation with HIV encephalitis. *Aids* 12:389-94

Craig-Schapiro R, Perrin RJ, Roe CM, Xiong C, Carter D, et al. 2010. YKL-40: a novel prognostic fluid biomarker for preclinical Alzheimer's disease. *Biol Psychiatry* 68:903-12

Dale RC, Brilot F. 2010. Biomarkers of inflammatory and auto-immune central nervous system disorders. *Curr Opin Pediatr*

De Milito A, Hejdeman B, Albert J, Aleman S, Sonnerborg A, et al. 2000. High plasma levels of soluble fas in HIV type 1-infected subjects are not normalized during highly active antiretroviral therapy. *AIDS Res Hum Retroviruses* 16:1379-84

Debiasi RL, Tyler KL. 2004. Molecular methods for diagnosis of viral encephalitis. *Clin Microbiol Rev* 17:903-25, table of contents

Denes E, Labach C, Durox H, Adoukonou T, Weinbreck P, et al. 2010. Intrathecal synthesis of specific antibodies as a marker of herpes simplex encephalitis in patients with negative PCR. *Swiss Med Wkly* 140:w13107

Dore GJ, Correll PK, Li Y, Kaldor JM, Cooper DA, Brew BJ. 1999. Changes to AIDS dementia complex in the era of highly active antiretroviral therapy. *AIDS* 13:1249-53

Ellis R, Langford D, Masliah E. 2007. HIV and antiretroviral therapy in the brain: neuronal injury and repair. *Nat Rev Neurosci* 8:33-44

Felderhoff-Mueser U, Herold R, Hochhaus F, Koehne P, Ring-Mrozik E, et al. 2001. Increased cerebrospinal fluid concentrations of soluble Fas (CD95/Apo-1) in hydrocephalus. *Arch Dis Child* 84:369-72

Felgenhauer K, Nekic M, Ackermann R. 1982. The demonstration of locally synthesized herpes simplex IgG antibodies in CSF by a Sepharose 4B linked enzyme immunoassay. *J Neuroimmunol* 3:149-58

Felgenhauer K, Reiber H. 1992. The diagnostic significance of antibody specificity indices in multiple sclerosis and herpes virus induced diseases of the nervous system. *Clin Investig* 70:28-37

Ferracci F, Carnevale A. 2006. The neurological disorder associated with thyroid autoimmunity. *J Neurol* 253:975-84

Fuchs D, Chiodi F, Albert J, Asjo B, Hagberg L, et al. 1989a. Neopterin concentrations in cerebrospinal fluid and serum of individuals infected with HIV-1. *AIDS* 3:285-8

Fuchs D, Spira TJ, Hausen A, Reibnegger G, Werner ER, et al. 1989b. Neopterin as a predictive marker for disease progression in human immunodeficiency virus type 1 infection. *Clin Chem* 35:1746-9

Gallo P, Frei K, Rordorf C, Lazdins J, Tavolato B, Fontana A. 1989. Human immunodeficiency virus type 1 (HIV-1) infection of the central nervous system: an evaluation of cytokines in cerebrospinal fluid. *J Neuroimmunol* 23:109-16

Ghika-Schmid F, Ghika J, Regli F, Dworak N, Bogousslavsky J, et al. 1996. Hashimoto's myoclonic encephalopathy: an underdiagnosed treatable condition? *Mov Disord* 11:555-62

Gisolf EH, Enting RH, Jurriaans S, de Wolf F, van der Ende ME, et al. 2000. Cerebrospinal fluid HIV-1 RNA during treatment with ritonavir/saquinavir or ritonavir/saquinavir/stavudine. *AIDS* 14:1583-9

Gultekin SH, Rosenfeld MR, Voltz R, Eichen J, Posner JB, Dalmau J. 2000. Paraneoplastic limbic encephalitis: neurological symptoms, immunological findings and tumour association in 50 patients. *Brain* 123 (Pt 7):1481-94

Hagberg L, Cinque P, Gisslen M, Brew BJ, Spudich S, et al. 2010. Cerebrospinal fluid neopterin: an informative biomarker of central nervous system immune activation in HIV-1 infection. *AIDS Res Ther* 7:15

Hartmann M, Schaner B, Scheglmann K, Bucking A, Pfister R. 2000. [Hashimoto encephalopathy: steroid-sensitive encephalopathy in Hashimoto thyroiditis]. *Nervenarzt* 71:489-94

Hasegawa S, Matsushige T, Inoue H, Shirabe K, Fukano R, Ichiyama T. 2011. Serum and cerebrospinal fluid cytokine profile of patients with 2009 pandemic H1N1 influenza virus-associated encephalopathy. *Cytokine*

Hayes EB, Gubler DJ. 2006. West Nile virus: epidemiology and clinical features of an emerging epidemic in the United States. *Annu Rev Med* 57:181-94

Henchey R, Cibula J, Helveston W, Malone J, Gilmore RL. 1995. Electroencephalographic findings in Hashimoto's encephalopathy. *Neurology* 45:977-81

Hosoya M, Nunoi H, Aoyama M, Kawasaki Y, Suzuki H. 2005. Cytochrome c and tumor necrosis factor-alpha values in serum and cerebrospinal fluid of patients with influenza-associated encephalopathy. *Pediatr Infect Dis J* 24:467-70

Ichiyama T, Morishima T, Isumi H, Matsufuji H, Matsubara T, Furukawa S. 2004. Analysis of cytokine levels and NF-kappaB activation in peripheral blood mononuclear cells in influenza virus-associated encephalopathy. *Cytokine* 27:31-7

Ichiyama T, Nishikawa M, Yoshitomi T, Hayashi T, Furukawa S. 1998. Tumor necrosis factor-alpha, interleukin-1 beta, and interleukin-6 in cerebrospinal fluid from children with prolonged febrile seizures. Comparison with acute encephalitis/encephalopathy. *Neurology* 50:407-11

Ichiyama T, Shoji H, Takahashi Y, Matsushige T, Kajimoto M, et al. 2008. Cerebrospinal fluid levels of cytokines in non-herpetic acute limbic encephalitis: comparison with herpes simplex encephalitis. *Cytokine* 44:149-53

Ichiyama T, Takahashi Y, Matsushige T, Kajimoto M, Fukunaga S, Furukawa S. 2009. Serum matrix metalloproteinase-9 and tissue inhibitor of metalloproteinase-1 levels in non-herpetic acute limbic encephalitis. *J Neurol* 256:1846-50

Iizuka T, Sakai F, Ide T, Monzen T, Yoshii S, et al. 2008. Anti-NMDA receptor encephalitis in Japan: long-term outcome without tumor removal. *Neurology* 70:504-11

Jarius S, Hoffmann L, Clover L, Vincent A, Voltz R. 2008. CSF findings in patients with voltage gated potassium channel antibody associated limbic encephalitis. *J Neurol Sci* 268:74-7

Kamei S, Taira N, Ishihara M, Sekizawa T, Morita A, et al. 2009. Prognostic value of cerebrospinal fluid cytokine changes in herpes simplex virus encephalitis. *Cytokine* 46:187-93

Kapoor H, Signs K, Somsel P, Downes FP, Clark PA, Massey JP. 2004. Persistence of West Nile Virus (WNV) IgM antibodies in cerebrospinal fluid from patients with CNS disease. *J Clin Virol* 31:289-91

Karkela J, Bock E, Kaukinen S. 1993. CSF and serum brain-specific creatine kinase isoenzyme (CK-BB), neuron-specific enolase (NSE) and neural cell adhesion molecule (NCAM) as prognostic markers for hypoxic brain injury after cardiac arrest in man. *J Neurol Sci* 116:100-9

Kawashima H, Oguchi M, Ioi H, Amaha M, Yamanaka G, et al. 2006. Primary biomarkers in cerebral spinal fluid obtained from patients with influenza-associated encephalopathy analyzed by metabolomics. *Int J Neurosci* 116:927-36

Kawashima H, Watanabe Y, Ichiyama T, Mizuguchi M, Yamada N, et al. 2002. High concentration of serum nitrite/nitrate obtained from patients with influenza-associated encephalopathy. *Pediatr Int* 44:705-7

Kawashima H, Watanabe Y, Morishima T, Togashi T, Yamada N, et al. 2003. NOx (nitrite/nitrate) in cerebral spinal fluids obtained from patients with influenza-associated encephalopathy. *Neuropediatrics* 34:137-40

Kelder W, McArthur JC, Nance-Sproson T, McClernon D, Griffin DE. 1998. Beta-chemokines MCP-1 and RANTES are selectively increased in cerebrospinal fluid of patients with human immunodeficiency virus-associated dementia. *Ann Neurol* 44:831-5

Kennard C, Swash M. 1981. Acute viral encephalitis: its diagnosis and outcome. *Brain* 104:129-48

Kirkpatrick RB, Emery JG, Connor JR, Dodds R, Lysko PG, Rosenberg M. 1997. Induction and expression of human cartilage glycoprotein 39 in rheumatoid inflammatory and peripheral blood monocyte-derived macrophages. *Exp Cell Res* 237:46-54

Kolb SA, Sporer B, Lahrtz F, Koedel U, Pfister HW, Fontana A. 1999. Identification of a T cell chemotactic factor in the cerebrospinal fluid of HIV-1-infected individuals as interferon-gamma inducible protein 10. *J Neuroimmunol* 93:172-81

Koskiniemi M, Piiparinen H, Mannonen L, Rantalaiho T, Vaheri A. 1996. Herpes encephalitis is a disease of middle aged and elderly people: polymerase chain reaction for detection of herpes simplex virus in the CSF of 516 patients with encephalitis. The Study Group. *J Neurol Neurosurg Psychiatry* 60:174-8

Kothbauer-Margreiter I, Sturzenegger M, Komor J, Baumgartner R, Hess CW. 1996. Encephalopathy associated with Hashimoto thyroiditis: diagnosis and treatment. *J Neurol* 243:585-93

Kusuhara T, Shoji H, Kaji M, Ayabe M, Hino H. 1994. [Non-herpetic acute limbic encephalitis]. *Rinsho Shinkeigaku* 34:1083-8

Leis AA, Stokic DS. 2005. Neuromuscular Manifestations of Human West Nile Virus Infection. *Curr Treat Options Neurol* 7:15-22

Leis AA, Stokic DS, Polk JL, Dostrow V, Winkelmann M. 2002. A poliomyelitis-like syndrome from West Nile virus infection. *N Engl J Med* 347:1279-80

Leis AA, Stokic DS, Webb RM, Slavinski SA, Fratkin J. 2003. Clinical spectrum of muscle weakness in human West Nile virus infection. *Muscle Nerve* 28:302-8

Lenzlinger PM, Marx A, Trentz O, Kossmann T, Morganti-Kossmann MC. 2002. Prolonged intrathecal release of soluble Fas following severe traumatic brain injury in humans. *J Neuroimmunol* 122:167-74

Linde A, Andersson B, Svenson SB, Ahrne H, Carlsson M, et al. 1992. Serum levels of lymphokines and soluble cellular receptors in primary Epstein-Barr virus infection and in patients with chronic fatigue syndrome. *J Infect Dis* 165:994-1000

Mastrangelo M, Mariani R, Menichella A. 2010. Eponym : Rasmussen syndrome. *Eur J Pediatr* 169:919-24

McGrath N, Anderson NE, Croxson MC, Powell KF. 1997. Herpes simplex encephalitis treated with acyclovir: diagnosis and long term outcome. *J Neurol Neurosurg Psychiatry* 63:321-6

Mijajlovic M, Mirkovic M, Dackovic J, Zidverc-Trajkovic J, Sternic N. 2010. Clinical manifestations, diagnostic criteria and therapy of Hashimoto's encephalopathy: report of two cases. *J Neurol Sci* 288:194-6

Miller JD, Ross CA. 1968. Encephalitis. A four-year survey. *Lancet* 1:1121-6

Mogi M, Harada M, Kondo T, Mizuno Y, Narabayashi H, et al. 1996. The soluble form of Fas molecule is elevated in parkinsonian brain tissues. *Neurosci Lett* 220:195-8

Monteiro de Almeida S, Letendre S, Zimmerman J, Kolakowski S, Lazzaretto D, et al. 2006. Relationship of CSF leukocytosis to compartmentalized changes in MCP-1/CCL2 in the CSF of HIV-infected patients undergoing interruption of antiretroviral therapy. *J Neuroimmunol* 179:180-5

Monteiro de Almeida S, Letendre S, Zimmerman J, Lazzaretto D, McCutchan A, Ellis R. 2005. Dynamics of monocyte chemoattractant protein type one (MCP-1) and HIV viral load in human cerebrospinal fluid and plasma. *J Neuroimmunol* 169:144-52

Morishima T, Togashi T, Yokota S, Okuno Y, Miyazaki C, et al. 2002. Encephalitis and encephalopathy associated with an influenza epidemic in Japan. *Clin Infect Dis* 35:512-7

Nash D, Mostashari F, Fine A, Miller J, O'Leary D, et al. 2001. The outbreak of West Nile virus infection in the New York City area in 1999. *N Engl J Med* 344:1807-14

Nath A, Sacktor N. 2006. Influence of highly active antiretroviral therapy on persistence of HIV in the central nervous system. *Curr Opin Neurol* 19:358-61

Navia BA, Jordan BD, Price RW. 1986. The AIDS dementia complex: I. Clinical features. *Ann Neurol* 19:517-24

Nixon ML, Prince HE. 2006. West Nile virus immunoglobulin A (WNV IgA) detection in cerebrospinal fluid in relation to WNV IgG and IgM reactivity. *J Clin Virol* 37:174-8

Oide T, Tokuda T, Yazaki M, Watarai M, Mitsuhashi S, et al. 2004. Anti-neuronal autoantibody in Hashimoto's encephalopathy: neuropathological, immunohistochemical, and biochemical analysis of two patients. *J Neurol Sci* 217:7-12

Ottervald J, Franzen B, Nilsson K, Andersson LI, Khademi M, et al. 2010. Multiple sclerosis: Identification and clinical evaluation of novel CSF biomarkers. *J Proteomics* 73:1117-32

Perrin RJ, Craig-Schapiro R, Malone JP, Shah AR, Gilmore P, et al. 2011. Identification and validation of novel cerebrospinal fluid biomarkers for staging early Alzheimer's disease. *PLoS One* 6:e16032

Peschen-Rosin R, Schabet M, Dichgans J. 1999. Manifestation of Hashimoto's encephalopathy years before onset of thyroid disease. *Eur Neurol* 41:79-84

Petersen LR, Marfin AA. 2002. West Nile virus: a primer for the clinician. *Ann Intern Med* 137:173-9

Petzold A, Groves M, Leis AA, Scaravilli F, Stokic DS. 2010. Neuronal and glial cerebrospinal fluid protein biomarkers are elevated after West Nile virus infection. *Muscle Nerve* 41:42-9

Pleasure D. 2008. Diagnostic and pathogenic significance of glutamate receptor autoantibodies. *Arch Neurol* 65:589-92

Pozo-Rosich P, Clover L, Saiz A, Vincent A, Graus F. 2003. Voltage-gated potassium channel antibodies in limbic encephalitis. *Ann Neurol* 54:530-3

Rehli M, Niller HH, Ammon C, Langmann S, Schwarzfischer L, et al. 2003. Transcriptional regulation of CHI3L1, a marker gene for late stages of macrophage differentiation. *J Biol Chem* 278:44058-67

Reiber H, Lange P. 1991. Quantification of virus-specific antibodies in cerebrospinal fluid and serum: sensitive and specific detection of antibody synthesis in brain. *Clin Chem* 37:1153-60

Romeo MJ, Espina V, Lowenthal M, Espina BH, Petricoin EF, 3rd, Liotta LA. 2005. CSF proteome: a protein repository for potential biomarker identification. *Expert Rev Proteomics* 2:57-70

Rosengren LE, Wikkelso C, Hagberg L. 1994. A sensitive ELISA for glial fibrillary acidic protein: application in CSF of adults. *J Neurosci Methods* 51:197-204

Rosler A, Pohl M, Braune HJ, Oertel WH, Gemsa D, Sprenger H. 1998. Time course of chemokines in the cerebrospinal fluid and serum during herpes simplex type 1 encephalitis. *J Neurol Sci* 157:82-9

Sabri F, De Milito A, Pirskanen R, Elovaara I, Hagberg L, et al. 2001. Elevated levels of soluble Fas and Fas ligand in cerebrospinal fluid of patients with AIDS dementia complex. *J Neuroimmunol* 114:197-206

Sabri F, Granath F, Hjalmarsson A, Aurelius E, Skoldenberg B. 2006. Modulation of sFas indicates apoptosis in human herpes simplex encephalitis. *J Neuroimmunol* 171:171-6

Sejvar JJ, Leis AA, Stokic DS, Van Gerpen JA, Marfin AA, et al. 2003. Acute flaccid paralysis and West Nile virus infection. *Emerg Infect Dis* 9:788-93

Sevigny JJ, Albert SM, McDermott MP, McArthur JC, Sacktor N, et al. 2004. Evaluation of HIV RNA and markers of immune activation as predictors of HIV-associated dementia. *Neurology* 63:2084-90

Sevigny JJ, Albert SM, McDermott MP, Schifitto G, McArthur JC, et al. 2007. An evaluation of neurocognitive status and markers of immune activation as predictors of time to death in advanced HIV infection. *Arch Neurol* 64:97-102

Sharief MK, Ciardi M, Thompson EJ, Sorice F, Rossi F, et al. 1992. Tumour necrosis factor-alpha mediates blood-brain barrier damage in HIV-1 infection of the central nervous system. *Mediators Inflamm* 1:191-6

Shaw PJ, Walls TJ, Newman PK, Cleland PG, Cartlidge NE. 1991. Hashimoto's encephalopathy: a steroid-responsive disorder associated with high anti-thyroid antibody titers--report of 5 cases. *Neurology* 41:228-33

Shoji H. 2010. [Clinical characteristics of non-herpetic limbic encephalitis]. *Brain Nerve* 62:853-60

Shoji H, Asaoka K, Ayabe M, Ichiyama T, Sakai K. 2004. Non-herpetic acute limbic encephalitis: a new subgroup of limbic encephalitis? *Intern Med* 43:348

Sidenius N, Nebuloni M, Sala S, Zerbi P, Price RW, et al. 2004. Expression of the urokinase plasminogen activator and its receptor in HIV-1-associated central nervous system disease. *J Neuroimmunol* 157:133-9

Sindic CJ, Kevers L, Chalon MP, Laterre EC, Masson PL. 1985. Monitoring and tentative diagnosis of herpetic encephalitis by protein analysis of cerebrospinal fluid. Particular relevance of the assays of ferritin and S-100. *J Neurol Sci* 67:359-69

Sivertsen B, Christensen PB. 1996. Acute encephalitis. *Acta Neurol Scand* 93:156-9

Skoldenberg B. 1991. Herpes simplex encephalitis. *Scand J Infect Dis Suppl* 80:40-6

Skoldenberg B, Forsgren M, Alestig K, Bergstrom T, Burman L, et al. 1984. Acyclovir versus vidarabine in herpes simplex encephalitis. Randomised multicentre study in consecutive Swedish patients. *Lancet* 2:707-11

Sonnerborg AB, von Stedingk LV, Hansson LO, Strannegard OO. 1989. Elevated neopterin and beta 2-microglobulin levels in blood and cerebrospinal fluid occur early in HIV-1 infection. *AIDS* 3:277-83

Studahl M, Rosengren L, Gunther G, Hagberg L. 2000. Difference in pathogenesis between herpes simplex virus type 1 encephalitis and tick-borne encephalitis demonstrated by means of cerebrospinal fluid markers of glial and neuronal destruction. *J Neurol* 247:636-42

Takahashi S, Mitamura R, Itoh Y, Suzuki N, Okuno A. 1994. Hashimoto encephalopathy: etiologic considerations. *Pediatr Neurol* 11:328-31

Takahashi Y, Kubota H, Fujiwara T, Yagi K, Seino M. 1997. Epilepsia partialis continua of childhood involving bilateral brain hemispheres. *Acta Neurol Scand* 96:345-52

Takahashi Y, Mogami Y, Takayama R, Ikeda H, Imai K. 2010. [Antibodies to glutamate receptor in limbic encephalitis]. *Brain Nerve* 62:827-37

Takahashi Y, Mori H, Mishina M, Watanabe M, Fujiwara T, et al. 2003. Autoantibodies to NMDA receptor in patients with chronic forms of epilepsia partialis continua. *Neurology* 61:891-6

Takahashi Y, Mori H, Mishina M, Watanabe M, Kondo N, et al. 2005. Autoantibodies and cell-mediated autoimmunity to NMDA-type GluRepsilon2 in patients with Rasmussen's encephalitis and chronic progressive epilepsia partialis continua. *Epilepsia* 46 Suppl 5:152-8

Thieben MJ, Lennon VA, Boeve BF, Aksamit AJ, Keegan M, Vernino S. 2004. Potentially reversible autoimmune limbic encephalitis with neuronal potassium channel antibody. *Neurology* 62:1177-82

Tilley PA, Fox JD, Jayaraman GC, Preiksaitis JK. 2007. Maculopapular rash and tremor are associated with West Nile fever and neurological syndromes. *J Neurol Neurosurg Psychiatry* 78:529-31

Togashi T, Matsuzono Y, Narita M, Morishima T. 2004. Influenza-associated acute encephalopathy in Japanese children in 1994-2002. *Virus Res* 103:75-8

Towfighi A, Skolasky RL, St Hillaire C, Conant K, McArthur JC. 2004. CSF soluble Fas correlates with the severity of HIV-associated dementia. *Neurology* 62:654-6

Vernino S, Geschwind M, Boeve B. 2007. Autoimmune encephalopathies. *Neurologist* 13:140-7

Vernino S, Lennon VA. 2004. Autoantibody profiles and neurological correlations of thymoma. *Clin Cancer Res* 10:7270-5

Vincent A, Buckley C, Schott JM, Baker I, Dewar BK, et al. 2004. Potassium channel antibody-associated encephalopathy: a potentially immunotherapy-responsive form of limbic encephalitis. *Brain* 127:701-12

Vitaliani R, Zoccarato M, Vianello M, Giometto B. 2008. Clinical, immunological and therapeutic aspects of autoimmune encephalitis. *Recent Pat CNS Drug Discov* 3:16-22

Voltz R. 2002. Paraneoplastic neurological syndromes: an update on diagnosis, pathogenesis, and therapy. *Lancet Neurol* 1:294-305

Wang GF, Li W, Li K. 2010. Acute encephalopathy and encephalitis caused by influenza virus infection. *Curr Opin Neurol* 23:305-11

Whitley RJ, Cobbs CG, Alford CA, Jr., Soong SJ, Hirsch MS, et al. 1989. Diseases that mimic herpes simplex encephalitis. Diagnosis, presentation, and outcome. NIAD Collaborative Antiviral Study Group. *JAMA* 262:234-9

Wiley CA, Achim CL, Schrier RD, Heyes MP, McCutchan JA, Grant I. 1992. Relationship of cerebrospinal fluid immune activation associated factors to HIV encephalitis. *AIDS* 6:1299-307

Wiley CA, Soontornniyomkij V, Radhakrishnan L, Masliah E, Mellors J, et al. 1998. Distribution of brain HIV load in AIDS. *Brain Pathol* 8:277-84

Williams KC, Hickey WF. 2002. Central nervous system damage, monocytes and macrophages, and neurological disorders in AIDS. *Annu Rev Neurosci* 25:537-62

Yamanaka G, Ishii C, Kawashima H, Oana S, Miyajima T, Hoshika A. 2008. Cerebrospinal fluid Diacron-Reactive Oxygen Metabolite levels in pediatric patients with central nervous system diseases. *Pediatr Neurol* 39:80-4

Yamanaka G, Kawashima H, Suganami Y, Watanabe C, Watanabe Y, et al. 2006. Diagnostic and predictive value of CSF d-ROM level in influenza virus-associated encephalopathy. *J Neurol Sci* 243:71-5

Zink MC, Suryanarayana K, Mankowski JL, Shen A, Piatak M, Jr., et al. 1999. High viral load in the cerebrospinal fluid and brain correlates with severity of simian immunodeficiency virus encephalitis. *J Virol* 73:10480-8

Zink MC, Uhrlaub J, DeWitt J, Voelker T, Bullock B, et al. 2005. Neuroprotective and anti-human immunodeficiency virus activity of minocycline. *JAMA* 293:2003-11

Zipp F, Weller M, Calabresi PA, Frank JA, Bash CN, et al. 1998. Increased serum levels of soluble CD95 (APO-1/Fas) in relapsing-remitting multiple sclerosis. *Ann Neurol* 43:116-20

2

Neuropathologic Diagnosis of Central Nervous System Viral Diseases

Kymberly A. Gyure
West Virginia University School of Medicine
U.S.A.

1. Introduction

The principal aim of this chapter is to provide an illustrated review of the neuropathologic features of common and recently emerging central nervous system (CNS) viral diseases. An overview of the histopathologic features common to most viral infections of the central nervous system will be provided. This will be followed by a description of the gross and microscopic findings characteristic of specific viral infections of the CNS. Conditions which can be accurately diagnosed via brain biopsy and their differential diagnosis will be emphasized. Where appropriate, ancillary studies including molecular diagnostic techniques will be covered.

2. Overview of neuropathologic findings in CNS viral diseases

The accurate diagnosis of viral meningoencephalitis is important in order to institute appropriate specific therapy to improve survival and reduce the extent of permanent brain injury. In many cases, a diagnosis can be made based on medical history and examination followed by a combination of cerebrospinal fluid (CSF) analysis, serology, and neuroimaging studies (Johnson & Power, 2008; Steiner et al., 2010). However, in clinically unusual and diagnostically difficult cases, brain biopsy may be performed.

Although the pathologic features of viral encephalitis vary somewhat depending on the specific infectious agent and the immunologic status of the patient, most viral infections of the CNS are characterized by a triad of findings including perivascular chronic inflammation, microglial nodules, and neuronophagia (Figure 1). The distribution of these findings as well as the presence of characteristic intranuclear or intracytoplasmic viral inclusions can lead to a specific diagnosis in an appropriate clinical setting. Ancillary techniques, including immunohistochemistry (IHC), in-situ hybridization (ISH), or polymerase chain reaction (PCR) amplification, are useful in some settings.

3. DNA Viruses

3.1 Herpesviruses

The herpesviruses are double-stranded DNA viruses which have the capacity to cause latent infections in the nervous system.

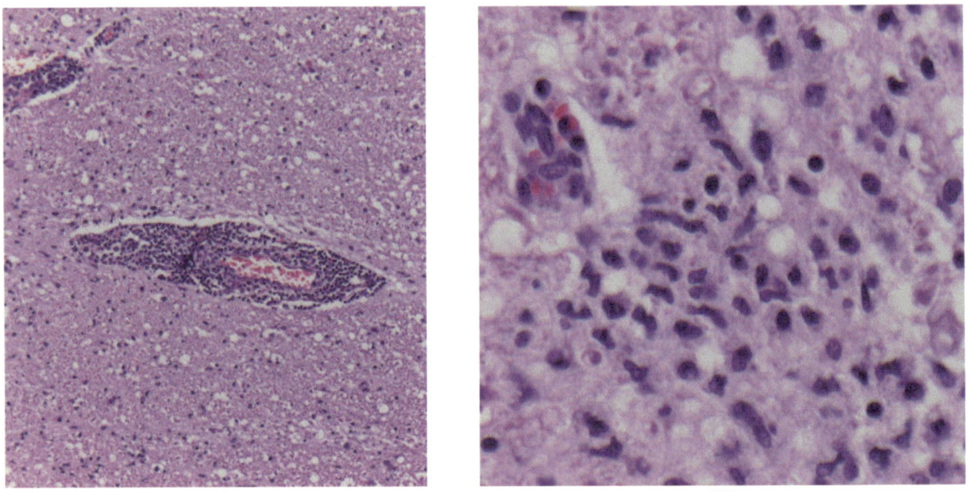

(A) (B)

Fig. 1. Viral encephalitis. Perivascular chronic inflammation (A) and microglial nodules (B) are characteristic findings.

3.1.1 Herpes Simplex Virus type 1

Herpes simplex virus (HSV) is the most common cause of sporadic, nonseasonal encephalitis and is most often caused by HSV type 1 (herpes labialis). It produces a clinical picture consisting of fever, headache, seizures, and mental status changes which may rapidly progress to coma and death. If not treated, the mortality ranges up to 70% (Baringer, 2008).

PCR amplification of viral DNA in the CSF has largely supplanted brain biopsy as the main diagnostic procedure in HSV encephalitis, however, brain biopsy may be performed in cases in which the diagnosis is not suspected or in patients who fail to respond to empiric antiviral therapy. In immunocompetent hosts, HSV encephalitis is characterized by hemorrhagic necrosis affecting the medial and inferior temporal lobes, the insulae, the cingulate gyri, and the posterior orbitofrontal cortices (Figure 2). In addition to perivascular chronic inflammation and microglial nodules, one sees necrosis associated with a macrophage-rich inflammatory infiltrate. Cowdry type A intranuclear inclusions, which are often difficult to identify, particularly in previously treated individuals, may be seen in both neurons and glial cells. Neurons with a homogeneous, stained-glass appearance may also be seen (Figure 3). In cases in which the characteristic inclusions are difficult to identify, IHC or ISH for viral antigens may be used to confirm the diagnosis.

3.1.2 Herpes Simplex Virus type 2

HSV type 2 (herpes genitalis) may also produce an encephalitis, particularly in neonates. These infections are the result of passage of the infant through an infected birth canal. Affected neonates typically have disseminated infection with vesicular skin lesions and signs of keratoconjunctivitis. Pathologic findings are similar to those of HSV type 1 encephalitis but are typically more diffuse.

3.1.3 Varicella-zoster Virus

Central nervous system disease can develop as part of primary varicella-zoster virus (VZV) infection (varicella/chickenpox) or after reactivation (zoster/shingles). The clinical and

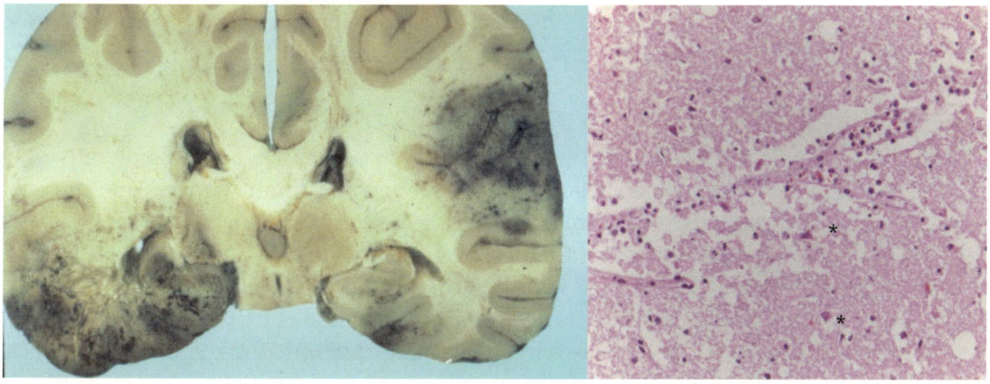

Figs. 2 & 3. HSV encephalitis. Grossly, one sees hemorrhagic necrosis affecting limbic structures. Microscopically, there is a macrophage-rich inflammatory infiltrate and neurons with a stained-glass appearance (asterisks).

pathologic features depend in part on the immune status of the patient. In immunocompetent patients, bulbar encephalitis or transverse myelitis can occur when the virus spreads centrally toward the brainstem or spinal cord. Immunocompromised patients are more likely to develop disseminated disease.

Vasculopathies caused by VZV can also occur during primary infection or after reactivation (Gilden et al., 2009). These affect both small and large arteries and lead to ischemic or hemorrhagic infarction. Useful diagnostic studies include magnetic resonance imaging and angiography with detection of anti-VZV IgG antibodies in cerebrospinal fluid. Pathologic findings are variable and include vasculitis, which may be granulomatous in large vessels, necrosis, and demyelination (Figure 4). Cowdry A intranuclear inclusions may be seen in glial cells.

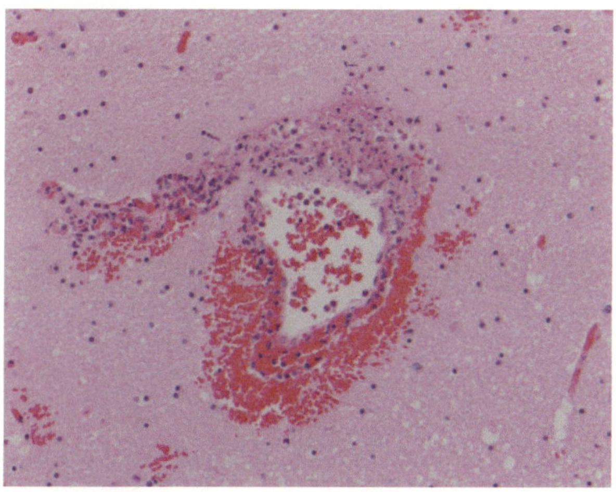

Fig. 4. VZV vasculitis. A small vessel with fibrinoid necrosis and a mural inflammatory infiltrate is present in white matter.

3.1.4 Epstein-Barr Virus

Encephalitis is a rare complication of Epstein-Barr virus (EBV) infection. In immunocompromised patients, this virus has been implicated in the development of primary brain lymphoma (Figure 5). In this clinical setting, these lesions need to be distinguished from encephalitis due to *Toxoplasma gondii* infection.

3.1.5 Cytomegalovirus

Cytomegalovirus (CMV) infection of the nervous system occurs most commonly in patients with the acquired immunodeficiency syndrome (AIDS). Other immunosuppressed patients, including transplant patients, may also be affected. Symptomatic CNS disease also occurs in neonates who are infected in utero. PCR detection of CMV DNA in the CSF is useful in confirming a diagnosis of CMV-related neurological disease (Griffiths, 2004).

The gross appearance of the brain in adults with CMV infection is variable. There may be no gross evidence of disease; in severe cases in which there is ventriculitis, ependymal necrosis may be evident. In neonates, the brain is usually small and may show porencephaly or polymicrogyria (Gyure, 2005).

Microscopically, most cases of CMV encephalitis are characterized by diffuse microglial nodules. These often contain the characteristic cytomegalic cells which have both intranuclear and intracytoplasmic viral inclusions (Figure 6). IHC for CMV antigens may be useful to identify these cells or to confirm the diagnosis in difficult cases (Figure 7).

3.1.6 Human Herpes Virus 6

Human herpes virus 6 (HHV6) is the cause of the childhood disease exanthem subitum (roseola infantum). It has recently been identified as a cause of encephalitis in immunocompetent adults and children and appears to be a major cause of post-transplant limbic encephalitis (Tyler, 2009a; Vinnard et al., 2009). Magnetic resonance imaging studies show bilateral T2 and FLAIR hyperintense lesions in the medial temporal lobes, and the diagnosis is confirmed by identifying HHV6 DNA by PCR in CSF (Tyler, 2009a). Described pathologic findings are rare and include multifocal lymphohistiocytic inflammation involving gray and white matter (Love & Wiley, 2008).

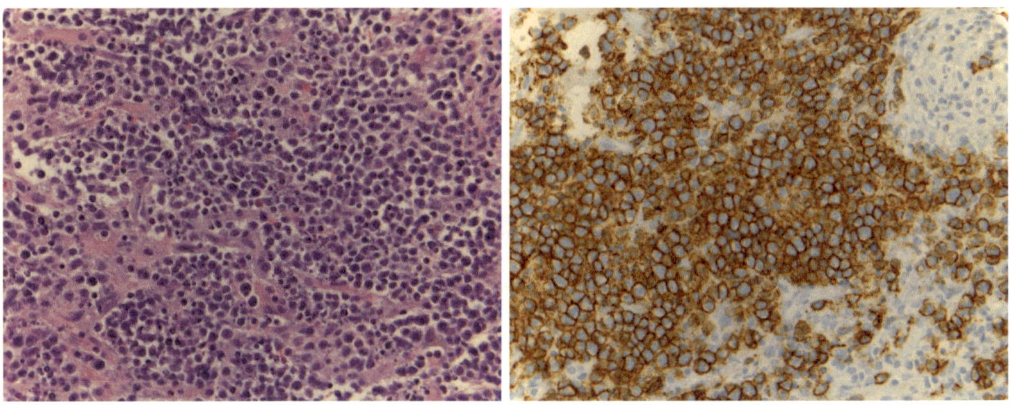

(A) (B)

Fig. 5. EBV-associated primary brain lymphoma. In most cases, these lesions are large B-cell lymphomas (A). This is confirmed with CD20 immunohistochemistry (B).

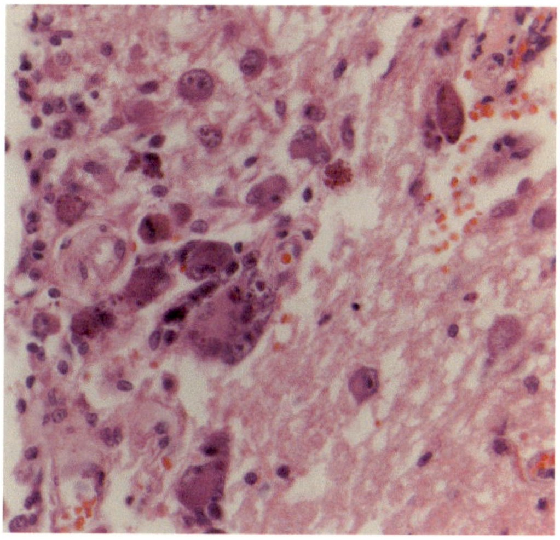

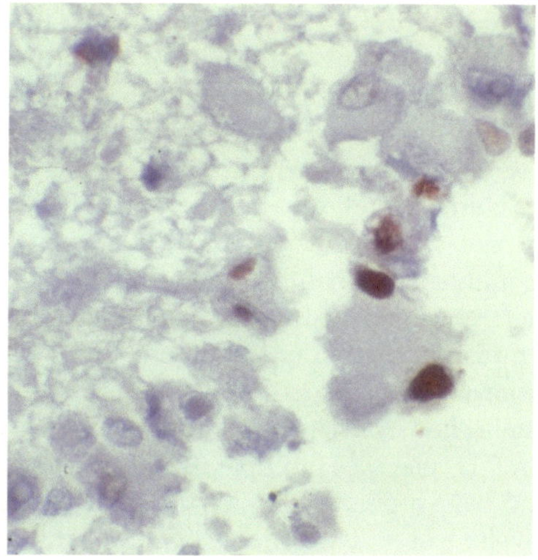

Figs. 6 & 7. CMV encephalitis. The characteristic cytomegalic cells contain both intranuclear and intracytoplasmic inclusions. IHC for CMV antigens highlights the intranuclear inclusions.

3.2 Adenovirus

Encephalitis is a rare complication of adenovirus infection which occurs predominantly in immunosuppressed patients. Findings include perivascular chronic inflammation and basophilic intranuclear inclusions (Figure 8).

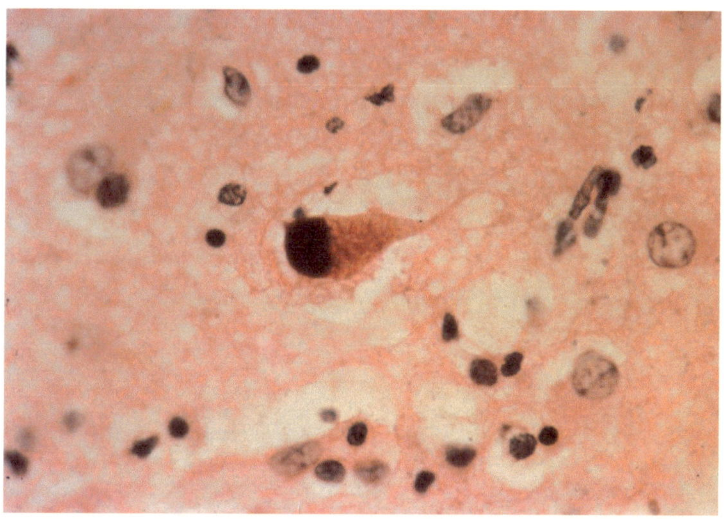

Fig. 8. Adenovirus encephalitis. Basophilic intranuclear inclusions are present in neurons and glial cells.

3.3 Papovaviruses

The papovavirus family includes the human polyomaviruses JC virus, BK virus, and simian virus 40.

3.3.1 JC virus

JC virus is the cause of progressive multifocal leukoencephalopathy (PML), a demyelinating disease that results from the infection of oligodendroglial cells by this virus. It occurs almost exclusively in immunocompromised patients, including those with AIDS. More recently, it has been associated with treatment with the monoclonal antibodies natalizumab, efalizumab, and rituximab (Tan & Koralnik, 2010; Tyler, 2009b; Weber, 2008). Patients present with non-specific symptoms including limb weakness, speech or visual deficits, cognitive abnormalities, and seizures. Therefore, the clinical differential diagnosis is broad and encompasses other AIDS-related illnesses including toxoplasmosis and CNS lymphoma. In multiple sclerosis (MS) patients treated with monoclonal antibodies, the lesions of PML must be distinguished from those of MS (Weber, 2008). The diagnosis is established by brain biopsy or by detection of JC virus DNA in the CSF by PCR.

Grossly, one sees multiple foci of demyelination which are typically subcortical in location and have a predilection for the parieto-occipital region (Figure 9). Microscopically, there is myelin loss with a variable degree of inflammation including macrophages (Shishido-Hara, 2010). Infected oligodendroglial nuclei are enlarged with a ground-glass appearance (Figure 10). Bizarre-appearing astrocytes with lobulated, hyperchromatic nuclei may also be present and can be confused with neoplastic astrocytes (Figure 11). The presence of viral inclusions within oligodendrocyte nuclei can be confirmed with IHC for JC virus or simian virus 40, which cross reacts with JC virus (Crowder et al., 2005).

3.3.2 Simian virus 40

Simian virus 40 (SV40) DNA sequences have been identified in a variety of human neoplasms including brain tumors (Love & Wiley, 2008). The significance of this finding in relationship to the development of these lesions remains unclear.

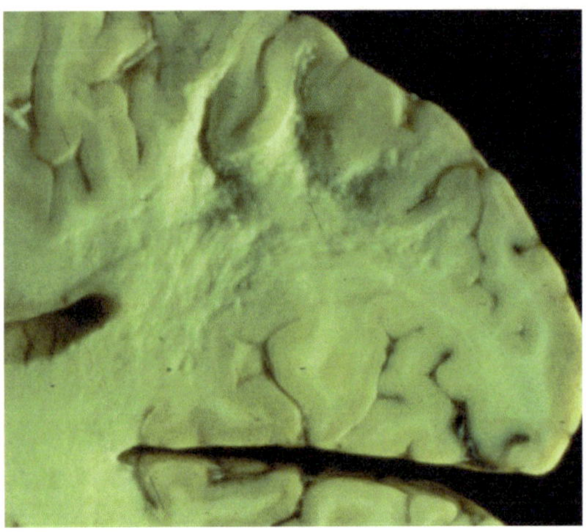

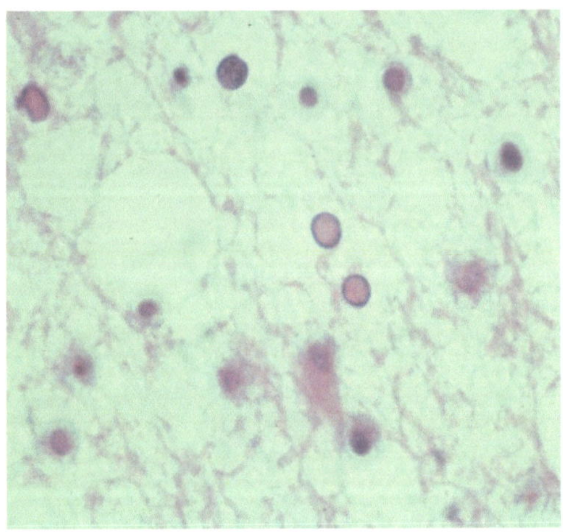

Figs. 9 & 10. Progressive multifocal leukoencephalopathy. Gross findings include subcortical foci of myelin loss. Microscopically, enlarged oligodendrocyte nuclei have a ground-glass appearance.

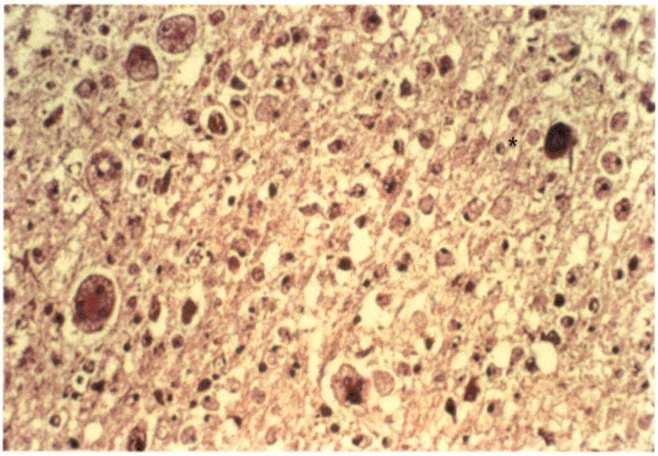

Fig. 11. Progressive multifocal leukoencephalopathy. Enlarged, hyperchromatic astrocytes (asterisk) are present in a background containing numerous macrophages.

4. RNA viruses

Numerous RNA viruses are capable of causing CNS disease including meningitis and encephalitis. An important subset of these viruses is the so-called arbovirus (*ar*thropod-*bo*rne *virus*) group; these viruses are responsible for most outbreaks of epidemic viral encephalitis. They have animal (horses and small mammals) or bird hosts and mosquito or tick vectors and belong to four main families: the reoviruses, the alphavirus subgroup of togaviruses, the flaviviruses, and the bunyaviruses.

4.1 Reoviruses

Reoviruses are double-stranded RNA viruses. The principal CNS pathogen in this family is the Colorado tick fever virus. Its naturally infected host species include squirrels, chipmunks, porcupines, deer mice, and wood rats; and the vector is the wood tick *Dermacentor andersoni* (Romero & Simonsen, 2008).

Colorado tick fever is an acute febrile illness which occurs most commonly in the Rocky Mountain region of North America. It is the second most common arboviral infection in the United States. Neurologic manifestations including encephalitis occur most commonly in children. The diagnosis is typically made serologically.

4.2 Retroviruses

The retroviruses are single-stranded RNA viruses possessing the enzyme reverse transcriptase. Human pathogens affecting the nervous system include the human immunodeficiency viruses (HIV-1 and HIV-2) and human T-cell lymphotropic virus I (HTLV-I).

4.2.1 Human Immunodeficiency Viruses

HIV is the cause of AIDS and has infected approximately 33 million individuals worldwide (Singer et al., 2010). Neurologic dysfunction develops in 40-70% of patients during the course of their illness, and neuropathologic changes can be demonstrated in up to 90%

brains from this patient population (Anthony & Bell, 2008; Boissé et al., 2008). These findings include opportunistic infections; primary CNS lymphomas; lesions thought to be directly related to the HIV virus including aseptic meningitis, HIV-associated neurocognitive disorders/HIV encephalitis, and vacuolar myelopathy; and disorders related to antiretroviral therapy.

Commonly seen opportunistic infections in AIDS patients include the viral infections PML and cytomegalovirus encephalitis (illustrated above), the fungal infection cryptococcosis (Figure 12), and parasitic infection due to *Toxoplasma gondii* (Figure 13). These must be distinguished from primary CNS lymphomas, also illustrated above.

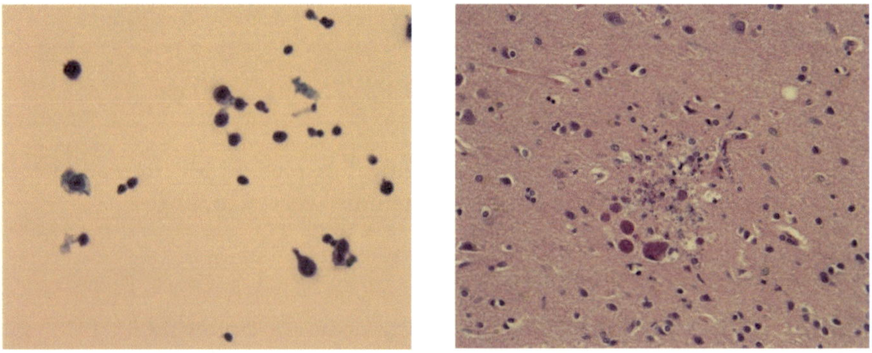

Figs. 12 & 13. Opportunistic infections in AIDS. Cryptococcal meninginitis may be diagnosed by finding budding yeasts in CSF. Toxoplasma encephalitis is characterized by cysts and trophozoites in a background containing microglial nodules.

A significant number of AIDS patients develop neurocognitive disorders that are not attributable to opportunistic infections. The term HIV-associated neurocognitive disorder (HAND) has been applied to a number of clinical syndromes including HIV-associated dementia (HAD, also referred to as AIDS dementia complex or HIV encephalopathy), mild neurocognitive disorder (MND), and asymptomatic neurocognitive impairment (Boissé et al., 2008; Letendre et al., 2010; Singer et al., 2010). Many individuals with cognitive and motor abnormalities exhibit a pathologic picture which has been termed HIV encephalitis that is characterized by diffuse or multifocal accumulations of microglia including ill-defined microglial nodules. Characteristic macrophage-derived multinucleated cells are diagnostic when observed in this setting (Figure 14).

Vacuolar myelopathy is an uncommon manifestation of AIDS. Patients present with leg weakness, spastic paraparesis, ataxia, and incontinence. Pathologic findings consist of vacuolation of white matter tracts in the lateral and posterior columns of the spinal cord. This disorder may be difficult to distinguish from subacute combined degeneration of the spinal cord associated with vitamin B_{12} deficiency.

The introduction of highly active antiretroviral therapy (HAART) in very immunosuppressed AIDS patients may result in an abrupt clinical deterioration termed the immune reconstitution inflammatory syndrome (IRIS). This syndrome is thought to be secondary to the sudden activation of and increase in CD4-positive T cells resulting in a heightened immune response with host-mediated inflammatory cell damage, resulting in new neurologic deficits or worsening of prior signs and symptoms (McCombe et al., 2009). Neuropathologic findings include widespread chronic inflammatory infiltrates in the brain adjacent to areas of pre-existing infection as well as demyelination.

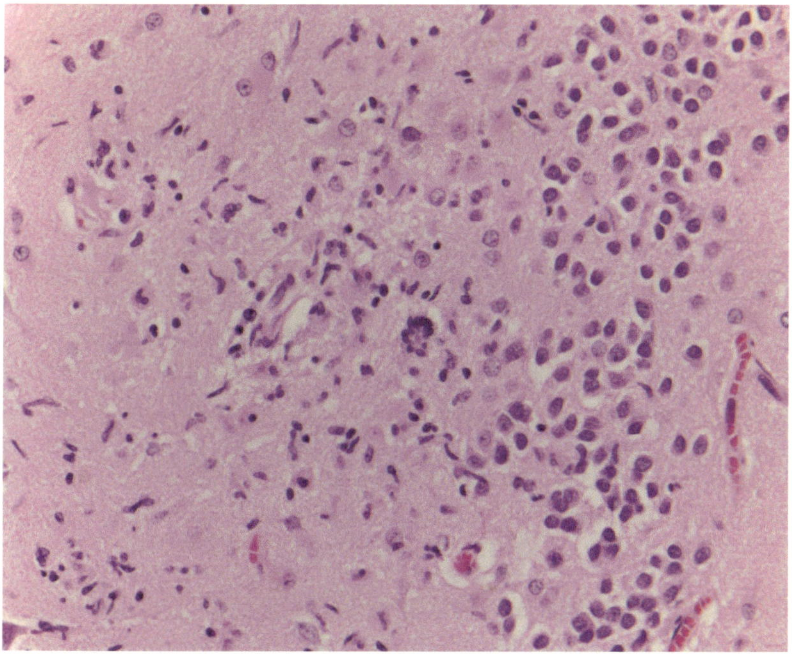

Fig. 14. HIV encephalitis. Characteristic multinucleated giant cells are present in a background containing ill-defined microglial nodules.

4.2.2 Human T-cell Lymphotropic Virus

HTLV-1 is the etiologic agent of tropical spastic paraparesis/HTLV-1 associated myelopathy. This virus, which is endemic in southern Japan, the Caribbean, parts of Africa, and South America, is best known for causing an aggressive T-cell leukemia. Tropical spastic paraparesis, which develops months to years after infection, develops in less than one percent of infected individuals and is characterized clinically by slowly progressive weakness of the lower limbs, sensory disturbances, and difficulties with bladder control (Love & Wiley, 2005). Grossly, there is atrophy of the spinal cord with thickening of the meninges. Microscopic findings include perivascular chronic inflammation and microglial nodules (Figure 15).

4.3 Togaviruses

Togaviruses are single-stranded RNA viruses. Clinically important members of this family of viruses include Rubivirus and the arboviruses Eastern equine encephalitis virus (EEEV), Western equine encephalitis virus (WEEV), and Venezuelan equine encephalitis virus (VEEV).

4.3.1 Rubivirus

Rubivirus is the cause of rubella (German measles), which has been largely eliminated by effective vaccination programs. Congenital rubella infection may result in neurologic abnormalities including sensorineural deafness and encephalitis. Vascular abnormalities including mineralization of vessels in the deep gray nuclei and white matter have been described in this setting (Rorke, 1973).

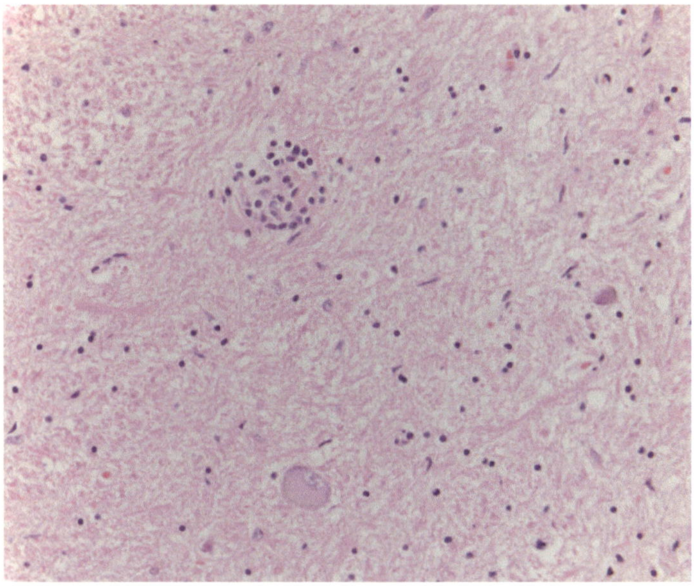

Fig. 15. Tropical spastic paraparesis. A proliferation of microglial cells and perivascular chronic inflammation involve the gray and white matter of the spinal cord.

4.3.2 Alphaviruses

The encephalitic alphaviruses (EEEV, WEEV, and VEEV) are neuroinvasive and can cause neurologic symptoms in humans and equines. They have a widespread distribution in North, Central, and South America.

EEEV has a bird host and a mosquito vector. Transmission to humans and horses occurs most commonly in the Atlantic and Gulf Coast states and in the Great Lakes region of the United States (Zacks & Paessler, 2010). Encephalitis in humans is characterized by fever, headaches, vomiting, seizures, and coma. The diagnosis is confirmed by the detection of IgM antibodies in serum and CSF. Pathologic findings are not specific and include perivascular chronic inflammation, microglial nodules, and neuronophagia with a predilection for the basal ganglia and brainstem (Love & Wiley, 2005). Vasculitis and hemorrhage may also be present (Zacks & Paessler, 2010).

WEEV also has passerine birds as its natural hosts and the mosquito as its arthropod vector. It causes epidemics of encephalitis in humans and horses in summer and early autumn in the western United States and Canada. In adults, WEEV infections tend to be asymptomatic or mild; but in children, a severe meningoencephalitis leading to coma and death can occur, and survivors may have severe neurologic sequelae (Zacks & Paessler, 2010). The diagnosis is usually confirmed using serological methods. Amplification of virus-specific RNA can also be performed using real-time PCR. Neuropathologic findings are similar to those seen in EEEV infection (Love & Wiley, 2005).

VEEV has a rodent host and a mosquito vector. It is transmitted to humans and horses in the Caribbean basin and South America. In adults, infection usually results in a flu-like illness, and encephalitis is rare. Neurologic symptoms including disorientation, ataxia, and convulsions are more common in children. Reported neuropathologic findings in fatal cases include edema, congestion, hemorrhage, vasculitis, meningitis, and encephalitis (Zacks & Paessler, 2010).

4.4 Flaviviruses

Flaviviruses are enveloped, single-stranded RNA viruses. Most are arboviruses that produce a variety of diseases in humans.

Japanese encephalitis virus (JEV) is the most common cause of acute viral encephalitis worldwide and causes 10,000 to 15,000 deaths annually (Granerod et al., 2010; Tyler, 2009a). The geographic area where it is endemic has been increasing, and encephalitis due to this virus is prevalent throughout Eastern and Southern Asia and the Pacific Rim (Misra & Kalita, 2010). Its hosts include water birds and pigs, and mosquitoes are its vector. In endemic areas, Japanese encephalitis is a disease of children. JEV may produce asymptomatic infections, a non-specific febrile illness, aseptic meningitis, or severe encephalitis. Grossly, lesions are mainly restricted to gray matter and consist of petechiae or focal hemorrhages. Microscopic findings, which are most prominent in the diencephalon and mesencephalon, include congestion and hemorrhage, thrombus formation with associated necrosis, and widespread chronic inflammation with neuronophagia (Love & Wiley, 2005; Misra and Kalita, 2010).

St. Louis encephalitis virus (SLEV) is present throughout the United States and produces infections in late summer and early autumn. It has a bird host and a mosquito vector. Most SLEV virus infections are subclinical; symptomatic encephalitis is most common in patients over the age of 60 years. Neuropathologic findings are those of a non-necrotizing encephalitis which may be particularly marked in the thalamus and midbrain (Love & Wiley, 2005).

West Nile virus (WNV) is the most common cause of epidemic meningoencephalitis in North America and the leading cause of arboviral encephalitis in the United States. Recent epidemics in Algeria, Morocco, Tunisia, Italy, France, Romania, Israel, and Russia have also been associated with severe human disease including neurologic complications (Rossi et al., 2010). WNV cycles between bird hosts and mosquito vectors; humans and horses are incidental hosts. Transmission may also occur via transfusion of blood products and via organ transplantation from infected donors. Approximately one of 150 patients develops CNS disease; risk factors for neuroinvasive disease are older age and immunosuppression. CNS manifestations include meningitis, encephalitis, and acute flaccid paralysis/poliomyelitis. The diagnosis in most cases is confirmed by detecting WNV-specific antibodies in serum or CSF. The brain and spinal cord are grossly normal in most cases of WNV meningoencephalitis. Microscopically, one sees perivascular chronic inflammation, microglial nodules, and variable neuronal loss (Figure 16). Neuronophagia and foci of necrosis are sometimes present. Gray matter is more severely affected than white matter, and the inflammatory infiltrate is typically most prominent in the brainstem (Gyure, 2009).

Tick-borne encephalitis virus (TBEV) is the cause of tick-borne encephalitis. This potentially fatal neurologic infection occurs predominantly in Europe and Asia. TBEV has wild mammalian hosts, particularly rodents, and its vector is the Ixodid tick. Symptoms of acute tick-borne encephalitis range from mild meningitis to a severe meningoencephalitis characterized by muscle weakness. The diagnosis is made by demonstrating TBEV-specific antibodies or by detecting viral RNA in serum and CSF (Mansfield et al., 2009). Neuropathologic findings in fatal cases include chronic inflammation with microglial activation affecting gray matter structures including those of the spinal cord, especially the anterior horns (Love & Wiley, 2005).

Other flaviviruses that can affect the nervous system include Murray Valley encephalitis virus, louping ill virus, Powasan virus, Kyasanur Forest disease virus, and Omsk hemorrhagic fever virus (LaSala & Holbrook, 2010; Romero & Simonsen, 2008).

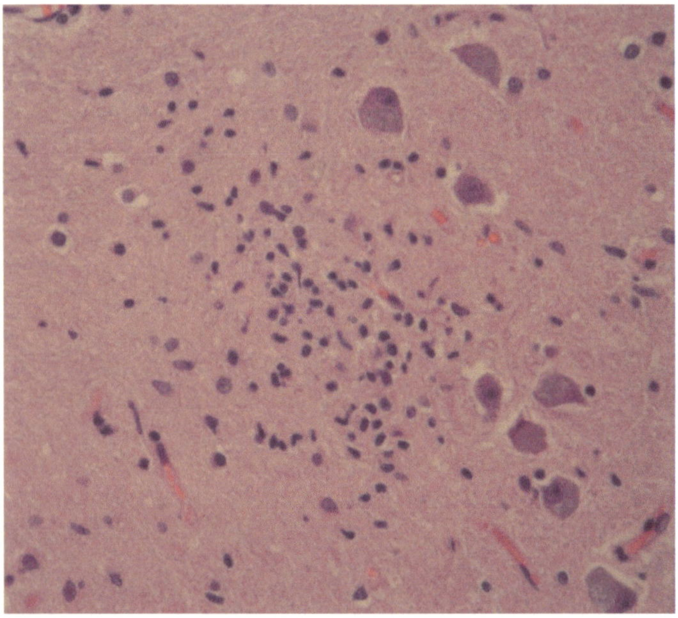

Fig. 16. WNV encephalomyelitis. Microglial nodules are associated with variable neuronal loss.

4.5 Picornaviruses

Picornaviruses are single-stranded RNA viruses. Important human pathogens include poliovirus and other enteroviruses.

4.5.1 Poliovirus

Despite the overall success of the Global Poliomyelitis Eradication Initiative of the World Health Organization, poliovirus remains endemic in Afghanistan, India, Nigeria, and Pakistan (Dutta, 2008). Polio outbreaks attributed to circulating vaccine-derived poliovirus have also occurred throughout the world (Tyler, 2009a). In most infected patients, a non-specific gastroenteritis develops. Paralytic disease occurs in one to two percent of patients and is characterized by a flaccid paralysis with muscle wasting and hyporeflexia. A late complication termed postpolio syndrome, which occurs 30-40 years after the acute illness, is characterized by progressive weakness associated with decreased muscle bulk and pain.

In most cases, the brain and spinal cord are grossly normal, but in severe cases, vascular congestion, petechial hemorrhages, and necrosis may be present. Chronically, there is atrophy of the anterior nerve roots. Microscopically, there is perivascular chronic inflammation and neuronophagia involving the anterior horns of the spinal cord. Neutrophils may be present in some cases.

4.5.2 Enteroviruses

Other enteroviruses have been associated with a poliomyelitis-like syndrome. Enterovirus 71, a cause of hand-foot-and-mouth disease, has caused numerous outbreaks of disease in the Southeast Asia and Pacific region (Johnson & Power, 2008; Tyler, 2009a). In addition to the poliomyelitis-like syndrome, neurologic manifestations include meningitis, cerebellitis, brainstem encephalitis, opsoclonus-myoclonus syndrome, Guillain-Barré syndrome, and transverse myelitis. Neuropathologic findings are non-specific and involve the brainstem and spinal cord (Figure 17).

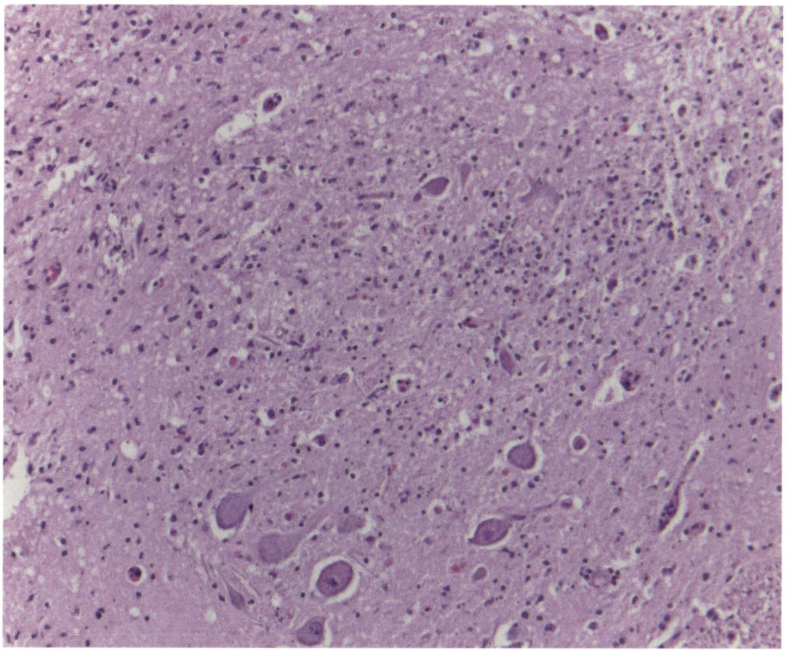

Fig. 17. Enterovirus myelitis. Chronic inflammatory cells including microglial cells involve the anterior horns.

4.6 Bunyaviruses

Bunyaviruses are negative-stranded RNA viruses. Human pathogens include the arboviruses La Crosse encephalitis virus and Toscana virus.

La Crosse encephalitis virus is endemic in the mid-Atlantic and midwestern United States. Small mammals are the host, and mosquitoes are the vector. La Cross encephalitis is predominantly a disease of children. Patients present with aseptic meningitis that may progress to encephalitis. Seizures are relatively common. Neuropathologic findings include meningitis, perivascular chronic inflammation, microglial nodules, and foci of necrosis (Love & Wiley, 2005).

Toscana virus is transmitted by the bite of the sandfly, which may be both the vector and the reservoir. It is the most common cause of summertime viral meningitis in central Italy and has spread within Europe to Spain, Portugal, and France (Tyler, 2009a). Most infections are mild with rare reports of severe encephalitis. The diagnosis is made by detecting IgM antibodies in CSF or by PCR amplification of viral RNA.

4.7 Arenavirus

The arenaviruses are enveloped, single-stranded RNA viruses. The principal human pathogen affecting the nervous system in this family is lymphocytic choriomeningitis virus (LCMV). Its principal reservoir is the mouse. LCMV infection is acquired by contact with contaminated fomites, via inhalation of aerosolized virus, via organ transplantation, or transplacentally when a pregnant woman acquires a primary infection (Bonthius, 2009; Tyler, 2009a). Typically, patients present with a non-specific viral syndrome followed by symptoms of an aseptic/viral meningitis. Some patients develop a more severe neurologic illness including transverse myelitis, Guillain-Barré syndrome, hydrocephalus, or encephalitis. Congenital LCMV leads to chorioretinitis with scarring, macrocephaly secondary to a non-communicating hydrocephalus, or microcephaly with periventricular calcifications. Other reported findings include periventricular cysts, porencephaly, encephalomalacia, intraparenchymal calcifications, cerebellar hypoplasia, and disturbances in neuronal migration (Bonthius, 2009).

4.8 Paramyxoviruses

Paramyxoviruses are single-stranded RNA viruses. Members of this family causing CNS disease are the measles virus (Morbillivirus) and the recently emerging henipaviruses, Hendra and Nipah.

4.8.1 Morbillivirus

Measles virus can cause CNS complications early after acute measles (acute postinfectious measles encephalitis) or after years of viral persistence (subacute sclerosing panencephalitis) (Reuter & Schneider-Schaulies, 2010). These disorders are rare in developed countries because of widespread immunization against measles.

Subacute sclerosing panencephalitis (SSPE) is caused by a persistent infection of the brain by a defective form of the measles virus. It typically affects children and adolescents and is characterized by personality changes, intellectual deterioration, seizures, myoclonus, and ocular changes (Garg, 2008). The brain in most cases of SSPE is atrophic with abnormally firm, mottled gray white matter (Figure 18). The microscopic findings are those of a chronic encephalitis including perivascular chronic inflammation, microglial nodules, and neuronophagia. Affected white matter is gliotic, and oligodendroglial nuclei exhibit a ground-glass appearance similar to those seen in progressive multifocal leukoencephalopathy (Figure 19). Eosinophilic inclusions may also be seen in neuronal nuclei, and subtle intracytoplasmic inclusions may also be present. Neurofibrillary tangles within glial cells have also been described (Garg, 2008).

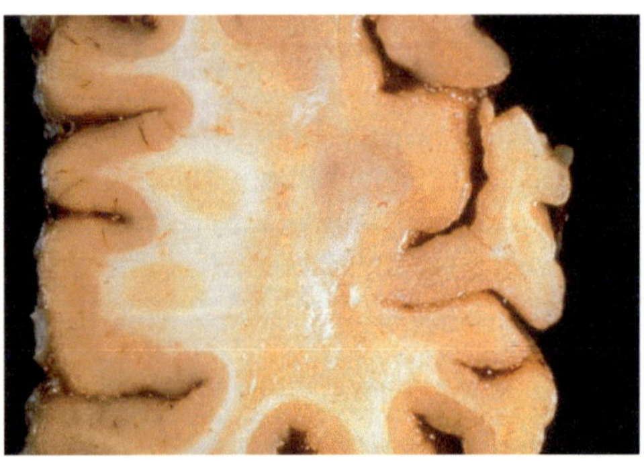

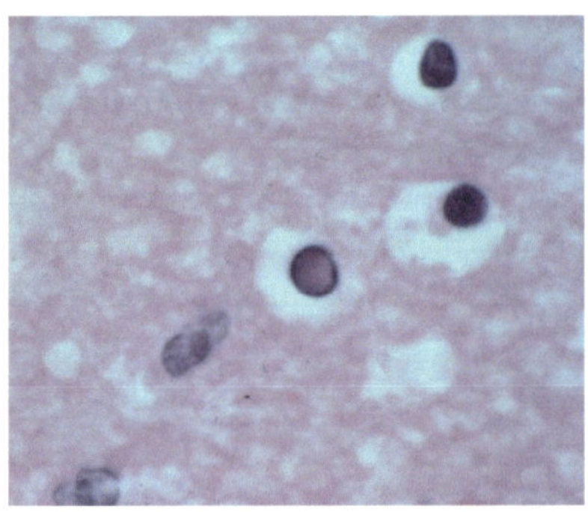

Figs. 18 & 19. SSPE. Grossly, there is grayish discoloration of the white matter. Microscopically, ground-glass inclusions are present in oligodendroglial cells.

4.8.2 Hendra and Nipah viruses

Hendra and Nipah viruses are relatively recently identified members of the genus *Henipavirus* causing outbreaks in Australia and Asia, respectively. Their natural host is the fruit bat. Bat-to-human transmission may be direct or via intermediate hosts such as the horse or pig (Wong, 2010).

Hendra virus infection may manifest as either a pulmonary or neurological syndrome consisting of confusion, motor deficits, and seizures. The diagnosis is based on the finding of IgM and IgG antibodies in the serum and CSF (Wong, 2010).

CNS disease in Nipah virus infection follows a prodrome of fever, nausea, myalgia, and dizziness. Neurologic signs and symptoms include reduced deep tendon reflexes, segmental myoclonus, nuchal rigidity, seizures, cerebellar ataxia, and brainstem signs. A relapsing or late-onset encephalitis occurs in some patients (Johnson & Power, 2008; Tyler, 2009b; Wong; 2010).

The neuropathologic findings in these two viral infections are similar and consist of vasculitis with associated vascular thrombosis and foci of necrosis. Perivascular chronic inflammation, microglial nodules, and neuronophagia are also present. Intranuclear and intracytoplasmic inclusions are seen predominantly in neurons near areas of vasculitis or necrosis (Tyler, 2009b; Wong, 2010).

4.9 Orthomyxoviruses

The orthomyxoviruses are single-stranded RNA viruses. The influenza viruses are part of this family and can cause CNS dysfunction via a number of different mechanisms including influenza-associated encephalopathy, febrile seizures, Reye syndrome, postinfluenzal encephalitic Parkinson disease, and encephalitis lethargica (Wang et al., 2010). Influenza A viruses have the potential to cause pandemics, as illustrated recently by the emergence of a novel influenza A (H1N1) virus of swine origin (Maritz et al., 2010).

Influenza-associated encephalopathy (IAE) is an uncommon complication with high mortality characterized by typical flu symptoms with associated CNS manifestations including seizure, alteration in consciousness, decreased cognitive function, abnormal behavior, and change in mental status that occurs most commonly in children. Imaging studies show a necrotizing encephalopathy with associated cerebral edema (Lyon et al., 2010; Wang et al., 2010; Webster et al., 2010). Risk factors for the development of severe disease in the recent H1N1 pandemic include age less than two years, pregnancy, chronic pulmonary disease, immunosuppression, and metabolic disorders including diabetes mellitus and obesity (Maritz et al., 2010). Most fatal cases are the result of pulmonary complications.

Gross brain findings in fatal cases of influenza H1N1 infection include cerebral edema, dusky discoloration of gray matter structures, and petechial hemorrhages (Figure 20). Microscopic findings include diffuse anoxic changes thought to be secondary to systemic disease; most patients do not have a meningoencephalitis (Milyani et al., 2010).

4.10 Rhabdoviruses

The principal human pathogen in the rhabdovirus family is rabies virus. It is usually transmitted from the bite of a rabid animal, but rare cases have been transmitted by aerosols in laboratories or caves with large numbers of bats and by organ transplantation (Jackson, 2008; Tyler, 2009a). There are two clinical forms of rabies. The more common form, encephalitic (furious) rabies is characterized by generalized arousal or hyperexcitability, disorientation, bizarre behavior, and hallucinations. Hydrophobia, or spasms of inspiratory muscles on attempts to drink, is characteristic but only seen in up to half of patients. Paralytic (dumb) rabies is characterized by motor weakness, often beginning in the bitten extremity, which progresses to quadriparesis with facial weakness (Mrak & Young, 1994; Jackson, 2008). Both types of rabies progress to coma with subsequent organ failure and death. The diagnosis can be confirmed by detecting viral RNA using reverse transcription-PCR of saliva, tears, and skin biopsies (Jackson, 2008).

The brain and spinal cord are usually grossly normal. Microscopic findings include a variable distribution of perivascular chronic inflammation, microglial nodules, and neuronophagia. Intracytoplasmic viral inclusions known as Negri bodies are diagnostic and may be best identified in the pyramidal neurons of the hippocampus and Purkinje cells of the cerebellum (Figure 21).

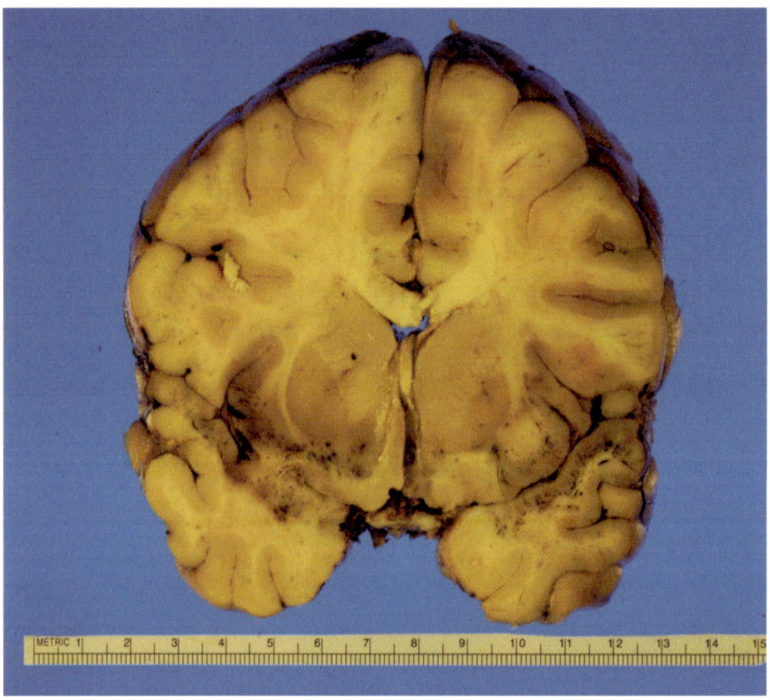

Fig. 20. Influenza H1N1. Cerebral edema and petechial hemorrhages are common in fatal cases.

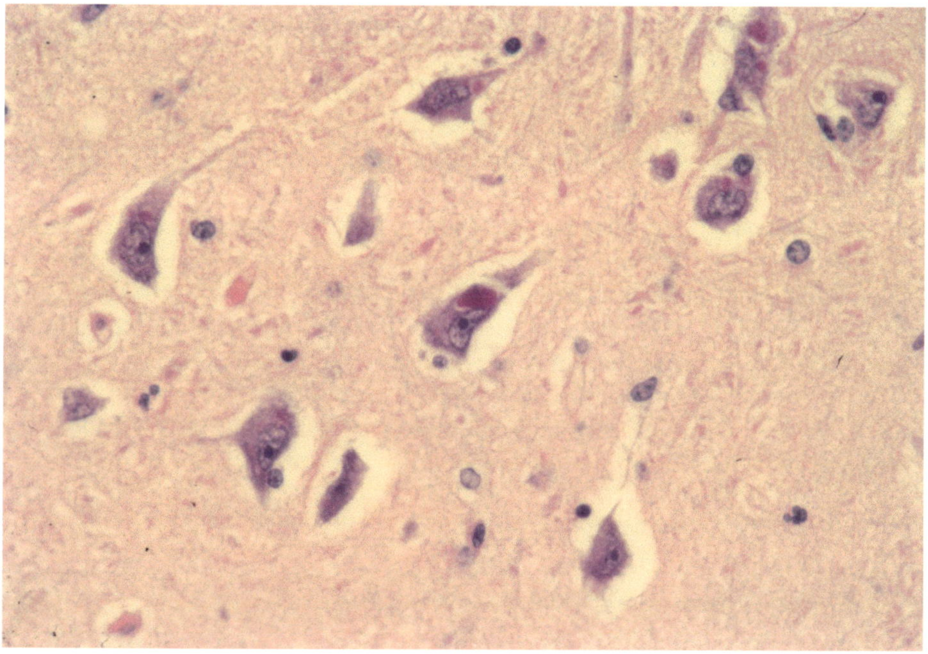

Fig. 21. Rabies. Intracytoplasmic inclusions termed Negri bodies are characteristic.

5. Conclusion

Viral infections of the central nervous system are most often diagnosed using a combination of clinical findings and serologic or molecular methods. In some instances, brain biopsy is performed as part of the diagnostic work-up. Viral infections which may be diagnosed on brain biopsy include herpes simplex virus encephalitis, varicella-zoster virus vasculopathy, and progressive multifocal leukoencephalopathy (JC virus). In immunocompromised patients, viral encephalitis, especially PML, must be distinguished from other causes of encephalitis including toxoplasmosis and from primary brain lymphoma.

6. References

Anthony, I.C. & Bell, J.E. (2008). The neuropathology of HIV/AIDS. *International Review of Psychiatry*. Vol. 20, No. 1, pp. 15-24, ISSN 0954-0262

Baringer, J.R. (2008). Herpes simplex infections of the nervous system. *Neurologic Clinics*. Vol. 26, pp. 657-674, ISSN 0733-8619

Boissé, L., Gill, J., & Power, C. (2008). HIV infection of the central nervous system: Clinical features and neuropathogenesis. *Neurologic Clinics*. Vol. 26, pp. 799-819

Bonthius, D.J. (2009). Lymphocytic choriomeningitis virus: A prenatal and postnatal threat. *Advances in Pediatrics*. Vol. 56, pp. 75-86, ISSN 0065-3101

Crowder, C.D., Gyure, K.A., Drachenberg, C.B., Werner, J., Morales, R.E., Hirsch, H.H., & Ramos, E. (2005). Successful outcome of progressive multifocal leukoencephalopathy in a renal transplant patient. *American Journal of Transplantation*. Vol. 5, pp. 1151-1158

Dutta, A. (2008). Epidemiology of poliomyelitis - Options and update. *Vaccine*. Vol. 26, pp. 5767-5773, ISSN 0264-410X

Garg, R.K. (2008). Subacute sclerosing panencephalitis. *Journal of Neurology*. Vol. 255, pp. 1861-1871

Gilden, D., Cohrs, R.J., Mahalingam, R., & Nagel, M.A. (2009). Varicella zoster virus vasculopathies: Diverse clinical manifestations, laboratory features, pathogenesis, and treatment. *Lancet Neurology*. Vol. 8, pp. 731-740

Granerod, J., Tam, C.C., Crowcroft, N.S., Davies, N.W.S., Borchert, M., & Thomas, S.L. (2010). Challenge of the unknown: A systematic review of acute encephalitis in non-outbreak situations. *Neurology*. Vol. 75. pp. 924-932

Griffiths, P. (2004). Cytomegalovirus infection of the central nervous system. *Herpes*. Vol. 11, pp. 95A-104A

Gyure, K.A. (2005). Infections, In: *Neuropathology*, Prayson, R.A. (ed.), pp.287-338, Elsevier Inc., ISBN 0-443-06658-2, Philadelphia, PA

Gyure, K.A. (2009). West Nile virus infections. *Journal of Neuropathology and Experimental Neurology*. Vol. 68, No. 10, pp. 1053-1060

Jackson, A.C. (2008). Rabies. *Neurologic Clinics*. Vol. 26, pp. 717-726, ISSN 0733-8619

Johnson, R.T. & Power, C. (2008). Emerging issues in neurovirology: New viruses, diagnostic tools, and therapeutics. *Neurologic Clinics*. Vol. 26, pp. 855-864, ISSN 0733-8619

LaSala, P.R. & Holbrook, M. (2010). Tick-borne flaviviruses. *Clinics in Laboratory Medicine*. Vol. 30, pp. 221-235, ISSN 0272-2712

Letendre, S.L., Ellis, R.J., Ances, B.M., & McCutchan, J.A. (2010). Neurologic complications of HIV disease and their treatment. *Topics in HIV Medicine*. Vol. 18, No. 2, pp. 45-55

Lo, M.K., & Rota, P.A. (2008). The emergence of Nipah virus, a highly pathogenic paramyxovirus. *Journal of Clinical Virology*. Vol. 43, pp. 396-400, ISSN 1386-6532

Love, S. & Wiley, C.A. (2008). Viral infections, In: *Greenfield's Neuropathology*, Love, S., Louis, D.N., & Ellison, D.W. (eds.), pp. 1275-1389, Edward Arnold (Publishers) Ltd, ISBN 978-0-340-90682-8

Lyon, J.B., Remigio, C., Milligan, T., & Deline, C. (2010). Acute necrotizing encephalopathy in a child with H1N1 influenza infection. *Pediatric Radiology*. Vol. 40, pp. 200-205

Mansfield, K.L., Johnson, N., Phipps, L.P., Stephenson, J.R., Fooks, A.R., & Solomon, T. (2009). Tick-borne encephalitis virus - A review of an emerging zoonosis. *Journal of General Virology*. Vol. 90, pp. 1781-1794

Maritz, J., Maree, L., Preiser, W. (2010). Pandemic influenza A (H1N1): The experience of the first 6 months. *Clinical Chemistry and Laboratory Medicine*. Vol. 48, No. 1, pp. 11-21

McCombe, J.A., Auer, R.N., Maingat, F.G., Houston, S., Gill, M.J., & Power, C. (2009). Neurologic immune reconstitution inflammatory syndrome in HIV/AIDS: Outcome and epidemiology. *Neurology*. Vol. 72, pp. 835-841

Milyani, W., Skitarelic, K., Bafakih, F., Gyure, K. (2010) Neuropathologic findings in a fatal case of H1N1 influenza virus infection (abstract). *Journal of Neuropathology and Experimental Neurology*. Vol. 69, p. 555

Misra, U.K. & Kalita, J. (2010). Overview: Japanese encephalitis. *Progress in Neurobiology*. Vol. 91, pp. 108-120, ISSN 0301-0082

Mrak, R.E., Young, L. (1994). Rabies encephalitis in humans: Pathology, pathogenesis and pathophysiology. *Journal of Neuropathology and Experimental Neurology*. Vol. 53, No. 1, pp. 1-10

Reuter, D. & Schneider-Schaulies, D. (2010). Measles virus infection of the CNS: Human disease, animal models, and approaches to therapy. *Medical Microbiology and Immunology*. Vol. 199, pp. 261-271

Romero, J.R. & Simonsen, K.A. (2008). Powassan encephalitis and Colorado tick fever. *Infectious Disease Clinics of North America*. Vol. 22, pp. 545-559, ISSN 0891-5520

Rorke, L. (1973). Nervous system lesions in the congenital rubella syndrome. *Archives of Otolaryngology*. Vol. 98, pp. 249-251

Rossi, S.L., Ross, T.M., & Evans, J.D. (2010). West Nile virus. *Clinics in Laboratory Medicine*. Vol. 30, pp. 47-65, ISSN 0272-2712

Singer, E.J., Valdes-Sueiras, M., Commins, D., & Levine, A. (2010). Neurologic presentations of AIDS. *Neurologic Clinics*. Vol. 28, pp. 253-275, ISSN 0733-8619

Shishido-Hara, Y. (2010). Progressive multifocal leukoencephalopathy and promyelocytic leukemia nuclear bodies: A review of clinical, neuropathological, and virological aspects of JC virus-induced demyelinating disease. *Acta Neuropathologica*. Vol. 120, pp. 403-417

Steiner, I., Budka, H., Chaudhuri, A., Koskiniemi, M., Sainio, K., Salonen, O., & Kennedy, P.G.E. (2010). Viral meningoencephalitis: A review of diagnostic methods and guidelines for management. *European Journal of Neurology*. Vol. 17, pp. 999-1009, ISSN 1468-1331

Tan, C.S. & Koralnik, I.J. (2010). Progressive multifocal leukoencephalopathy and other disorders caused by JC virus: Clinical features and pathogenesis. *Lancet Neurology*. Vol. 9, pp. 425-437

Tyler, K.L. (2009). Emerging viral infections of the central nervous system: Part 1. *Archives of Neurology*. Vol. 66, No. 8, pp. 939-948

Tyler, K.L. (2009). Emerging viral infections of the central nervous system: Part 2. *Archives of Neurology*. Vol. 66, No. 9, pp. 1065-1074

Vinnard, C., Barton, T., Jerud, E., & Blumberg, E. (2009). A report of human herpesvirus 6-associated encephalitis in a solid organ transplant recipient and a review of previously published cases. *Liver Transplantation*. Vol. 15, pp. 1242-1246

Wang, G.F., Weizhong, L., & Li, K. (2010). Acute encephalopathy and encephalitis caused by influenza virus infection. *Current Opinion in Neurology*. Vol. 23, pp. 305-311, ISSN 1350-7540

Weber, T. (2008). Progressive multifocal leukoencephalopathy. *Neurologic Clinics*. Vol. 26, pp. 833-854, ISSN 0733-8619

Webster, R.I., Hazelton, B., Suleiman, J., Macartney, K., Kesson, A., & Dale, R.C. (2010). Severe encephalopathy with swine origin influenza A H1N1 infection in childhood: Case reports. Neurology. Vol. 74, pp. 1077-1078.

Wong, K.T. Emerging epidemic viral encephalitides with a special focus on henipaviruses. (2010). *Acta Neuropathologica*. Vol. 120, pp. 317-325

Zacks, M.A. & Paessler S. (2010). Encephalitic alphaviruses. *Veterinary Microbiololgy*. Vol. 140, pp. 281-286, ISSN 0378-1135

3

The Neuropsychiatric Consequences of Childhood Encephalitis: A Review of Cases from Middle-Eastern Countries

Ali Evren Tufan, Tugba Guven, Banu Aslantas-Ertekin and Irem Yalug Ulubil
Abant Izzet Baysal University Medical Faculty
Elazig Hospital for Mental Disorders
Kocaeli University Medical Faculty
Turkey

1. Introduction

Encephalitis is an acute inflammation of the brain which can arise after infections such as septicemia or by primary extension of the inflammation in cases of cerebral abscess or meningitis. In a more restricted sense, it refers to a primary disease in which inflammation of the brain is caused by viral agents. Especially in children it may also arise via autoimmune or hypersensitivity reactions. Although, laboratory processes have sufficiently developed to isolate and demonstrate offending agents in most of the cases, a number of sporadic cases remain in which a viral etiology is suspected on account of general presentation. The symptoms of encephalitis include headache, fever, drowsiness tremors, vomiting and photophobia along with those arising from involvement of the central nervous system (Lishman, 2003; Maria & Bale JR, 2006).

The principal feature of cerebral involvement is disturbance of consciousness. Delirium may figure prominently in some varieties. Seizures are common especially in children and can be the presenting feature. Focal neurological signs depend on the site of inflammation and may vary. Changes in pupils and in deep tendon reflexes, ocular palsies, nystagmus, ataxia, pathological reflexes, and paresis of limbs are common. Dysphasia may denote involvement of the temporal lobe while urinary retention or paraparesis may reveal involvement of the spinal cord. Occasional cases may present with neuropsychiatric symptoms such as hallucinations, psychosis, changes in personality, dementia, delirium, delusions, affective changes, paraphilias, amnesia and parkinsonism. Those attracted attention in early epidemics of encephalitis lethargica and examples may still occur with other varieties (Lishman, 2003; Maria and Bale JR, 2006).

Although encephalitis may be an important cause of delirium and dementia as well as other psychopathology in childhood, those diagnoses present a diagnostic challenge to most child and adolescent psychiatrists leading to missed diagnoses (Cepeda, 2000; Jha, 2004; Nunn, Williams & Ouvrier, 2002, Schieveld et al., 2007). Also, encephalitis may be associated with significant childhood morbidity and mortality worldwide, however not much is known about the contemporary epidemiology and outcome (Galanakis et al., 2009).

The review and comparison of psychological consequences of various causes of childhood encephalitis may have the potential to elucidate the mechanisms of development of the human brain as well as improving our knowledge of child and adolescent neuropsychiatry. Up to now, publications tend to be isolated case histories or case series, from separate centers and this may preclude generalizations. The authors have also noted that, up to now no research group has attempted a collected presentation of cases published in Middle Eastern countries. Considering the potentially rewarding nature of this condition a critical review, especially using information from cases reported from the said countries, was deemed to benefit clinicians. In this review, first the classical accounts of neuropsychiatric consequences of encephalitis throughout the lifespan will be reviewed and augmented with the results of studies conducted to determine the neuropsychiatric consequences of childhood encephalitis, then a collected presentation of cases published in Middle Eastern countries will be attempted, lastly targets for future research and intervention will be delineated.

2. Methods

A literature search was conducted by using the PubMed search engine (http://www.ncbi.nlm.nih.gov/sites/entrez) and "childhood encephalitis" was entered as key-word. The data from the results of this search is combined with those from text-books to provide a "standard" description. Thereafter, the names of the countries in Middle-East were added to this key-word (i.e. "Turkey", "Syria", "Lebanon", "Israel", etc.) and separate searches were conducted. Data for cases were extracted. A search of the database yielded that 309 publications from Turkey and 409 from Israel were conducted on Encephalitis. Iran (n=37) and Lebanon (n=30) followed those countries. Lastly, targets for future research and intervention will be delineated.

3. Types of encephalitis and their consequences throughout the life span

3.1 Arthropod borne encephalitis

This group of illnesses, including Eastern Equine, Western Equine and St. Louis encephalitis as well as Japanese B encephalitis causes seasonal, recurrent epidemics in various parts of the world. Transmission is by insect bites which may include mosquitoes, ticks and mites. The illnesses especially affect the very young and the elderly. The onset is with fever, headache and gastrointestinal disturbances. Signs of meningeal irritation often accompany these with seizures and reduced consciousness. Delirium may be rarer in those cases. Focal motor signs may include cranial nerve palsies (especially the occulomotor nerve) and upper motor neuron pareses in limbs. Approximately 70 % of cases may result in severe neurological damage or death (Lishman, 2003; Stone and Hawkins, 2007).

The sequels are directly related to the length of coma in the acute stage and inversely related to the age at infection. Residual deficits are reported in approximately 50 % of infants less than one year of age while the rate is 20 % for adults. Sequels in infants may include mental retardation, spastic paralysis, motor abnormalities and seizures. In adults, the sequels may include depressed mood and lethargy during recovery, occasional changes in personality and intelligence, and, rarely; ataxia, dysarthria and hemiparesis. Post-encephalitic parkinsonism is thought to be rare. Adult patients frequently report multiple, vague, somatic complaints. Depression, irritability, insomnia, forgetfulness, reduced concentration, and tremors may also be reported (Lishman, 2003; Stone and Hawkins, 2007). Recent studies conducted in Turkey and Middle-Eastern countries revealed that, Tick-borne and other arthropod related encephalitis may be commoner than thought before (Ergunay et al., 2007).

3.2 Enterovirus encephalitis

This group of viruses mostly produces aseptic meningitis rather than encephalitis. For poliomyelitis, spinal cord is the main target with usually slight encephalitis while coxackie and ECHO viruses can occasionally produce encephalitis. Outbreaks are commonest in summer and autumn. Children affected while they were less than one year old may occasionally be left with neurological impairment and seizures. Other serious sequels are reported to be rare. Muscle weakness may be marked however, true paralysis is rare. Very rarely, a mild post-encephalitic parkinsonism may be seen after those infections (Lishman, 2003; Stone and Hawkins, 2007).

3.3 Encephalitis lethargica

This atypical form of encephalitis, which was first reported by Von Economo in 1917, caused epidemics with chronic and severe sequels throughout 1918-1920 (Lishman, 2003). Although the epidemic has not recurred since then, isolated cases continue to be reported (Reid et al., 2001). The symptoms arise after a flu-like prodrome and include, fever, sore throat, headache, diplopia, alterations in consciousness, sleep inversion, catatonia and lethargy (Dale et al., 2004; Lishman, 2003). Akinetic mutism, oculogyric crises, parkinsonism, paresis, muscle pains, tremors, nuchal rigidity, and behavioral changes including psychosis are also reported (Vilenksy et al., 2006). Sequels include tics, psychosis, personality changes and post-encephalitic parkinsonism, the latter even arising years after the initial infection. The disease is polymorphic, although each epidemic was reported to share some features within itself. Reportedly, most epidemics had a seasonal pattern with peaks in winter (Lishman, 2003).

The cause is still not known for certain, although recent research suggests an autoimmune reaction (Dale et al., 2004; McCall et al., 2008). Alternatively, some authors posit that the offending agent might be a variant of influenza (Vilensky et al., 2007). A recent study revealed that influenza infection in mice may trigger an autoimmune response which destroys dopaminergic neurons, thereby bridging these two views (Jang et al., 2009).

Regardless of cause, the disease was reported to have distinct forms; including a somnolent-ophtalmoplegic variety along with hyperkinetic, parkinsonian and psychotic forms. The somnolent-ophtalmoplegic variety or the basic form was reported mainly in sporadic cases and demonstrated somnolence after a prodrome of mild meningeal irritation, movement and ocular abnormalities and cranial nerve palsies. Initial presentation was with drowsiness, sometimes with mild delirium. This stage may be followed by recovery or a long term sleep which may even last for months. The sleep problems persisted even after recovery. Seizures, aphasias which may be temporary and cerebellar signs were also reported in those patients (Lishman, 2003).

In contrast, the hyperkinetic form was characterized by motor restlessness after the prodrome. Myoclonic twitches, chorea, anxiety were reported along with compulsive, tic-like movements, torticollis, torsion spasms, occulomotor symptoms and seizures. Delirium could be marked. This acute phase lasted for a few days, and followed by sleep abnormalities after recovery. Some patients may develop into somnolent-ophtalmoplegic or parkinsonian types after the acute stage, illustrating the polymorphic character of the disease (Lishman, 2003).

In the parkinsonian form; rigidity and akinesis are seen from the outset. The patient displays psychomotor retardation, hypophonia and increased latency of speech. While he/ she was reported to be mentally intact, the muscle tone was increased and there were coarse tremors in their hands. Also, festinating gait, hypersalivation, catatonia, somnolence, sleep inversion and occulomotor symptoms can be seen. Many of those patients were reported to progress into chronic parkinsonian forms (Lishman, 2003).

Psychotic forms, which initially present with isolated psychopathology are rare and the presentation is with an acute organic reaction with stupor, depression, hypomania and catatonia. Impulsive and bizarre behavior with bewildered/ fearful affect may be the only finding for several days. Controversially, it was posited that some cases might have occurred as isolated psychoses without somatic symptoms and they were called as "cerebral forms" (Lishman, 2003). There may also be other forms with bulbar palsies or involving isolated cases of chorea, neuritis and hiccoughs (Lishman, 2003).

During recovery, patients report fatigue, depression and sleep problems. Focal neurological problems may also persist after recovery. Motor abnormalities and seizures were also reported to persist, albeit rarely. Hypothalamic damage may lead to endocrine abnormalities. According to earliest resources, 40 % of the cases were fatal while 20 % demonstrated complete recovery. The remainder had residual deficits, of which the most important were parkinsonism and personality changes. Also, among the patients with residual problems, approximately one half were permanently disabled, mostly due to progressive parkinsonism. As a result, the most important chronic sequels reported were parkinsonism, personality changes and mental retardation. Severe psychopathologies were also seen in varying numbers. The sequels mentioned depended on the age at infection with adults developing parkinsonism and subcortical dementia, children personality changes and infants mental retardation. They were not related with the severity of the initial infection (Bruneau, 2005; Lishman, 2003). Parkinsonism may develop gradually from the acute stage onwards or may arise after full recovery (Lishman, 2003).

Post-encephalitic parkinsonism after encephalitis lethargica was the most common sequel, which developed insidiously. Typical pill-rolling tremor in this type of parkinsonism was reported to be rarer, with occasional coarse tremors and athetosis. Apathy was more striking with rigidity developing later.. Stereotypies were also distinctive, developing in advanced cases. Within this picture, compulsive elements were observed in speech, thought and motor behavior. In some cases, reportedly, compulsive thoughts and urges may arise independently of motor phenomena. Oculogyric crises were also seen along with changes in the function of the autonomic nervous system. As reported in classical resources, suggestibility played a role in this picture. Punding, that is compulsive/ impulsive behavior and interests arising after infection may be seen and be related with oculogyric crises (Bruneau, 2005; Lishman 2003).

Post-encephalitic personality change was mostly observed in children and adolescents. It was frequently accompanied by parkinsonism, sleep changes, obesity and endocrine abnormalities. The personality changes included emotional lability, hyperactivity and impulsive behavior. Some of those patients improved with puberty while 50 % developed parkinsonism in their later years (Lishman, 2003).

Post-encephalitic psychoses after encephalitis lethargica were usually affective in nature. Paranoid-hallucinatory states were reported in 15 to 30 % of patients while 10 % displayed schizophrenia like psychoses. Severe cases of hypochondriasis were also reported. (Lishman, 2003).

As for current cases, it can be said that the diagnosis is mainly clinical with a high index of suspicion for patients with parkinsonism and sleep changes developing after an encephalitis along with oculogyric crises, ocular/ pupillary abnormalities, involuntary movements and psychopathology. Sporadic cases may be milder than those described in epidemics and psychiatric symptoms may be prominent in the clinical picture (Lishman, 2003). Lopez-

Alberola et al., 2009). Cases which arose after seasonal influenza infections as well as infections with Ebstein-Barr virus have also been reported, therefore supporting the position that encephalitis lethargica may be a heterogenous presentation of infections affecting the circuits between frontal lobes and basal ganglia (Alarcón et al., 2011; Toovey et al., 2011).

3.4 Encephalitis due to herpesviridiae

This group involves encephalitis due to Herpes simplex, Ebstein Barr and Varicella Zoster viruses.

3.4.1 Herpes Simplex Virus Encephalitis (HSVE)

HSV is the commonest single cause of severe sporadic encephalitis with a high mortality and marked psychopathology both in the acute presentation and as sequels. It affects especially medial temporal and orbital lobes and causes sporadic encephalitis without seasonal variation among all age groups. It may be primary or due to reactivation. There is typically a rapid onset with fever, seizures, meningeal irritation, drowsiness/ confusion, and focal neurological signs. A study conducted at a pediatric tertiary treatment center in Turkey found that 40 % of the patients applying for treatment with status epilepticus had either meningitis or encephalitis, underlying the pre-eminence of seizures in HSVE (Saz et al., 2011). Sometimes, psychiatric symptoms may be prominent at the onset. Hallucinations as part of psychiatric symptoms or part of delirium are typically vivid and colorful with marked emotional reactions. Restlessness and hyperactivity may be seen after recovery. Additionally, anosmia, olfactory and gustatory hallucinations, amnesia, symptoms of elevated intracranial pressure could be seen. Rarely, benign aseptic meningitis or recurrent organic psychoses may be seen. The sequels involve mental retardation in children, dementia in adults, seizures, dysphasia, personality changes, severe amnestic states, and bizarre behavior resembling Kluver-Bucy Syndrome throughout the life span (Arciniegas and Anderson, 2004; Lishman, 2003; Stone and Hawkins, 2007).

Even among recovered patients, subtle neuro-psychological deficits are observed, especially involving language and memory. Calculation, facial recognition and visuo-spatial abilities were also reported to be affected. (Ku et al. 1996; Ward et al. 2011).

3.4.2 Encephalitis due to EBV (Infectious Mononucleosis)

The most distinctive feature of this type of encephalitis is its picture of depression and fatigue in the recovery period. Reportedly, the two phenomena are not related (Lishman, 2003). However, in isolated cases more severe presentations and neuropsychological sequelae may occur (Dagdemir et al., 2008).

3.4.3 Varicella Zoster Virus (VZV)

Although the introduction of live attenuated VZV vaccine in 1995 helped to reduce the incidence and complications of varicella infections and sequels with this virus continue to be reported, mainly involving meningitis (Pahud et al. 2011). Although an eight year old male patient was reported to develop acute hemiplegia and obsessive-compulsive disorder secondary to a lesion of lentiform nuclei after a varicella infection and that he was reported to respond to sertraline treatment and to make a full-recovery, studies and/ or case series involving larger samples from both genders may be needed to elucidate the neuropsychological consequences of VZV infection (Yaramiş et al., 2009).

4. Other types of sporadic, viral encephalitis

This group includes mumps, adenoviruses, infectious hepatitis, rabies and influenza. Among those, mumps is the most important one, it may cause encephalitis even without overt disease. The virus can itself invade the central nervous system. It usually causes aseptic meningitis, with only occasional cases of encephalitis. Therefore, if encephalitis due to mumps is present then as a rule, co-morbid meningitis and sometimes myelitis is also present. The symptoms occur 2-10 days after parotitis or in some cases, may precede it (Lishman, 2003).

5. Long term consequences of childhood encephalitis

Studies conducted on the long term consequences of childhood encephalitis are scarce. However, it was reported that childhood encephalitis between 0-16 years at the time of infection caused mortality at a rate of 2.8 % while the rate increased to one third if the patients were less than three years of age (Lishman, 2003). The risk of mortality may be especially pronounced in patients less than one years old, those who are unconscious at the time of admission, within the first month and with infections by HSV (Lishman, 2003). After a follow-up of 10 years it was reported that 40 % of patients may have problems with motor functions/ academic achievement, 20 % may have epilepsy and a further 20 % displayed behavioral problems, mostly hyperactivity (Lishman, 2003).

5.1 Studies conducted on childhood encephalitis in Middle-Eastern countries

When the results of studies conducted on childhood encephalitis in Middle-Eastern countries were reviewed it was observed that they focused mostly on cases of HSVE, reflecting the international literature (Ibrahim et al., 2005; Yildirim 2008). Pediatric complications associated with Influenza and results of West Nile encephalitis were reported in studies conducted in Israel (Landau et al. 2011). Also, reflecting the 2009 pandemic of influenza, cases of meningitis and meningo-encephalitis in children were reported with influenza A (H1N1) infections from Turkey (Ozdemir et al., 2011, Yildizdas et al., 2011). However, neuropsychiatric and neurobehavioral consequences of childhood encephalitis were reported only in limited studies (Yildirim, 2008). According to those; pediatric HSVE caused deficits in IQ, short term memory and in language functions while deficits due to mumps meningoencephalitis were slight (Yildirim, 2008), though results of another study from Turkey may contradict the latter position (Aygun et al., 2001, Yildirim, 2008). Aygun and colleagues (2001), investigated the viral etiology of 36 children at a regional medical center in eastern Turkey in between 1995 and 1999 and reported that mumps was the most common pathogen in their sample (47.1 %) and that mental and/ or focal neurological deficits were observed in 52.9 % (Aygun et al. 2001). Isolated cases of neuropsychological consequences with VZV are also reported (Yaramiş et al., 2009).

6. Conclusion

Although encephalitis may be associated with significant childhood morbidity and mortality worldwide, our knowledge about its contemporary epidemiology and outcome are limited, especially for the long term (Galanakis et al., 2009). Therefore, future multi-centre studies conducted on patients who recovered from childhood encephalitis may be necessary. Elucidation of neuropsychological deficits caused by varieties of childhood encephalitis may help us determine potential remedial methods for rehabilitation (Dewar and Gracey, 2007).

7. References

Alarcón F, Dueñas G, Lees A. (2011) Encephalitis lethargica due to Epstein-Barr virus infection. Mov Disord; Vol., 26, No.,11, pp 2132-4.

Arciniegas DB, Anderson CA. (2004) Viral encephalitis: neuropsychiatric and neurobehavioral aspects. *Curr Psychiatr Rep*; Vol., 6, pp. 372-379

Aygün AD, Kabakuş N, Çelik İ, Turgut M, Yoldaş T, Gök Ü, Güler R. (2001) Long-term neurological outcome of acute encephalitis. *Trop Pediatr;* 47, pp. 243-247.

Bruneau M-A. (2005) Obsessionality. In: Parkinson's Disease and Non-motor dysfunction. Pp. 29, Humana Press, e-ISBN 1-59259-859-5, New Jersey

Cepeda C. (2000) The Neuropsychiatric Interview and Examination, In: *Concise Guide to The Psychiatric Interview of Children and Adolescents*. Pp. 219-282, American Psychiatric Press, ISBN 0-88048-330-X, Washington D.C.

Dagdemir A, Tasdemir HA, Dilber C, Gok F, Kubar A. (2006). Increased intracranial pressure due to chronic active Epstein-Barr virus infection. *J Child Neurol.* Vol. 21, pp.820-2.

Dale RC, Church AJ, Surtees RA, Lees AJ, Adcock JE, Harding B, Neville BGR, Giovannoni G. (2004). Encephalitis lethargica syndrome: 20 new cases and evidence of basal ganglia autoimmunity". *Brain* Vol., 127, Pt., 1, pp. 21–33

Dewar B-K, Gracey F. (2007). "Am not was": Cognitive-behavioral therapy for adjustment and identity change following herpes simplex encephalitis. *Neuropsychol Rehabil;* Vol., 17, No., 4, pp. 602-620

Ergunay K, Ozer N, Us D, Ozkul A, Simsek F, Kaynas S, Ustacelebi S. (2007) Seroprevalence of West Nile virus and tick-borne encephalitis virus in southeastern Turkey: first evidence for tick-borne encephalitis virus infections. *Vector Borne Zoonotic Dis.*; Vol. 7, pp. 157-61.

Galanakis E, Tzoufi M, Katragkou A, Nakou I, Roilides E. (2009) A prospective multicenter study of childhood encephalitis in Greece. *Pediatr Infect Dis J*; Vol. 28, No: 8, pp. 740-742.

Ibrahim AI, Obeid MT, Jouma MJ, Roemer K, Mueller-Lantzsch N, Gärtner BC. (2005). Prevalence of Herpes Simplex Virus (Types 1 and 2), Varicella-Zoster Virus, Cytomegalovirus, and Human Herpesvirus 6 and 7 DNA in Cerebrospinal Fluid of Middle Eastern Patients with Encephalitis. *J Clin Microbiol*; Vol., 43, No., 8, pp. 4172-414

Jang H;Boltz D, Sturm-Ramirez K,Shepherd KR, Jiao Y, Webster R, Smeyne RJ. (2009).Highly pathogenic H5N1 influenza virus can enter the central nervous system and induce neuroinflammation and neurodegeneration. *Proc Nat AcadSci; Vol.,* 106, No., 33, pp. 14063

Jha S, Patel R, Yadav RK, Kumar V. (2004). Clinical spectrum, pitfalls in diagnosis and therapeutic implications in herpes simplex encephalitis. *J Assoc Physicians India;* Vol. 52, No. 1, pp. 24-26.

Ku A, Lachmann EA, Nagler W. (1996). Selective language aphasia from herpes simplex encephalitis. Pediatr Neurol; Vol., 15, No., 2, pp. 169-71.

Landau YE, Grisaru-Soen G, Reif S, Fattal-Valevski A. (2011). Pediatric neurologic complications associated with Influenza A H1N1. *Pediatr Neurol*; Vol., 44, pp. 47-51

Lishman WA. (2003) Intracranial Infections. In: *Organic Psychiatry: The Psychological Cansequences of Cerebral Disorder*. Third Edition. Pp. 346-365, Blackwell Science, ISBN 0-86542-842-5, Oxford.

Lopez-Alberola R, Georgiou M, Sfakianakis GN, Singer C, Papapetropoulos S. (2009). Contemporary Encephalitis Lethargica: phenotype, laboratory findings and treatment outcomes. J Neurol; Vol. 256, No. 3, pp. 396-404.

Maria BL, Bale JR JF.(2006). Infections of the Nervous System. In: *Child Neurology*. Menkes JH, Sarnat BH, Maria BL (Eds). Seventh Edition. Pp. 433-555, Lippincott Williams & Wilkins. ISBN 0-78175-104-7 Philadelphia.

McCall S, Vilensky JA, Gilman S, Taubenberger JK. (2008). The relationship between encephalitis lethargica and influenza: a critical analysis. *J. Neurovirol.; Vol.,* 14, No., 3, pp. 177–85.

Nunn K, Williams K, Ouvrier R. (2002). The Australian Childhood Dementia Study. *Eur Child Adolesc Psych;* Vol. 11, No. 2, pp. 63-70.

Ozdemir H, Karbuz A, Ciftçi E, Ince E, Doğru U. (2011) Aseptic meningitis in a child due to 2009 pandemic influenza A (H1N1) infection. *Turk J Pediatr.;* Vol. 53, pp.91-3

Pahud BA, Glaser CA, Dekker CL, Arvin AM, Schmid DS. (2011). Varicella zoster disease of the central nervous system: epidemiological, clinical, and laboratory features 10 years after the introduction of the varicella vaccine. J Infect Dis. Vol., 203, No., 3, pp. 316-23.

Reid AH, McCall S, Henry JM, Taubenberger JK (2001).Experimenting on the past: the enigma of von Economo's encephalitis lethargica. *J. Neuropathol. Exp. Neurol;* Vol. 60, No. 7, pp.663–70.

Saz EU, Karapinar B, Ozcetin M, Polat M, Tosun A, Serdaroglu G, Gokben S, Tekgul H. (2011). Convulsive status epilepticus in children: etiology, treatment protocol and outcome. *Seizure.;* Vol. 20, pp.115-8.

Schieveld JN, Leroy PL, van Os J, Nicolai J, Vos GD, Leentjens AF. (2007). Pediatric delirium in critical illness: phenomenology, clinical correlates and treatment response in 40 cases in the pediatric intensive care unit. *Intensive Care Med;* Vol. 33, No. 6, pp. 1033-40.

Stone MJ, Hawkins CP. (2007). A medical overview of encephalitis. *Neuropsychol Rehabil;* Vol., 17, No., 4/ 5, pp. 429-449.

Toovey S, Jick SS, Meier CR. (2011). Parkinson's disease or Parkinson symptoms following seasonal influenza. Influenza Other Respi Viruses; Vol., 5, No., 5, pp.328-33

Vilensky JA, Goetz CG, Gilman S. (2006). Movement disorders associated with encephalitis lethargica: a video compilation. *Mov. Disord.;* Vol.,21, No., 1, pp.1–8.

Vilensky JA, Foley P, Gilman S (2007). Children and encephalitis lethargica: a historical review. *Pediatr. Neurol;* Vol.,37, No., 2, pp. 79–84.

Ward KN, Ohrling A, Bryant NJ, Bowley JS, Ross EM, Verity CM. (2011). Herpes simplex serious neurological disease in young children: incidence and long-term outcome. Arch Dis Child. [In Press], PMID: 21685219

Yaramiş A, Hergüner S, Kara B, Tatli B, Tüzün U, Ozmen M. (2009). Cerebral vasculitis and obsessive-compulsive disorder following varicella infection in childhood. Turk J Pediatr; Vol., 51, No., 1, pp. 72-5.".

Yildirim I. (2008) Children followed with the diagnosis of Herpes Simplex encephalitis: clinical presentations, laboratory findigs and neuro-psychometric evaluation. Hacettepe Faculty of Medicine Thesis in Pediatric Infectious Diseases. Ankara.

Yildizdaş D, Kendirli T, Arslanköylü AE, Horoz OO, Incecik F, Ince E, Ciftçi E. (2011) Neurological complications of pandemic influenza (H1N1) in children. *Eur J Pediatr.;* Vol. 170, pp.779-88.

4

Encephalitis in Elderly Population

Şerefnur Öztürk[1] and Fahrettin Ege[2]
[1]*Selçuk University, Selçuklu Faculty of Medicine, Neurology Department*
[2]*Cihanbeyli State Hospital, Neurology Department*
Turkey

1. Introduction

The elderly population is increasing worldwide. Population of people above 65 years old was 420 million in the year 2000, and is estimated to be 973 million in 2030 (Centers for disease control and prevention [CDCP], 2003). Mortality rate related to infectious diseases decreased after the discovery of anibiotics, particularly in the second half of the twentieth century, however it is stil being a problem in elderly age group.

Several immun alterations arise with aging and these alterations make elderly people more vulnerable to infections. In addition, body composition changes with aging, chronic diseases such as hypertension, diabetes mellitus and cardiac failure are more frequent in elderly age group, so this multi-factorial situation also reduces the immunological resistance to infections. For all these reasons, encephalitis is more frequent in elderly people as compared to younger individuals and it usually causes clinically a more severe course.

Encephalitis in elderly deserves a more sensitive approach. The disease may be difficultly perceived by clinicians for some reasons. Premorbid brain disorders such as dementia and stroke especially, may lead to diagnostic delay. Numerous co-morbid situations in this age group may lessen the efficiency of treatment and may bring about seconder problems. Therefore encephalitis in elderly may result in severe central nervous system damage, high morbidity and mortality.

2. Etiological agents

Defined etiological agents in elderly encephalitis are not fairly different than those in younger patients. However frequency of encepahlitis caused by some pathogenes and disease severity is dissimilar in elderly age group

Herpes simplex virus is the main cause of encephalitis in adult population including individuals above 60 years old (Lee et al., 2003). However herpes simplex encephalitis is dramaticaly frequent in aged population (Hjalmarsson et al., 2007). The incidence of the disease is significantly higher in population above 60 years as compared to 3-60 age group (Puchhammer-Stöckl et al., 2001). In addition, clinicians encounter herpes simplex type 1 as the main etiological agent of elderly herpes simplex encephalitis, that is similar to ratios defined in other age groups (Jouanny et al., 1994).

Besides herpes simplex, viral and bacterial, lots of agents have been reported as a cause of elderly encephalitis. Some of these agents are associated with regional/geographical factors, and a portion with immunological status of patients. West nile virus (WNV) is a considerable etiological agent in aged population as the encephalitis caused by west nile virus is more frequent and more severe in elderly people as compared to younger adults (Berner et al., 2002, 2005, Cook et al., 2010, Roos, 2005). Elderly cases related to St. Louis encephalitis virus (Roos, 2005), Tick borne encephalitis virus (Logar et al., 2000), enteroviruses (EV) (Frantzidou et al., 2008), Ebstein Barr virus (EBV) (Hu & Chan, 2000), Varisella zoster virus (VZV) (Granerod et al., 2010, Gillanders et al., 1994) and Cytomegalovirus (CMV) (Lee et al., 2003) have been reported as far. Encephalitis caused by mycobacterium tuberculosis (Granerod et al., 2010, Lee et al., 2003) and other bacterial agents (Granerod et al., 2010) have also been defined in this age group. Etiological spectrum of elderly encephalisit is shown on Table 1.

<table>
<tr><td rowspan="10">HERPES SİMPLEX</td><td>West Nile Virus</td><td rowspan="10">UNDEFINED ETİOLOGY</td></tr>
<tr><td>Ebstein Barr virus</td></tr>
<tr><td>Cytomegalovirus</td></tr>
<tr><td>Herpes Zoster</td></tr>
<tr><td>Enterovirus</td></tr>
<tr><td>Tick Borne Encephalitis</td></tr>
<tr><td>Mycobacterium Tuberculosis</td></tr>
<tr><td>Japan Encephalitis</td></tr>
<tr><td>St. Louis Encephalitis</td></tr>
<tr><td>Other bacterial agents</td></tr>
</table>

Table 1. Etiological spectrum of elderly encephalitis

As the clinical utilization of serological methods and PCR technique become widespread, number of etiological agents in elderly population is increasing. However, it should be borne in mind that, cases with undefined etiology is more frequent in elderly age group as compared to younger adults (Lee et al., 2003).

3. Immune alterations

It is claimed that immune system progresively deteriorates with aging and elderly people are more vulnerable to infectious diseases (Sansoni et al., 2008). Several changes occur in immunity system of elders. The major proportion of these changes are involved in the quantity and the configuration of circulating lymphocytes. Numerical changes appear both in T cell and B cell compartments, thus effectiveness of cellular and humoral responses alter. The most prominent immune alteration is occured in T cell comparment. Response of T cells to mitogens weakens and T cell quantity in circulation decreases (Fahey et al., 2000). It is indicated that both circulating CD 4 (+) and CD 8 (+) T cells diminish with aging (Provinciali et al., 2009). Quantity of CD 4 (+) T cells is proportionally higher in normal immunity, however inverted CD 4 (+) / CD 8 (+) ratio (less than 1.00) is significantly more frequent in elderly individuals as compared to younger individuals (Wikby et al., 2008). Inverted ratio is reflecting the dominancy of suppresor activity in elderly age group. Similar numerical changes have also been occured in B cell compartment. Quantity of CD 5 (+) and CD 19 (+) B cells lessens with aging (Sansoni et al., 2008). Besides the changes in cellular level, several alterations appear in cytokin synthesis, which IL-6 levels increase and IL-2 levels decrease in aged individuals (Lesourd & Mazari, 1999). Immune alterations of elderly is shown on Table 2

As a consequence of age related immune alterations, antibody production dimishes and immunological memory shortens (Fahey et al., 2000). Immunologic response to antigens weakens, infections tend to be frequent and heavier with increased age.

T Cells
CD 4 (+) Reduction CD 8 (+) Reduction Inverted ratio of CD 4 (+)/CD 8 (+) Suppressor activity
B Cells
CD 5 (+) Reduction CD 19 (+) Reduction
Cytokines
IL-6 increase IL-2 decrease

Table 2. Immune alterations in elderly age group

Several clinical and laboratory observations concordant with the above mentioned immune alterations in increased age are present in the literature. These observations are related especially with the infections caused by viral etiology and closely linked with the pathogenesis of encephalitis. For instance, skin infection of herpes zoster is more frequent in aged population (Schmader & Dworkin, 2008) and with situations which impair cellular immunity (Schmader, 1999). Latent Herpes simplex virus existance in trigeminal ganglion is significantly more frequent in elderly individuals as compared to younger adults, which is concordant with the fact that herpes simplex encephalitis frequency is higher in aged population (Liedtke et al., 1993). This data is reflecting the poor immunological response to herpes simplex virus with increased age. (Figure 1)

It is considered that insufficient pleocytosis and low IgG activity in a case with herpes simplex type 2 encephalitis, is asssociated with age related immune disregulation (Reuter et al., 2007). Another clinical observation is the high frequency of re-infection or endogen virus activation in elderly herpetic meningoencephalitis as compared to primary infection (Jouanny et al., 1994), which may also reflects the age related immune alterations.

Furthermore, chronic diseases are seen more frequently in elderly population and some of these diseases lessen the immunological resistance to antigens. Immune alterations related to both aging and underlying chronic disorders make elderly people more vulnerable to infectious disorders and complications of infections (Yoshikawa, 2002). For instance esential hypertension and diabetes mellitus presence are found to be associated with the severity of west nile virus encephalitis, moreover they were reported as risk factors for persistancy of symptoms in elderly patients (Cook et al., 2010)

As concordant with the data about immunity alterations in elderly individuals, herpes simplex encephalitis is seen more frequently in elderly age group, makes a more severe clinical course, and mortality is significantly higher in individuals above 70 years old (Hjalmarsson et al., 2007). Increased age is found to be associated with the outcome of herpes encephalitis (Whitley et al., 1986, Kamei et. al., 2005). Also west nile virus leads to a more severe clinical course in elderly patients as compared to younger adults (Cook et al., 2010, Berner et al., 2002). Increased age is an independent risk factor for fatality of west nile virus encephalitis (Berner et al., 2002). Such that mortality in patients above 70 years old increases 40-50 fold, as compared to younger patients (O'Leary et al., 2002). Also Tick borne encephalitis makes a more severe clinical course in elderly age group (Logar et al., 2000).

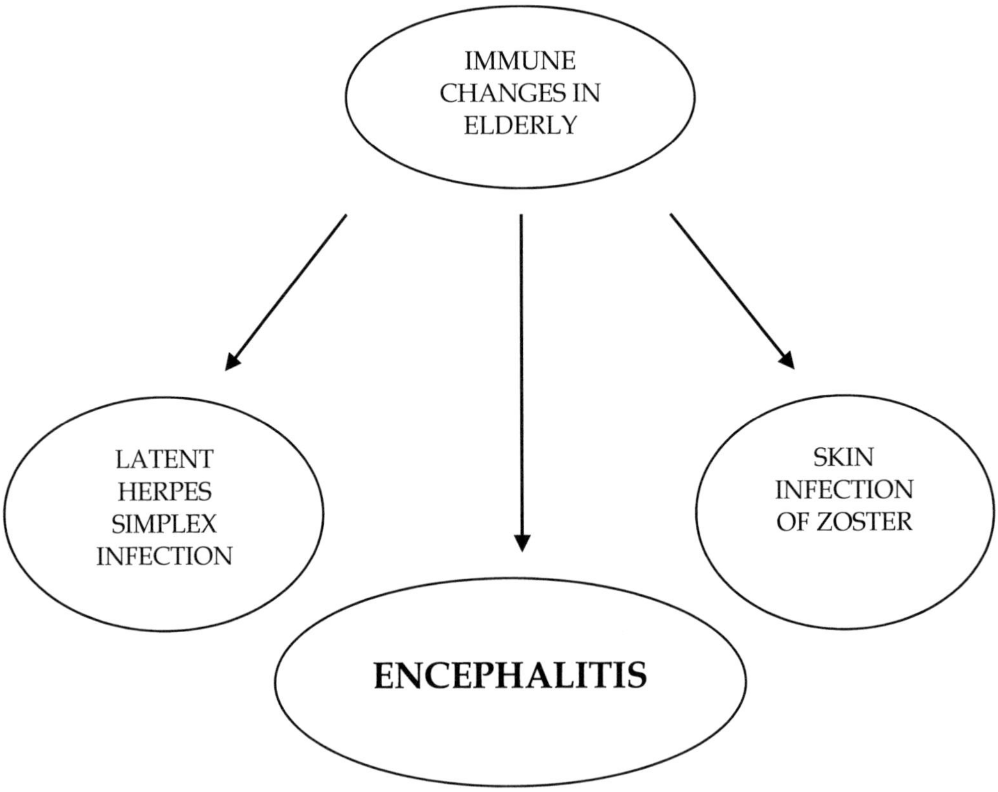

Fig. 1. Clinical entities related to immune alterations of elderly

4. Clinical course

Clinical symptoms of herpes simplex encephalitis are fever, headache, meningeal signs, alteration of consciousness, focal and generalised seizures and long tract signs. Mortality and morbidity of untreated herpes simplex encephalitis is high. Yet, morbidity and mortality are seen less frequently with today's spesific antiviral therapy. Currently, clinicians easily perceive and diagnose herpes encephalitis unless co-morbid conditions which may lead to a diagnostic confusion accompany, and if typical signs and spesific laboratory and imaging findings are present; thus spesific antiviral and symptomatic therapy is perfomed in the early phase of the disease.

However, herpes simplex encephalitis in elderly mostly presents with atypical clinical symptoms, and may difficultly be perceived by clinicians. Encephalitis in elderly, may present with more subtle symptoms such as progresive amnestic cognitive disorder or behaviroual changes, which are fairly different from typical symptoms in younger adults (Wong & Yau, 2007). These clinical signs, may frequently be confused with neurodegenerative processes, metabolic delirium or stroke. Fever accompanied with progresive receptive aphasia may be a symptom of herpes encephalitis (Lester et al., 1988). As an atypical clinical presentation, progresive dysartria and hypersalivation with no cognitive impairment in a 65 years old patient has also been defined (Almekhlafi et al., 2010). Short-term memory deficit has been defined as a clinical sign of herpes encephalitis (Reuter et al., 2007).

Encephalitis should be considered in all elderly individuals with progresive mental confusion (Lester et al., 1988, Reuter et al., 2007, Fernandes et al., 2010). Furthermore, progresive mental confusion seems to be the most considerable sign of early phase of elderly encephalitis, and should not be neglected in emergency services (Jouanny et al., 1994). Atypical clinical presentations of elderly encephalitis is shown on Table 3

Herpes simplex encephalitis	Progresive amnestic cognitive disorder Behaviroual changes Progresive receptive aphasia Progresive mental confusion Frontal lobe syndrome Progresive dysartria + hypersalivation
Herpes zoster encephalitis	Confusion Deteriorating confusion (premorbid illness)
EBV encephalitis	Intermittant confusion
Enterovirus encephalitis	Cognitive + behaviroual impairment
WNV encephalitis	Focal neurological deficits mimicking stroke Febril attacks

Table 3. Atypical clinical presentation of encephalitis in elderly

Herpes simplex encephalitis usually affects the temporo-frontal grey matter and typical clinical symptoms of the disease is closely associated with this localisation. However, atypical localisations of herpes simplex encephalitis have also been reported both in elderly and non-elderly patients and currently, with the widespread clinical utilization of MRI, it is considered that atypical herpes simplex encephalitis localisations are more common than it's supposed to be (Fernandes et al., 2010). Clinicians may encounter cases with exclusively frontal lobe involvement with relatively sparing of the temporal lobes (Taylor et al., 2007). Frontal lobe syndrome in an elderly patient characterised by Bruns ataxia, incontinence and confusion may associated with herpes encephalitis (Ege et al., 2010). (Figure 2) Cerebellum, brain stem, parietal cortex, occipital cortex, thalamus and even white matter lesions due to herpes simplex encephalitis have been reported thus far. This condition however, has been seen more frequently in pediatric population and immun-compromised adults (Taylor et al., 2007). Similarly, aging is associated with several immun alterations, therefore may predispose to atypical localisations which may be confused with neoplasia and stroke. Herpes encephalitis should not be excluded when atypical clinical symptoms and extratemporal localisations appear, and be investigated with advanced diagnostic technices. Atypical localisations is shown on Table 4.

Atypical anatomical localisations of herpes simplex encephalitis reported thus far	Frontal cortex
	Occipital cortex
	Parietal corex
	Brain stem
	Thalamus
	White matter
	Cerebellum

Table 4. Atypical anatomcal localisations of herpes simplex encephalitis

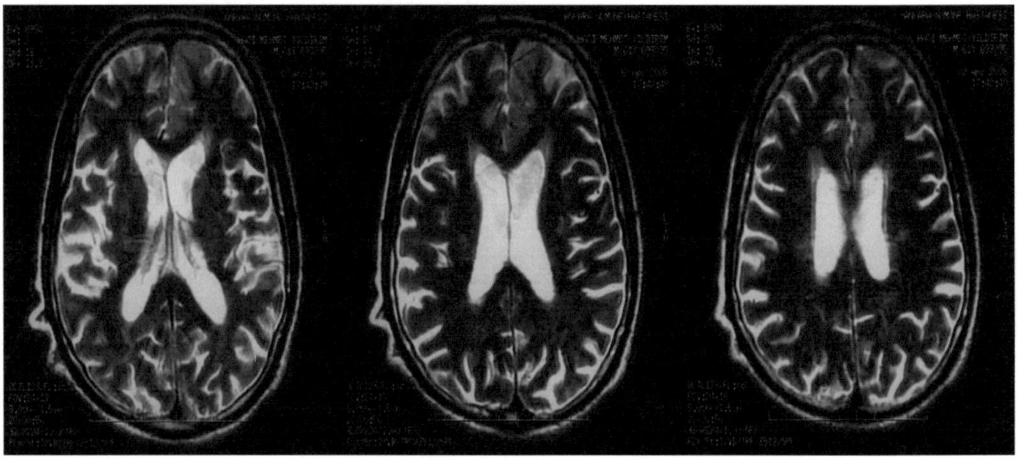

Fig. 2. Frontal lobe cortex involvement in herpes encephalitis

Atypical clinical presentations have also been defined in herpes zoster encephalitis. Confusion which is not accompanied with focal neurological deficits in an elderly patient or gradually deteriorating confusion in a patient with neurodegenerative dementia may be symptoms of zoster encephalitis (Gillanders et al., 1994). Similarly EBV encephalitis in an elderly patient may presents with intermittant confusion and febril attacks (Hu & Chan, 2000). An elderly case with enteroviral meningoencephalitis which is presented with cognitive and behavioural impairment has also been reported in the literature (Valcour et al., 2008)

Regardless of etiology, in patients over 60 years old, meningeal signs are less frequent as compared to non-elderly patients; and motor weakness is seen more frequently. Clinical course of the disease in elderly patients is more severe and outcome is worse than in non-elderly patients (Lee et al., 2003). Despite the fact that encephalitis in the elderly may presents with atypical clinical symptoms in the early phase, typical symptoms frequently arise as the disease progresses.

5. Prognosis

Encephalitis causes a severe central nervous sytem damage, and may result in morbidity and mortality. Altough the outcome can be changed by utilizing infection markers and modern treatment strategies in the early phase, the prognosis of the disease is also associated with several defined clinical factors. Old age and severity of clinical course are the most important prognostic factors. Old age, as well as the deterioration of consicoussness are found to be the major risk factors for mortality in herpes encephalitis (Whitley et al., 1986, Kamei et. al., 2005). Once again mortality in west nile virus encephalitis is clustered in elderly individuals as compared to younger adults (Berner et al., 2002). Regardless of etiology, encephalitis causes a poorer outcome in elderly population (Lee et al., 2003).

Another considerable problem in elderly patients is the persistency of neurological symptoms. Persistent symptoms not only deteriorate the life quality of patients but also cause secondary medical problems. The frequency of persistent neurological symptoms following west nile virus encephalitis has been found to be associated with diabetes mellitus and hypertension, and not with old age (Cook et al., 2010). However, it is known that chronic diseases are seen more frequently in elderly individuals. Rehabilitation programmes are currently taken into account for patients who have persistant neurological symptoms (Berner et al., 2005). Mortality and persistant neurological symptoms are frequent also in patients over 75 years old in Japan encephalitis (Berner et al., 2005 as cited in Tsai, 2000). Morbidity in herpes encephalitis is still being a problem despite the modern antiviral treatment in elderly patients (Whitley et al., 1986). Cerebellar encephalitis is reported both in elderly and non-elderly patients. However, dissimilar from outcome of younger patients, the disease may lead to a persistent and more severe cerebellar ataxia (Klockgether et al., 1993).

6. Differential diagnosis

Elderly encephalitis may mimic several clinical situations, as the disease presentation in elderly age group is atypical and accompanying vascular and neurodegenerative disorders may disguise markers of encephalitis. In addition, atypical localisations in herpes encephalitis demonstrated by magnetic resonance imaging may increase the confusion. Such that atypical localisations may be confused with ischeamic lesions and neoplasias. Encephalitis may mimic stroke, by causing unilateral motor weakness and other focal neurological deficits; furthermore it is reported that the disease may be presented as deterioration of motor weakness in patients having motor sequela of stroke (Berner et al., 2002).

In addition, many disorders in elderly may be presented with clinical symptoms mimicking encephalitis. If so, encephalitis should be differentiated from clinical situations causing mental confusion and delirium in aged individuals.

1. Metabolic encephalopathies (hepatic and renal failure, elcetrolyte disturbance, hypoglicemia, hyperglicemia)
2. Hypertensive encephalopathy
3. Cerebrovascular disorders
4. Head trauma
5. Bronchopneumonia, urinary tract infections, sepsis
6. Drug adverse effects
7. Paraneoplastic syndromes
8. Space occupying lesions
9. Neurodegenerative disorders, dementia
10. Hydrocephalus
11. Epilepsy

Metabolic encephalopathies in elderly individuals are imitating encephalitis by giving rise to confusion and disorientation; electrolyte disturbances, diabetic coma and uremia should be differentiated. Fever of any cause is a considerable situation in elderly patients and may lead to excaberation of symptoms of demented patients. Urinary tract, lung, upper respiratory tract and skin infections may cause fever and delirium, so be easily confused with encephalitis. Hypertensive encephalopathy presents with headache, seizures and consicoussness impairment and may mimic central nervous system infections. Fluctuations and excaberations of neurodegenerative disorders, Lewy body dementia in particular, may give rise to diagnostic confusion. Space occupying lesions in frontal and temporal lobes should be differentiated from infectious disorders, as they are presented with cognitive impairment, focal neurological deficits and seizures. Non-convulsive seizures in elderly population are seen both in epileptic patients and symptomatically, and with their clinical symptoms and EEG changes, may bring central nervous infections to mind. Briefly, encephalitis may mimic several conditions such as stroke and dementia, also numerous systemic and neurological disorders may present with symptoms resembling encephalitis in old age. For this reason, multi-disciplinary approach is required at times, in emergency services, for the elderly patients who have fever and mental deterioration.

7. Diagnostic tools

Diagnosis of encephalitis in elderly is based on high index of suspicion in the early course of the disease, as the presentation is atypical. For this reason, MRI and cerebro-spinal fluid examination should be performed in all patients with probable encephalitis. Altough MRI is an effective tool for demonstrating the encephalitis lesions, it may reveal negative results in the early course of the disease. Anatomically atypical encephalitis lesions is another problem and clinicians should not exclude the disease in the presence of such lesions.

CSF protein levels increase mild to moderataly in the course of viral encephalitis with accompanying mononuclear pleocytosis. Polymorphonuclear pleocytosis may be seen however in WNV encephalitis. CSF is normal in 10% of the cases of viral encephalitis. CSF glucose level is normal in viral encephalitis, nevertheless may found to be decreased in bacterial, fungal and parasitic encephalitis (Tunkel et al., 2008).

PCR tecnique which detects the nucleic acids of pathogenes is fairly benefical in elderly patients when findings of MRI and CSF examination are non-spesific or insufficient for diagnosis. CSF protein and lymphocyte levels may not increase in the early course of herpes encephalitis, therefore PCR should be performed in all patients. PCR should also be executed for agents such as EBV, CMV, VZV, WNV in suspected cases of encephalitis. Specifity and sensivity of PCR in herpes simplex encephalitis is high, despite false negative results may rarely be obtained. The test should be repeated after few days in suspected cases. Investigation of CSF IgM anti-bodies is useful in some cases. Detection of virus spesific IgM anti-bodies can be utilized so as to diagnose flavivirus infection. 4 fold increase in spesific serum IgG anti-body level is also an important marker for determining lots of viral and bacterial agents (Tunkel et al., 2008, Roos, 2005).

Electroencephalogram (EEG) is adjunctive and sensitive method in encephalitis, however its specifity is partially decreased in aged population. Frequent disorders in old age such as vascular lesions, metabolic disturbances and neurodegenerative diseases cause EEG changes, slow wave activity in particular. Still, it is found to be beneficial for demonstrating the periodic activity in herpes encephalitis. (Jouanny et al., 1994) Efficiency of diagnostik tools in elderly encephalitis is shown on Table 5.

Numerous disorders which may be confused with encephalitis have been defined in elderly patients. For instance bronchopneumonia may cause high fever and progresive mental confusion in elderly patients. Even an urinary tract infection may lead to delirium and be easily confused with encephalitis (Eriksson et al., 2011). For that reason, blood samples should be obtained for studying blood glucose, electrolytes, liver functions (SGPT, SGOT), renal funtions (BUN, creatinin), thyroid homones, blood count, C-reactive protein (CRP) and erythrocyte sedimentation rate (ESR). Urinary Ph, protein, nitrite and leucocyte number should also be determined. Blood and urinary cultures and chest roentgen examination are beneficial so as to scan localised and systemic infections.

Still, it should be borne in mind that, localised and systemic infections, co-morbid metabolic disturbances and chronic diseases may accompany encephalitis in elderly patients. Moreover, metabolic and systemic disorders may also be induced by encephalitis in elderly patients. For example confusion due to viral encephalitis may inhibit drug use in a diabetic elderly individual, so may secondarily causes extreme high glucose levels. Similarly a central nervous sytem infection leading to high fever and dehidratation may secondary impair renal functions. Once again, hyponatremia may be caused by inappropriate ADH syndrome secondary to encephalitis.

Alterations on mental level may mistakenly be related to metabolic disturbances in above mentioned examples, therefore indirect influence of encephalitis should also be remembered. As a consequence, encephalitis should be considered in elderly patients who have confusion and disorientation, yet investigations should be carried out for determining metabolic disturbances and systemic infections.

CLINICAL SYMPTOMS	Atypical presentations are frequent
CT SCAN	Non-spesific, sensitivity is low
MR IMAGING	Sensitive, may reveal atypical lesions
PCR	Sensitivity and specifity is high, beneficial
CSF EXAMINATION	Sensitive, specifity is low, negative in 10%
SEROLOGY	Beneficial for some agents, specifity is high
EEG	Specifity is low, sensitive

Table 5. Diagnostic tools for elderly encephalitis

8. Management of elderly patients

Amprical antibiotic treatment should be performed in suspected elderly cases before the confirmation of diagnosis. Today, parenteral acyclovir (10mg/kg iv q8h x 14-21 days, if renal functions are normal) is recommended for herpes simplex virus encephalitis. However, other ampirical antibiotic options should be initiated considering the epidemyological data. For instance, doxycycline can be given if there is clinical suspecion of ricetsial or erlichial encephalitis in risky regions (Tunkel et al., 2008).

Parenteral acyclovir is well tolerated in elderly patients, nevertheless nephrotoxic and neurotoxic adverse effects are reported rarely. BUN and creatinin levels should be studied more frequently in elderly patients than in younger individuals, to determine the nephrotoxicity. Neurotoxic side effects are seen more frequently in elderly population and patients having impaired renal functions and malignency. Neurotoxicity of acyclovir is a neuropsyhciatric disorder which consciousness is altered. Confusion, delirium, lethargia and tremor may appear in patients, so differentiation of this situation from mental changes due to encephalitis is crucial for maintaining the treatment and considering alternative options. Fever and headache do not accompany acyclovir associated neurotoxicity, and finding of lateralisation is not seen in EEG (Rashiq et al., 1993) (Figures 3 & 4)

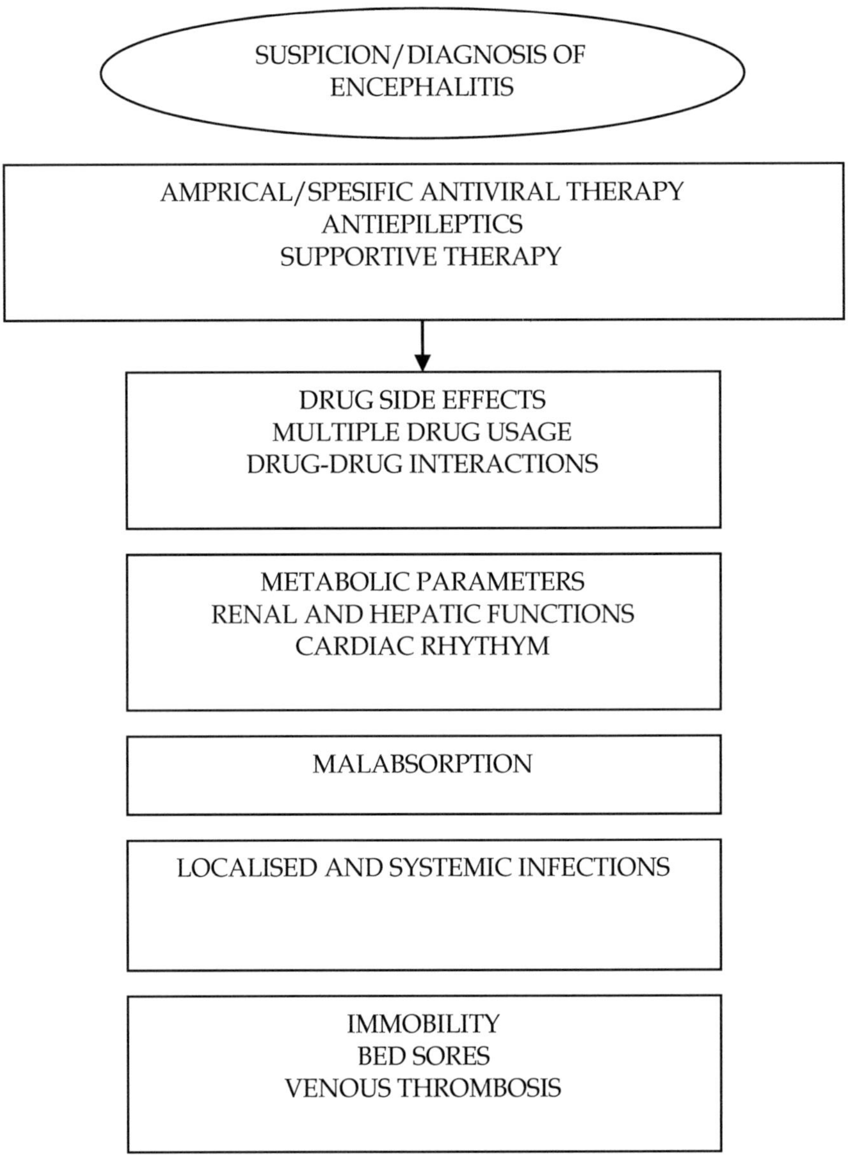

Fig. 3. Problems in management of encephalitis in elderly

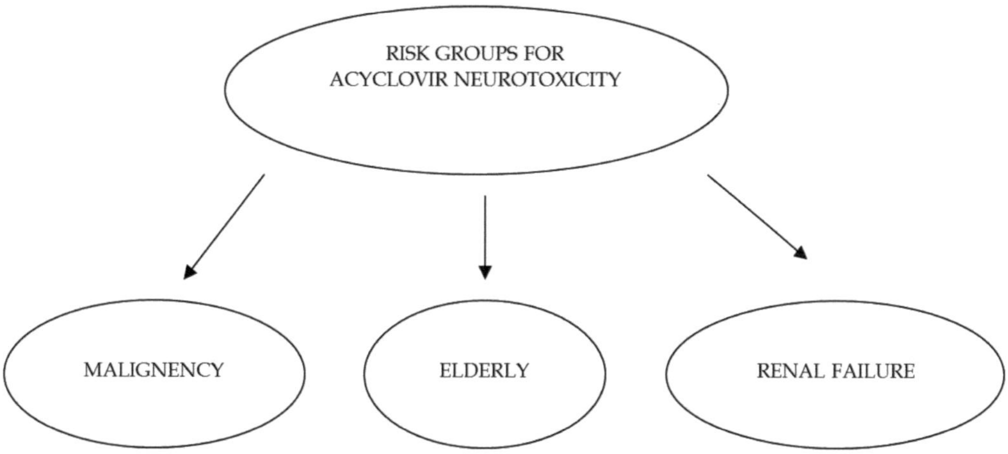

Fig. 4. Risk groups for acyclovir neurotoxicity

Acyclovir or gancyclovir for VZV encephalitis, and gancyclovir (5mg/kg q12h) + foscarnet (60mg/kg q8h) for CMV and HHV type 6 encephalitis can be prefered. Acyclovir can also be attempted in EBV encephalitis. Valacyclovir (1 gr oral 8qh) or acyclovir (10-15mg/kg iv 8qh) can be chosen for B virus encephalitis. However treatment in encephalitis due to other agents is still being a problem; currently supportive therapy strategies preserve their importance as spesific antiviral medications do not exist (Tunkel et al., 2008, Roos, 2005).

Renal and hepatic parameters as well as electrolytes should be closely monitored in elderly patients and drug doses should be adjusted to renal and hepatic functions. Metabolic conditions have to be considered in aged group, when initiating anti-epileptic agents, and clinicians should be aware of drug adverse effects in elderly. Hepatic and renal functions, blood count and cardiac rhythm have to be more closely monitored.

Drug-drug interactions is a crucial problem in old age. Elderly patients usually use multiple drugs as they possess chronic disorders. Drug interactions should be considered when choosing antibiotics and antiepileptics and dosing of these medications. Determination of blood levels is beneficial to minimise the drug interactions.

Insufficient alimentation and malabsorption is frequent in demented patients for both sociobiological and pathological reasons. Since malabsorption complicates the treatment of infectious diseases, probability of malabsorption should be evaluated in intensive care units and nutiritional support should be supplied in the early couse of the disease.

Since old age causes a predisposition to infections, clinicians should be aware of respiratory and urinary tract infections in intensive care units. Development of hospital infections and their complications are easier in elderly patients. Localised and systemic infections should be investigated if deterioration despite antiviral treatment has been perceived or persistency of high fever occurs.

Immobility due to dementia, stroke or other reasons is frequent in elderly population, in addition encephalitis may cause or worsen immobility for causing conscioussness impairment and long tract injury. It is better to take earlier measures for bed sores: patients position should be changed frequently and protein nutrition should be supplied. Abrasions and erythematous lesions have to be treated as soon as they noticed. Prophylactic anti-coagulant therapy should be given to all immobilised patients unless there is clear contraindication.

Briefly, management of encephalitis in elderly also includes sensitive approach to co-morbid situations, drug-drug interactions, premorbid chronic disorders and their excaberations. Vital signs and metabolic parameters should be more closely monitored and nutritional support should be given beginning from the early course of the disease.

9. References

Almekhlafi, MA.; Couillard, PL.; Patry, DG. & Jette, N. (2010), Herpes encephalitis presenting with an opercular syndrome and epilepsia partialis contunia, *The neurologist*, 16, 208-210

Berner, YN.; Lang, R. & Chowers, MY. (2002) Outcome of West Nile Fever in older adults, *Journal of American geriatrics society*, 50, 1884-1846

Berner, Y.; Feldman, J.; Spigel, D.; Chowers, M. & Finckeltov, B. (2005) Rehabilitation of West Nile Fever (WNF) encephalitis in elderly, *Archives of Gerontology and Geriatrics*, 41, 15-21

Centers for Disease Control and Prevention (2003) Public health and aging: Trends in aging-United States and worldwide. *JAMA*, 289, 1371-1373

Cook, RL.; Xu, X.; Yablonsky, EJ.; Sakata, N.; Tripp, JH.; Hess, R.; Piazza, P. & Rinaldo, CR. (2010) Demographic and clinical factors associated with persistent symptoms after west nile virus infection, *American society of tropical medicine and hygiene*, 83 (5), 1133-1136

Ege, F.; Gülünay, A.; Öztürk, Ş.; Karadağ, Y. & Özbakır, Ş. (2010), Herpes encephalitis with frontal localisation in an elderly patient, *Turkish journal of geriatrics*, 13 (2), 129-132

Eriksson, I.; Gustafson, Y.; Fagerström, L. & Olofsson B. (2011) Urinary tract infection in very old women is associated with delirium, *International psychogeriatrics*, 23(3), 496-502

Fahey, JL.; Schnelle, JF., Boscardin, J.; Thomas JK.; Gorre, ME., Aziz, N.; Sadeghi, H. & Nishanian, P. (2000) Distinct categories of immunologic changes in frail elderly, *Mechanisms of ageing and development*, 115, 1-20

Fernandes, AF.; Lange, MC.; Novak, FT.; Zavala, JA.; Zamproni, LN.; Germiniani, FM.; Piovesan, EJ. & Teive, HA. (2010) Extra-temporal involvement in herpes simplex encephalitis, Journal of clinical neurosciences, 17 (9) 1221-1223

Frantzidou, F.; Kamaria, F.; Dumaidi, K.; Skoura, L.; Antoniadis, A. & Papa, A. (2008) Aseptic meningitis and encephalitis because of herpesviruses and enteroviruses in an immunocompetent adult population, *European journal of neurology*, 15, 995-997

Gillanders, I.; MacKay, J.; Campbell, F.; MacLennan, WJ. Herpes zoster encephalitis in the elderly (1994), *Postgraduate medical journal*, 70 (830), 940

Granerod, J.; Ambrose, HE.; Davies, NWS.; Clewley, JP.; Walsh, AL.; Morgan, D.; Cunningham, R.; Zuckerman, M.; Mutton, KJ.; Ward, KN.; Lunn, MPT.; Irani, SR.; Vincent, A.; Brown, DWG. & Crowcroft, NS., on behalf of the UK Health Protection agency (HPA) Aetiology of encephalitis study group (2010) Causes of encephalitis and differences in their clinical presentation in England: a multicentre, population-based prospective study, *Lancet infectious diseases*, 10, 835-844

Hjalmarsson, A.; Blomqvist, P. & Sköldenberg, B. (2007), Herpes simplex encephalitis in Sweden, 1990-2001: Incidence, morbidity, and mortality, *Clinical infectious diseases*, 45, 875-880

Hu, E. & Chan, DKY. Possible Ebstein-Barr virus encephalitis in an elderly patient, *Australian and New Zealand journal of medicine*, 30, 282

Jouanny, P.; Vespignani, H.; Gerard, A.; Jeandel, C.; Ducrocq, X.; Penin, F.; Weber, M.; Dureux, JB.; Cuny, G. & Canton, P. (1994) Herpetic meningoencephalitis in the elderly, Apropos of 13 cases, *La reveue de medecine interne*, 15 (8), 504-509

Kamei, S.; Sekizawa, T.; Shiota, H.; Mizutani, T.; Itoyama, Y.; Takasu, T.; Morishima, T. & Hirayanagi, K. (2005), Evaluation of combination therapy using aciclovir and corticosteroid in adult patients with herpes simplex virus encephalitis, Journal of neurology neurosurgerey psychiatry, 76, 1544-1549

Klockgether, T.; Döller, G.; Wüllner, U.; Petersen, D. & Dichgans, J. (1993) Cerebellar encephalitis in adults, *Journal of Neurology*, 240, 17-20

Lee, TC.; Tsai, CP.; Yuan, CL.; Wei, CY.; Tsao, WL.; Lee, RJ.; Cheih, SY.; Huang, IT. & Chen, KW. (2003) Encephalitis in Taiwan: A prospective hospital-based study, *Japanese journal of infectious diseases*, 56, 193-199

Lesourd, B. & Mazari, L. Nutrition and immunity in the elderly (1999), *Proceedings of the nutrition society*, 58, 685-695

Lester, JW.; Carter, MP. & Reynolds, TL. (1988) Herpes encephalitis: MR monitoring of response to acyclovir therapy, *Journal of computer assisted tomography* 12 (6), 941-943

Liedtke, W.; Opalka, W.; Zimmermann, CW. & Lingitz, E. (1993) Age distribution of latent herpes simplex virus 1 and varicella-zoster virus genome in human nervous tissue, *Journal of neurological sciences*, 116(1), 6-11

Logar, M.; Arnez, M.; Kolbl, J.; Avsic-Zupanc, T. & Strle, F. (2000) Comparison of the epidemiological and clinical features of Tick-Borne Encephalitis in children and adults, *Infection*, 28, 74-77

O'Leary, DR.; Marfin, AA.; Montgomery, SP.; Kipp, AM. & Lehman, JA.; Biggerstaff, BJ.; Elko, VL.; Collins, PD.; Jones, JE. & Campbell, GL. (2004) The epidemic of west nile virus in the United States, *Vector borne zoonotic diseases*, 4, 61-70

Provinciali, M.; Moresi, R.; Donnini, A. & Lisa, RM. (2009) Reference values for CD4+ and CD8+ T lymphocytes with naive or memory phenotype and their association with mortality in the elderly, *Gerontology*, 55, 314-321

Puchhammer-Stöckl, E.; Presterl, E.; Croy, C.; Aberle, S.; Popow-Kraupp, T.; Kundi, M.; Hofmann, H.; Weninger, U. & Gödl, I. (2001), Screening for possible failure of herpes simplex virus PCR in cerebrospinal fluid for the diagnosis of herpes simplex encephalitis, *Journal of medical virology*, 64, 531-536

Rashiq, S.; Briewa, L.; Money, M.; Giancarlo, T.; Khatib, R. & Wilson, FM. (1993) Distinguishing acyclovir neurotoxicity from encephalomyelitis, *Journal of internal medicine*, 234, 507-511

Reuter, MD.; Manian, FA.; Kershaw, MA & Alpert, MA. (2007) Herpes simplex virus type 2 encephalitis in an elderly immunocompetent male, Southern medical journal, 100 (11), 1143-1146

Roos, KN. (2005) Encephalitis, In: *Principles of neurologic infectious diseases*, Roos KN., 65-76, McGraw-Hill, ISBN 0-07-140816-9, United States of America

Sansoni, P.; Vescovini, R.; Fragnoni, F.; Biasini, C.; Zanni, F.; Zanlari, F.; Telera, A.; Lucchini, G.; Passeri, G.; Monti, D.; Franceschi, C. & Passeri M. (2008) The immune system in extreme longevity, *Experimental gerontology*, 43, 61-65

Schmader, K. (1999) Herpes zoster in the elderly: issues related to geriatrics, *Clinical infectious diseases*, 28, 736-739

Schmader, KE. & Dworkin, RH. (2008) Natural history and treatment of Herpes zoster, *The journal of pain*, 9(1), 53-59

Taylor, SW.; Lee, DH. & Jackson, AC. (2007) Herpes simplex encephalitis presenting with exclusively frontal lobe involvement, *Journal of NeuroVirology*, 13, 477-481

Tunkel, AR.; Glaser, CA.; Bloch, KC.; Sejvar, JJ.; Roos, KL.; Hartman, BJ.; Kaplan, SL.; Scheld, WM. & Whitley, RJ. (2008) The Management of Encephalitis: Clinical Practice Guidelines by the Infectious Diseases Society of America, *Clinical infectious diseases*, 47 (3), 303-327

Valcour, V.; Haman, A.; Cornes, S.; Lawall, C.; Parsa, AT.; Glaser, C.; Yagi, S.; Tihan, T.; Bhatnagar, J. & Geschwind, M. (2008) A case of enteroviral meningoencephalitis presenting as rapidly progressive dementia, *Nature clinical practice neurology*, 4, 399-403

Whitley, RJ.; Alford, CA.; Hirsch, MS.; Schooley, RT.; Luby, JP.; Aoki, FY.; Hanley, D.; Nahmias, AJ.; Soong, SJ. & The NIAID Colloborative antiviral study group (1986), Vidarabine versus acyclovir therapy in herpes simplex encephalitis, *The New England journal of medicine*, 314(3), 144-149

Wikby, A.; Mansson, IA.; Johansson, B.; Strindhall, J. & Nilsson, SE. (2008) The immune risk profile is associated with age and gender: findings fron three Swedish population studies of individuals 20-100 years of age, *Biogerontology*, 9, 299-308

Wong, TW. & Yau T. (2007) Acute delirium in a 65-year-old-man, *Asian journal of gerontology & geriatrics* 2, 161-163

Yoshikawa, TT. (2002) Antimicrobial resistance and aging: Beginning of the end of the antibiotic era? *Journal of the American geriatric society*, 50, 226-229

5

Language and Cognitive Impairments Associated with Encephalitis

Raphiq Ibrahim
The Edmond J. Safra Brain Research Center for the Study of Learning Disabilities, Department of Learning Disabilities, University of Haifa, Israel

1. Introduction

Although the gross deficits of diseases of the brain have been extensively characterized, few studies have examined their associated cognitive impairments. Interest has focused recently on the language and cognitive impairments that develop following encephalitis. The symptoms of impairments following the disease were determined mainly by examining hospital records of those previously admitted with cerebral inflammation, who were assessed at least 20 months after discharge to detect motor, speech and language, and other cognitive (attention, memory, and non-verbal ability) impairments. This chapter deals with language and cognitive disturbances based on the literature and a published case study of a proficient bilingual man suffering from brain damage following intracranial hemorrhage and epileptic seizures related to herpes encephalitis (Ibrahim, 2009a). This case showed somewhat different symptomatologies on language ability measures in first language and second languages.

2. Background

Encephalitis is an inflammation of the brain usually caused by a virus, or, in rare cases, by bacteria. It is typically caused by one of three groups of viruses: the herpes viruses including chickenpox, Epstein-Barr (that causes mononucleosis), and herpes simplex (that causes cold sores); viruses transmitted by insects, like West Nile virus, and the germs that cause Lyme disease and Rocky Mountain Spotted Fever; and viruses that cause childhood infections like measles, mumps, and German measles.

Widespread immunization against encephalitis and other diseases has brought a marked decrease in their occurrence, but they continue to appear, sporadically and in mini-epidemics. While most cases of encephalitis are mild and symptoms last for only a short time, severe life-threatening cases can develop. Symptoms of mild cases include fever, headache, poor appetite, loss of energy, and/or a general feeling of malaise. In more severe cases patients develop high fever, severe headache, sensitivity to light, nausea and vomiting, stiff neck, confusion, sleepiness, difficulty waking, and/or unconsciousness. As encephalitis affects the brain, severe cases can sometimes develop epileptic seizures and intracranial hemorrhages that lead to difficulties with muscle movement and coordination, speech disorders, cognitive deficits and learning disabilities. These symptoms of encephalitis may last months or longer.

Risk factors for the development of language (speech) and cognitive deficits after illnesses of the brain have been described (Holding, Stevenson, et al., 1999; Carter, Murira, et al., 2003), but the studies generally classified patients as having impairments or not, rather than differentiating between impairments of different functions.

2.1 Language and cognitive impairments

Cognitive and language impairments following encephalitis have not been extensively described in the literature. Language and speech impairments develop mostly in children with severe encephalopathy (generally those with hypoglycaemia or elevated intracranial pressure), and in cases of long-term nutritional deprivation (Walther & Ramaekers, 1982). These deficits might be a manifestation of global cerebral damage rather than injury to a specific area of the brain, given the wide range of risk factors associated with language. In these cases, language deficits overlap with impairments in other cognitive abilities and motor functions, and impairment in one ability may affect the others. For example, because language, cognitive abilities, memory and attention overlap, impairments in language and other cognitive functions may arise as side-effects of impaired memory and attention (which has sizeable verbal components in terms of instructions, teaching elements, or response formats), while other language difficulties may stem from impaired motor function (Pennington, et al., 2004).

With regard to cognitive impairment after encephalitis, researchers suggested that only episodes of epileptic seizures increased the risk of cognitive impairment (Holding et al., 1999; Boivin, 2002). Based on clinical and epidemiological studies, they concluded that only in cases of hypoglycaemia and absence of hyperpyrexia is there impairment of cognition (Holding et al., 1999).

Idro and colleagues (2006) also reported this finding, stating that "hypoglycaemia was associated with impairment of non-verbal functioning but instead of absence of hyperpyrexia, we observed that children who failed to mount a febrile response (no history of fever before admission) had an increased risk of developing memory impairment" (p.146). Researchers described in detail the neurological and cognitive assessments: tests of attention (visual search), memory tests based on the Rivermead Behavioural Memory Test for Children (Wilson & Aldrich, 1991), non-verbal functioning (construction tasks such as copying shapes using drawings, blocks, or sticks to assess the coordination of complex cognitive tasks), and a parental rating of behaviour problems (Holding et al., 1999). Speech and language assessments included all major areas of language: receptive grammar and vocabulary, lexical semantics (expressive vocabulary), syntax/morphology, pragmatics (language use), phonology, higher level language, and word finding (Carter, et al., 2003). A classification of "speech and language impairment" was defined as an impairment level score on two or more of the language assessments, while a designation of "impairment in other cognitive functions" described children with impairment level performance in any one of attention, memory, or non-verbal functioning (Carter, et al., 2005a; Carter, et al., 2005b).

Idro et al. (2006) found that seizures are common precipitators of admission. Thus, it is possible that each episode cumulatively increases the risk of focal neurological damage, and that on subsequent visits, patients present with multiple seizures, focal neurological signs, and motor impairment (Ido, et al., 2004). Due to their diffuse nature, deficits are likely to involve more than one function (Holding et al., 1999), and survivors of the more severe forms are likely to suffer greater neuronal damage. Some cognitive functions such as language may be affected by external factors such as the child's nutritional state at the time of the encephalopathy (Neumann, et al., 1992; Johnston, et al., 1987).

In a systematic review of neurological and cognitive impairments associated with common central nervous system infections, Carter, Neville and Newton (2003) found those exposed to acute bacterial meningitis (ABM) had a higher prevalence of long-term impairments. The risk of impairments after ABM was greatest for, but not confined to, those who had acute neurological complications such as coma. This chapter presents the performance of a bilingual patient (M.H.) suffering from brain damage following intracranial hemorrhage related to herpes encephalitis disease (Ibrahim, 2009a). His performance on several linguistic tasks in his first language (L1-Arabic) and second language (L2-Hebrew) displayed somewhat different symptomatologies in the two languages. There was a dissociation between the two languages in terms of the magnitude of the errors and the error types, suggesting aphasic symptoms in the two languages, with Hebrew (L2) being more impaired. As we will see, this dissociation was better explained by damage at the lexical level rather than at the semantic level of representation. We further explore whether this specific impairment is also present in the patient's L2 in order to elucidate the organization of a second language in the brain.

3. Case report

M.H. is a 41-year-old, right-handed male high school biology teacher. He is a native speaker of Arabic, was born in Israel, and acquired Hebrew language in 4th grade. He used Hebrew in his academic, professional and private settings, and before contracting encephalitis at the age of 39, his Hebrew competence was reported by his bother to be very high. He was a university graduate, where the language of instruction was Hebrew, and had passed the Hebrew proficiency exam required at enrollment.

In May, 2004, M.H. was brought to the hospital with sudden onset of fever and confusion. Following an initial examination in which he was found to be febrile, confused and disoriented, he was sent to a regional hospital (Rambam Medical Center). A cereberal spinal fluid specimen was positive for herpes simplex virus type 1 (HSV-1) by polymerase chain reaction testing on the third day of hospitalization, and antiviral therapy (acyclovir) was begun. Two days later he suddenly developed a severe headache, vomiting and disturbance of consciousness. Radiological investigations showed severe, massive intracranial hemorrhage in the left temporal lobe, compressing the central line of the brain contralaterally. On the same day, he underwent left temporal craniotomy for removal of the lesion mass, following which a CT scan demonstrated moderate hemorrhage and encephalomyelitis in the left temporal lobe and right frontal subdural hemorrhage. His fever returned to normal 12 hours after surgery but he became lethargic. He was sent to Bet Levenstein Rehabilitation Hospital where he stayed two months, during which he developed an acute onset of a neurological deficit, epileptic status with left temporal focus, and amnestic aphasia.

Upon admission to Bet Levenstein, M.H. was active, cooperative, and oriented to place, situation and time. His visual fields and auditory abilities were intact. His spontaneous language production was non-fluent, with grammatical disruptions and common anomic states. The subtest from the Western Aphasia Battery (WAB; Kertesz, 1982) and the Boston

Naming Test (BNT; Kaplan, et al., 1983) in Arabic and Hebrew yielded results consistent with mild to moderate amnestic aphasia (Albert, et al., 1981). Throughout this period he received intensive language therapy.

3.1 Neuropsychological tests

Neuropsychological tests were conducted in January 2006, 32 months after hospitalization in Bet Levenstein, and included visual and language abilities.

3.1.1 Visual abilities

To rule out the possibility that the patient's symptoms were caused by the right frontal hemorrhage, his performance was assessed on tasks that tap visuospatial and frontal difficulties. The results showed normal visual ability good copying and construction abilities on the Rey Complex Figure test (Meyers & Meyers, 1995). Cognitive flexibility was measured by a Wisconsin Card Sorting Test (WCST) (Heaton, et al., 1993). His capacity for non-verbal abstraction was close to normal for his age, consistent with his intact visual perception and reasoning skills.

3.1.2 Language abilities

3.1.2.1 Phonological/phonetic abilities

M.H. was given three auditory tasks, as described by Luria (1970): (a) counting the letters in individual spoken words, (b) counting syllables in an individual spoken word, and (c) synthesizing words from individually pronounced letters (i.e., recognizing an auditorally spelled word). His performance on these tasks was found to be dependent on word length, with better performance on short words (three to five letters). Both Arabic and Hebrew are languages with deep orthography: they do not have one-to-one correspondence between letters and sounds, because most Arabic and Hebrew vowels are not instantiated as letters. This is probably reflected in the relatively similar performance by M.H. in the two languages. It was observed that M.H. counted phonemes instead of letters. Interestingly, in naming Hebrew phonemes, M.H. used the Arabic terms, referring to the sounds rather than the real names of these letters. For example, when presented with the letter he said [*ba*] instead of [*bet*]. Also, in many cases he counted syllables instead of sounds or letters. His ability to count the number of syllables was intact.

3.1.2.2 Reading and writing

When reading aloud in Arabic, M.H. demonstrated two strategies. In some cases of single and short words he seemed to use a direct visual strategy, immediately recognizing the word. In other cases this strategy was not successful and he turned to letter-by-letter reading, resulting in literal paralexias (for example, the word *a'melat*, "workers," was read as *a'lamat*, which is not a meaningful word), but often he recognized this immediately and corrected himself. His strategy for reading in Hebrew was similar, but his performance was poor, probably because of the general inappropriateness of letter-by-letter reading for unvoweled Hebrew (see Birnboim, 1995). His spontaneous writing (in Arabic) was good at the level of single words and word combinations without literal paragraphias. In Hebrew, he was able to write to dictation only at the level of words with literal paragraphias (for example, the word *mapa*, "map," was written as *maba*, which is not a meaningful word).

As can be seen from the tests administered in two languages, M.H. displayed different symptomatologies in the two languages, with the language impairment significantly more prominent in Hebrew. This was an interesting development. Arabic is structurally not very distant from Hebrew, especially in morphology and syntax. It is important to remember that, although Arabic is M.H.'s native language, he had nearly equivalent proficiency in the two languages prior to his illness. During the period of language therapy, the various tests administered to determine the nature of his impairments yielded an initial diagnosis of amnestic aphasia.

One of the important pieces of information in M.H.'s case is the localization of the brain injury. He had apparently suffered at least three distinct neurological insults during his hospitalization - herpes encephalitis with intraparenchymal hemorrhage into the left temporal lobe, right frontal subdural hematoma, and epileptic seizures - in addition to undergoing emergency surgical craniotomy of the presumably dominant hemisphere. As each insult involves distinct language networks, a detailed account of the patient's clinical language deterioration as it relates to these insults will illuminate the complex representation of more than one language in the brain, and the process of speech perception and production.

Herpes encephalitis is known to involve the bilateral temporal lobes. Among other functions, these lobes are critical in short-term memory consolidation (hippocampus) and naming functions (dominant hemisphere middle and superior temporal gyrus) (Gleissner, et al., 1997). The timing and the nature of the patient's language deterioration (detailed above) support the involvement of bilateral temporal lobes. This conclusion is in line with studies on the language organization of the temporal lobe, particularly with respect to the anatomy of the superior and middle temporal gyrus (Janszky, et al., 2004). The potentially aneurismal subrachnoid hemorrhage M.H. suffered may be associated with delayed ischemic deficits, vasospasm, and distal thromboembolic events, and might be related to the language symptoms.

Attempts have been made to explain the major aphasia syndromes, such as that seen in our patient. Evidence has accumulated over the past 30 years in support of the dissociation between languages (Caramazza & Zurif, 1976; Dehaene, Dupoux & Mehler, 1997; Green & Price, 2001): that is, that the performance of aphasic patients on some linguistic tasks may vary across languages. Researchers have turned to the nature of language representation in an attempt to explain this finding. One approach suggests that L1 and L2 representations are, to some extent, sustained by different brain areas. Another suggests that L2 representations are organized according to exactly the same principles as those governing L1 organization, which means that the two representations are sustained by the same brain areas.

Because the lexical representations of the two languages would be governed by variables such as grammatical class and semantic category regardless of language membership, this approach does not rule out the possibility that a bilingual aphasic may selectively recover one language and lose the other (see Green, 2005; Green & Price, 2001). M.H.'s performance on the naming tasks suggests that his naming difficulties probably stemmed from damage to a lexical retrieval mechanism. However, not all linguistic components (like naming) are similar in the two languages. As described above, once the target lexical node is selected, the next step in speech production is the selection of the word's phonological segments. The dynamics of the activation and selection of the phonological component of words vary widely between models. One of the major differences is the extent to which the models implement the spreading activation principle between the lexical layer and the phonological layer. Although the principle has been widely adopted when characterizing the dynamics of processing between the semantic level and the lexical level, it is not as widely employed when characterizing processing at the segmental phonological level. According to discrete stage models of lexical access (Levelt, 1989; Levelt et al., 1999), the activation of phonological properties is restricted to those of the selected lexical node. Furthermore, the activation of the phonological properties of words begins only after the target lexical node has been selected. In contrast, the cascaded models of lexical access (Caramazza, 1997; Dell et al., 1997) assume that all the lexical nodes activated from the semantic level send proportional activation to their phonological segments. Furthermore, the activation of the phonological properties of words occurs before lexical selection takes place.

4. Conclusions

This chapter shows how encephalitis can induce different types of damage to the cognitive system. In the context of the bilingual brain, and according to previous findings from behavioral cognitive studies (Ibrahim & Aharon-Peretz, 2005; Ibrahim, 2009b), the different impairments in L1 and L2 seen in our bilingual patient suggest that representations of LI and L2 are, to some extent, sustained by different brain areas, and that a common semantic system is connected to two independent lexical systems corresponding to each of the two languages known by the bilingual. Given that M.H. had residual brain damage, and evinced more deficits in L2 perception and production than L1, the data support this position. This study of a bilingual native Arab speaker who acquired Hebrew (also a Semitic language), together with experimental neurolinguistic data gathered from both the patient and the literature, is a valuable combination for elucidating the relationship between language and mechanisms of neurobiology. Further, the combination provides psycholinguistic evidence by which to understand the dynamics of processing two languages in bilingual patients.

Our findings raise a number of questions: Does this specific mechanism function very early during language acquisition? Does the availability of this mechanism depend on the age of L2 acquisition (in childhood or adulthood)? These and other questions remain to be addressed in the study of representation of more than one language in the brain, and of the mechanisms of speech perception and production.

5. References

Albert, M. L., Goodglass, H., Helm, N. A., Runens, A. B., & Alexander, M. P. (1981). *Clinical Aspects of Dysphasia*. New York: Springer-Verlag.

Birnboim, S. (1995). Acquired surface dyslexia: the evidence from Hebrew. *Applied Psycholinguistics*, 16, 83-102.

Boivin M.J. (2002). Effects of early cerebral malaria on cognitive ability in Senegalese children. *Journal of Developmental Behavioral Pediatrics*, 23(5), 353–364.

Caramazza, A. (1997). How many levels of processing are there in lexical access? *Cognitive Neuropsychology*, 14, 177-208.

Caramazza, A., and E. B. Zurif. (1976). Dissociation of algorithmic and heuristic processes in sentence comprehension: evidence from aphasia. *Brain & Language*, 3, 572 -582.

Carter, J A, Murira, G M, Ross, A J., Mung'ala-Odera, V., & Newton, C.R. (2003). Speech and language sequelae of severe malaria in Kenyan children. *Brain Injury,* 17(3),217–224.

Carter, J.A, Neville, B.G., & Newton, C.R. (2003). Neuro-cognitive impairment following acquired central nervous system infections in childhood: a systematic review. *Brain Research Brain Research Reviews,* 43(1), 57–69.

Carter, J.A., Mung'ala-Odera, V., Neville, B.G., Murira, G., Mturi, N., Musumba, C., & Newton, C.R. (2005a). Persistent neurocognitive impairments associated with severe falciparum malaria in Kenyan children. *Journal of Neurology, Neurosurgery and Psychiatry,* 76(4), 476–481.

Carter, J.A., Ross, A.J., Neville, B.G., Obiero, E., Katana, K., Mung'ala-Odera, V., Lees, J.A., & Newton, C,R, (2005b). Developmental impairments following severe falciparum malaria in children. *Tropical Medicine & International Health,* 10(1), 3–10.

Dehaene. S., Dupoux. E., & Mehler. J. (1997). Anatomical variability in the cortical representation of first and second language. *Neuroreport,* 8(17), 3809–3815.

Dell, G. S., Schwartz, M. F., Martin, N. M., Saffran, E. M., & Gagnon, D. A. (1997). Lexical access in aphasic and nonaphasic speakers. *Psychological Review,* 104(4), 801-838.

Green, D. W. (2005). The neurocognition of recovery patterns in bilingual aphasics. In J. F. Kroll, & A. M. B. de Groot (Eds.), *Handbook of Bilingualism: Psycholinguistic Approaches* (pp. 516–530). New York: Oxford University Press.

Green, D. W., & Price, C. J. (2001). Functional imaging in the study of recovery patterns in bilingual aphasia. Bilingualism. *Language and Cognition,* 4, 191–201.

Gleissner, U., Helmstaedter, C., Kurthen, M., & Elger C. E. (1997). Evidence of very fast memory consolidation: an intracarotid amytal study. *Neuroreport,* 8(13):2893-6.

Heaton, R. K., Chelune, G. J., Talley, J. L., Kay, G. G., & Curtis, G. (1993). *Wisconsin Card Sorting Test Manual: Revised and Expanded.* Odessa, FL: Psychological Assessment Resources.

Holding, P A, Stevenson, J, Peshu, N, Marsh, K (1999). Cognitive sequelae of severe malaria with impaired consciousness. *Transactions of the Royal Society of Tropical Medicine and Hygiene,* 93(5), 529–534.

Ibrahim, R. & Aharon-Peretz, J. (2005). Is literary Arabic a second language for native Arab speakers?: Evidence from a semantic priming study. *The Journal of Psycholinguistic Research,* 34(1),51-70.

Ibrahim, R. (2009a). Selective deficit of second language: A case of Arabic-Hebrew bilingual brain-damaged patient. *Behavioral and Brain Functions.* 5 (17).1-10.

Ibrahim, R. (2009b). The cognitive basis of diglossia in Arabic: Evidence from a repetition priming study within and between languages. *Psychology Research and Behavior Management.* 12, 95-105.

Idro, J.A, Carter, G., Fegan, B. G., Neville, G.R., & Newton, C.R.J.C. (2006). Risk factors for persisting neurological and cognitive impairments following cerebral malaria. *Archive of Disease in Childhood,* 91(2), 142-148.

Idro, R., Karamagi, C., & Tumwine, J. (2004). Immediate outcome and prognostic factors for cerebral malaria among children admitted to Mulago Hospital, Uganda. *Annals of Tropical Paediatrics,* 24(1), 17–24.

Janszky, J., Jokeit, H., Heinemann, D., Schulz, R., Woermann, F. G., & Ebner, A. (2004). Epileptic activity influences the speech organization in medial temporal lobe epilepsy. *Brain,* 127(7): 1518 - 1525

Johnston, F.E., Low, S.M., de Baessa, Y., & MacVean, R.B. (1987). *Interaction* of nutritional and socioeconomic status as determinants of cognitive development in disadvantaged urban Guatemalan children. *American Journal of Physical Anthropology*, 73, 501–506.

Kaplan, E., Goodglass, H., & Weintraub, S. (1983). *Boston Naming Test*. Philadelphia: Lea and Febiger.

Kertesz, A. (1982). *Western Aphasia Battery*. New York: Grune and Stratton.

Levelt, W. J. M. (1989). *Speaking: From Intention to Articulation*. Cambridge, MA: MIT Press.

Levelt, J. M. W., Roelofs, A., & Meyer, A. S. (1999). A theory of lexical access in speech production. *Behavioural and Brain Sciences*, 22(1), 1-75.

Luria, A. R., (1970). *Traumatic Aphasia: its Syndromes, Psychology, and Treatment*. The Hague: Mouton.

Meyers, J.E, & Meyers, K. R. (1995). *Rey Complex Figure Test and Recognition Trial:Professional Manual*. Odessa. FL: Psychological Assessment Resources.

Neumann, C., McDonald, M.A., Sigman, M., & Bwido, N. (1992). Medical illness in school-age Kenyans in relation to nutrition, cognition, and playground behaviors. *Journal of Developmental and Behavioral Pediatrics*, 13(6), 392–398.

Pennington, L., Goldbart, J., & Marshall, J. (2004). Speech and language therapy to improve the communication skills of children with cerebral palsy. *Cochrane Database System Review*, CD003466.

Walther, F.J., & Ramaekers, L.H. (1982) Language development at the age of 3 years of infants malnourished in utero. *Neuropediatrics*, 13(2),77–81.

Wilson, B. I.-C. R., & Aldrich, F. (1991) *The Rivermead Behavioural Memory Test for Children*, 2nd edn. Bury St Edmunds: Thames Valley Test Company.

6

The Value of Standardized Case Definitions in Encephalitis Clinical Research

Barbara Rath
Department of Pediatrics, Division of Pneumonology-Immunology,
Charité University Medical Center, Berlin
Germany

1. Introduction

Encephalitis is a poorly defined disease entity. Encephalitic symptoms may be vague and unspecific, especially in the neonatal and pediatric age groups. Early signs and symptoms such as fever, malaise, headache and fatigue are fairly common and shared with many disease entities, infectious and non-infectious. Even if neurologic symptoms prevail and an encephalitis diagnosis has moved to the top of the list of differential diagnoses, overlap with other disease entities remains a possibility - in particular with meningitis, cerebellitis, myelitis and acute disseminated encephalomyelitis (ADEM).

Encephalitis appears to be under-diagnosed and in the majority of cases of encephalitis, the pathogen or cause remain unknown.[1-5] Furthermore, surveillance programs in Scandinavia revealed that 60% of the children with encephalitis had persisting symptoms at the time of discharge. Systematic evidence-based research and prospective surveillance are warranted to learn more about the clinical spectrum, underlying causes, and prognostic factors of encephalitis. The ultimate goal of encephalitis clinical research should be to improve treatment modalities and disease outcomes in all patients, regardless of age and geographic background.

Meaningful epidemiologic investigations of encephalitis disease outcomes, incidence and prevalence require large-scale studies, multi-centric approaches, and the pooling and meta-analysis of significant amounts of data from different parts of the world. For data comparability purposes, pre-defined standards should be used for the inclusion of patients into encephalitis surveillance cohorts. Inclusion criteria for encephalitis studies should be based on observer-independent, widely accepted clinical case definitions and ideally, international consensus.

This paper aims to raise awareness of the challenges of defining and diagnosing encephalitis as a disease entity, while presenting a number of practical approaches to facilitate encephalitis screening for pediatric clinical research and public health purposes.

2. Problem

Very few large-scale studies have been conducted to date monitoring the incidence and prevalence of encephalitis, and even fewer targeting the paediatric age group. Usually, these studies are set up as laboratory-based investigations or with a specific disease entity or pathogen in mind such as West Nile Virus[6], Japanese Encephalitis Virus (JEV), tick borne encephalitis (TBE), rotavirus, varicella and other herpesviruses.

Examples of key topics in encephalitis studies in recent years are:

- The early detection of congenital encephalitis and TORCH infections
- Regional and periodic epidemiologic surveillance of arbovirus infections
- Polio surveillance (WHO)
- Baseline prevalence of vaccine preventable disease
- Monitoring of adverse events following immunization (AEFI)

Example 1: The discussion around Rotavirus Encephalitis/ Encephalopathy

Ever since the first cases of CNS involvement in rotavirus disease were reported, it has been discussed if and when one of the most common pathogens causing gastroenteritis in children under the age of 4 may also cause neurologic symptoms and complications. Table 1 illustrates a summary of the first case reports of rotavirus encephalitis in the medical literature.

Case, Reference	Location	Year	Age	Sex	Neurological Diagnosis	Stool	CSF	Blood	Outcome
1. Salmi et al. [7]	Finland	1978	2 yr	F	Seizures	EM			Patient died
2. Salmi et al. [7]	Finland	1978	3 yr	F	Seizures	EM		NCDV	Slow recovery
3. Wong et al. [8]	USA	1984	6 mo	M	Aseptic meningitis	EIA, IEM	EIA, IEM, pleocytosis		Healthy
4. Ushijima et al. [9]	Japan	1986	9 mo	M	Acute encephalitis	PAGE, Latex agglutination (LA), EM, RV IgA	RV IgG, IgA, IgM	RV IgG, IgA, IgM, CFT	Coma x 10 d, infantile spasms, developmental delay
5. Keidan et al. [10]	Israel	1992	2 yr	M	Encephalopathy	EIA	EM		Healthy
6. Keidan et al.[10]	Israel	1992	21 mo	M	Encephalopathy	EIA			Healthy
7. Yoshida et al.[11]	Japan	1995	2 yr	F	Encephalitis	Latex agglutination (LA)	RT-PCR, pleocytosis		Healthy
8. Pang et al. [12]	Finland	1996	9 mo	F	Febrile seizures	EIA, RT-PCR	RT-PCR	RT-PCR, RV IgG, IgA	Healthy
9. Makino et al. [13]	Japan	1996	21 mo	F	Encephalopathy	EIA, RT-PCR	RT-PCR	RT-PCR, CFT	Hemiparesis, mental retardation
10. Hongou et al.[14]	Japan	1998	2 yr	M	Encephalitis	LA	RT-PCR, RV IgG, pleocytosis	CFT	Healthy
11. Pager et al.[15]	South Africa	2000	1yr	M	Seizures	LA	RT-PCR		Pat. died first day of life
12. Lynch et al. [16]	USA	2001	6 yr	M	Seizures	EIA	RT-PCR	RV IgA	Pat. died after 5 mo
13. Lynch et al. [16]	USA	2001	2.5 yr	F	Encephalitis	EIA	RT-PCR		Healthy
14. Goldwater et al. [17]	Australia	2001	2.5 yr	M	Encephalitis	EIA	PCR, RT-PCR		Slow recovery, sequelae (hypotonia, unclear speach)
15. Goldwater et al. [17]	Australia	2001	13 mo	M	Encephalopathy	EIA	RT-PCR		Moderate hemiparesis
16. Nigrovic et al. [18]	USA	2002	3 yr	F	Cerebellitis	RT-PCR	RT-PCR		Wide-base gait, moderate expressive aphasia

Case, Reference	Location	Year	Age	Sex	Neurological Diagnosis	Stool	CSF	Blood	Outcome
17. Morrison[19]	USA	2001	4 yr		Encephalitis, cerebral edema, uncal herniation		CNS in situ RT-PCR, in situ hybridization		Patient died
18. Kobata et al.[20]	Japan	2002	2 yr	F	Encephalopathy	Immunochromatography, EM, RT-PCR			Healthy
19. Iturriza-Gomarra et al.[21]	UK	2002	2 yr	M	Seizures	LA, RT-PCR	RT-PCR		Healthy
20. Kehle et al.[22]	Germany	2003	9 mo	F	Meningo-encephalitis	EIA	RT-PCR, pleocytosis	IgM	Healthy
21. Rath et al.[23]	USA	2004	8 mo	M	Encephalitis	EIA	RT-PCR, probe hybridization		Mental retardation, dystonia, developmental delay
22. Nakagomi et al.[24]	Japan	2005	1.5 yr	M	Not reported in detail. Manifestations included encephalitis, encephalopathy, convulsions or seizures.	ELISA or LA		ELISA	Not reported
23. Nakagomi et al.[24]	Japan	2005	0.5 yr	M		ELISA or LA		ELISA	
24. Nakagomi et al.[24]	Japan	2005	4 yr	F		ELISA or LA		ELISA	
25. Nakagomi et al.[24]	Japan	2005	3 yr	F		ELISA or LA		ELISA	
26. Nakagomi et al.[24]	Japan	2005	2.5 yr	M		ELISA or LA		ELISA	
27. Nakagomi et al.[24]	Japan	2005	1.5 yr	F		ELISA or LA	RT-PCR		
28. Nakagomi et al.[24]	Japan	2005	9 yr	F		ELISA or LA	RT-PCR		
29. Nakagomi et al.[24]	Japan	2005	2 yr	F		ELISA or LA	RT-PCR		
30. Kirton et al.[25]	Canada	2005	15 mo	F	Necrotizing encephalopathy	EIA			Patient died
31. Shiihara et al.[26]	Japan	2007	2.5 yr	F	Encephalitis, Cerebellitis	Immunochromatography, RT-PCR	Pleocytosis (RT-PCR -)		Slow speech and dysarthria
31. Shiihara et al.[26]	Japan	2007	4.5 yr	M	Encephalitis, Cerebellitis	Immunochromatography			Slow speech, dysarthria, hand tremor
32. Furuya et al.[27]	Japan	2007	3.5 yr	F	Encephalitis	RT-PCR	RT-PCR		Not reported

Table 1.

Notably, thirty-three cases of rotavirus disease with CNS involvement had been reported up until the time when the new rotavirus vaccines were introduced in the United States.[16-22,25-28] Among these 32 cases, less than half (10/24; 42%) of the patients with reported outcomes recovered completely. Five children (21%) died from the disease, whereas the remaining 37% experienced neurological sequelae.[23]

With increased awareness evidence has since grown further, and CNS involvement is slowly being recognized as a rare but potentially serious complication in rotavirus gastroenteritis.[29-38] Over time, in addition to viral diagnostics radiological features of rotavirus encephalitis are better understood, which may help in directing clinicians to the correct diagnosis. [23 37]

During and prior to the time of rotavirus vaccine introduction in different parts of the world, large rotavirus surveillance programs have been instituted. Despite the size and number of such programs, meta-analysis is difficult as very little information can be obtained on rare complications of rotavirus disease. Studies were designed measuring different endpoints and inconsistent criteria and definitions have been applied (if any) for CNS complications.

An exception for surveillance studies of seizures in rotavirus disease:

A subanalysis of a 5- year rotavirus surveillance in Salt Lake City, Utah (2002-6) is a rare exception specifically focusing of CNS complications. Investigators retrospectively identified 34/59 children with laboratory-confirmed rotavirus infection and >=1 seizure without an alternative medical explanation. They reported one child with cerebral edema on neuroimaging and abnormal EEG and 2 children (7%) who required chronic anticonvulsant therapy concluding "…that seizures associated with rotavirus infection are a relatively benign neurologic condition in young children. With few exceptions, neurodiagnostic studies do not influence management or outcome."[39].

Precise data and incidence rates with respect to encephalitis/ encephalopathy in large-scale rotavirus surveillance programs are sill lacking. In the meantime, CNS complications have also been reported in gastroenteritis due to other viruses such as norovirus [40] and adenovirus [41].

Example 2: Encephalitis as a vaccine preventable disease

A number of recent encephalitis surveillance studies have been focusing on vaccine preventable disease, such as tick borne encephalitis (TBE) and Japanese encephalitis virus (JEV).

Systematic tick born encephalitis studies have recently been conducted in Eastern European countries where the disease is endemic, such as Slovenia [42], Poland [43], and Latvia [44]. A common European approach has been sought by VENICE (http://venice.cineca.org/final_report_TBE_19-01-2011.pdf) and several others [45, 46, 47] however, universal criteria for the clinical assessment and grading of encephalitis still remain to be implemented.

With respect to Japanese Encepahlitis Virus (JEV), surveillance has recently been extended to many Asian countries including Bangladesh [48], Nepal [49], Japan [48], to name only a few. New WHO criteria for JEV have been defined and evaluated. [50] More recently, general systemativ surveillance programs and monitoring activities preparing the introduction of JEV vaccine have been developed by PATH in Vietnam, and Nepal (http://www.path.org/publications/detail.php?i=1523).

With the introduction of varicella vaccine, varicella zoster virus (VZV) has become the first vaccine preventable disease caused by herpesviridae. Complications of VZV disease include CNS involvement with the clinical picture of encephalitis/cerebellitis. Neurologic complications in VZV infection are common in, but not restricted to immuno-compromized patients [51] and may even occur in the context of reactivation (varicella zoster). [52]

A 1-year surveillance of hospitalizations for VZV complications was conducted in 1997 in 485 German pediatric hospitals including neurologic complications, bacterial superinfections, and hematologic complications (with multiple entries permitted in the surveillance questionnaire). Notably, neurologic complications were among the most common with 61.3% (in comparison to infectious complications with 38.6%). Among CNS complications, cerebellitis was predominant with 40.3%, followed by encephalitis (18.4%) and meningitis (1.7%) and facial palsy (0.8%). [53] Similar studies have recently been conducted in Italy [54, 55], UK, Ireland, [56] and Saudi Arabia [57].

Parallel to increased efforts in developing a cytomegalovirus (CMV) vaccine [58-61], attention has also shifted to further understanding the neurologic sequelae and disease burden of congenital CMV disease and non-immunocompromised hosts. [62-22]

In addition, influenza has been increasingly recognized as a vaccine preventable cause of encephalitis, especially in children and adolescents. [67] Initial reports emerged from Japan and the United States [68-75] and recently, a number of case reports as well as surveillance reports by CDC have been issued on neurologic complications of Influenza A (in particular pandemic H1N1) disease. [76-88]

Example 3: Encephalitis as an adverse event following immunization (AEFI)

Encephalitis has not only been described as a viral and/or immunological illness, but also as an adverse event following immunization (AEFI)[89]. The British Pediatric Surveillance Unit conducted a 3-year prospective surveillance aiming to investigate encephalitis as an AEFI in the UK and Ireland[90]

By nature, AEFI are rare events requiring large-scale studies, meta-analyses, or extensive (ideally active) surveillance programs to be detected. Reporting bias and awareness are major obstacles to the systematic assessment of AEFI. Resent research revealed that physicians are more likely to report a specific AE if the AE constitutes an event a vaccine in designed to prevent. Interestingly, this "reverse placebo effect" also applied to non-live vaccines. [91]

When data have to be pooled from a number of different studies, the use of uniform diagnostic criteria is warranted allowing comparability among studies conducted at different sites. This demand has been met by the Brighton Collaboration, who published a clinical case definition for encephalitis as an AEFI in 2007. [89] The diagnostic criteria for encephalitis as an AEFI are listed in Table 2, below. The Brighton Collaboration criteria are designed to capture an adverse event independent from any potential triggers, but also to differentiate reliably and consistently between different kinds of CNS involvement, including meningitis, meningo-encephalitis, myleitis, ADEM and the like.

The Brighton Collaboration case definitions for aseptic meningitis, encephalitis, myelitis and ADEM have since been evaluated in a retrospective analysis of 255 clinical cases of CNS disease in a Swiss children's hospital. [93] This evaluation study revealed that unless predefined clinical criteria are applied consistently, the demarcation of closely related but distinct CNS disease entities will be missed. ICD-10 coding and diagnoses mentioned in hospital discharge summaries are insufficient and all too often observer-dependent. [93]

Brighton Collaboration Case Definition for Encephalitis as an AEFI [89]
"Case definitions: encephalitis, myelitis, and ADEM"[1]

Encephalitis - Level 1 of diagnostic certainty:[2]

(a) Demonstration of acute inflammation of central nervous system parenchyma (± meninges) by histopathology.

Encephalitis - Level 2 of diagnostic certainty:[3,4]

(a) Encephalopathy (e.g. depressed or altered level of consciousness, lethargy, or personality change lasting >24 h),

AND INCLUDING

(b) **ONE OR MORE** of the following:
1. Decreased or absent response to environment, as defined by response to loud noise or painful stimuli,
2. Decreased or absent eye contact,
3. Inconsistent or absent response to external stimuli,
4. Decreased arousability,
5. Seizure associated with loss of consciousness.[92]

OR

(c) Focal or multifocal findings referable to the central nervous system, including one or more of the following:
1. Focal cortical signs (including but not limited to: aphasia,alexia, agraphia, cortical blindness),
2. Cranial nerve abnormality/abnormalities,[5]
3. Visual field defect/defect(s),
4. Presence of primitive reflexes (Babinski's sign, glabellar reflex, snout/sucking reflex),
5. Motor weakness (either diffuse or focal; more often focal)[5]
6. Sensory abnormalities (either positive or negative; sensory level),
7. Altered deep tendon reflexes (hypo- or hyperreflexia, reflex asymmetry),
8. Cerebellar dysfunction, including ataxia, dysmetria, cerebellar nystagmus.

AND (for both possibilities to reach Level 2)

(d) TWO OR MORE[6] of the following indicators of inflammation of the CNS:
1. Fever (temperature ≥38° C),
2. CSF pleocytosis (>5WBC/mm3 in children >2 months of age; >15WBC/mm3 in children <2 months of age),
3. EEG findings consistent with encephalitis,[7] or
4. Neuroimaging consistent with encephalitis.[8]

Encephalitis - Level 3 of diagnostic certainty:[3,4]

(a) Encephalopathy (e.g. depressed or altered level of consciousness, lethargy, or personality change lasting >24 h),

AND INCUDING

(b) **ONE OR MORE** of the following:
1. Decreased or absent response to environment, as defined by response to loud noise or painful stimuli,
2. Decreased or absent eye contact,
3. Inconsistent or absent response to external stimuli,

4. Decreased arousability, or
5. Seizure associated with loss of consciousness. [92]

OR

(c) Focal or multifocal findings referable to the central nervous system, including one or more of the following:
1. Focal cortical signs (including but not limited to: aphasia, alexia, agraphia, cortical blindness),
2. Cranial nerve abnormality/abnormalities,[5]
3. Visual field defect/defect(s),
4. Presence of primitive reflexes (Babinski's sign, glabellar reflex, snout/sucking reflex),
5. Motor weakness (either diffuse or focal; more often focal),[5]
6. Sensory abnormalities (either positive or negative; sensory level),
7. Altered deep tendon reflexes (hypo- or hyperreflexia, reflex asymmetry), or
8. Cerebellar dysfunction, including ataxia, dysmetria, cerebellar nystagmus.

AND (for both possibilities to reach Level 3)

(d) **ONE**[7] of the following indicators of inflammation of CNS:
1. Fever (temperature ≥38°C),
2. CSF pleocytosis (>5WBC/mm3 in children >2 months of age; >15WBC/mm3 in children <2 months of age),
3. EEG findings consistent with encephalitis,[7] or
4. Neuroimaging consistent with encephalitis.[8]

Encephalitis - Level 3A of diagnostic certainty:[7,9]

(a) Insufficient information is available to distinguish case between acute encephalitis or ADEM; case unable to be definitively classified.

Encephalitis - Exclusion criterion for levels 2 and 3 of diagnostic certainty:

(a) Other diagnosis for illness present.[10]

[2] If the lowest applicable level of diagnostic certainty of the definition for a definitive category (i.e., Level 3, excluding Level 3A) is met and there is evidence that the criteria of the next higher level of diagnostic certainty (Level 2) are met, the event should be classified in the next category. This approach should be continued until the highest level of diagnostic certainty for a given event can be determined. Thus, if a case fits diagnostic criteria for both categories (encephalitis and ADEM), but reaches a higher level of diagnostic certainty in one, the higher level supercedes, and the case should be classified according to the category in which the higher diagnostic certainty level is reached. TheWorking Group recognizes that under this paradigm, it is possible to reach a higher level of diagnostic certainty forADEMwith less stringent criteria than it is for encephalitis e.g., Level 1 diagnostic certainty for encephalitis requires histopathologic diagnosis, whilst ADEM Level 1 does not require this. However, in the absence of a biological marker, the diagnosis of ADEM rests upon the proper neuroimaging findings in the appropriate clinical context, and the combination of appropriate neuroimaging and a monophasic pattern of illness are as close to a gold standard as exist for this clinical entity. Thus, one may have a higher level of diagnostic certainty of ADEM than of encephalitis, in the absence of other biologic data. When Level 1 ADEM and Level 2 encephalitis, or Level 2 ADEM

and

Level 3 encephalitis are met, the best category to choose would be ADEM.

[3] The encephalitis/ADEMWorking Group recognizes that, in most cases, histopathologic examination of tissue will not be practicable as a method of diagnosis; this may particularly be the case in developing countries. However, histopathologic demonstration of cerebral inflammation remains the "gold standard" for the diagnosis of encephalitis, and as such, the group has determined that this should be Level 1 for determination of encephalitis.

[4] Levels 2 and 3 of diagnostics certainty have been especially designed for adults and children older than or equal to 2 years of age. For children under the age of 2 years (and, in particular, those under the age of 6 months) the nervous system and, as such, the neurologic examination is continually in flux (e.g., what is normal in a 28-day old is not necessarily normal in a 2- month old child). The evaluation of encephalopathy and neurologic deficits in infants and young children will need to be done in an age-appropriate fashion, taking into account the age and level of development of the child.

[5] Levels 2 or 3 of encephalitis are met if criteria (a+b+d) or (c+d) from the respective levels are fulfilled, and no exclusion criteria are met.

[6] Note that only criteria 2 and 5 may be applicable in all age groups; other criteria for focal/mulitfocal neurologic signs may be age-dependent, and will not be applicable to all age groups.

[7] Note that Level 2 of diagnostic certainty requires at least 2 of the listed criteria for inflammation, while Level 3 required only 1 criteria. This is in recognition that, in some cases of encephalitis, all listed criteria will either not be present, or such data will be unavailable. Thus, a clinical diagnosis of encephalitis should still be applicable, but will be of less diagnostic certainty than if sufficient criteria were present.

[8] Electroencephalographic (EEG) findings consistent with encephalitis:EEG findings consistent with encephalitis include, but are not limited to: Diffuse or multifocal nonspecific (nonphysiologic) background slowing; periodic discharges or other encephalographic abnormalities may or may not be present.

[9] Neuroimaging findings consistent with encephalitis: Neuroimaging findings consistent with encephalitis include, but are not limited to: head computed tomography (CT) displaying areas of hypodensity; contrast images demonstrating meningeal and parenchymal enhancement indicating meningeal and parenchymal inflammation, or gyral enhancement, brain/spine magnetic resonance imaging (MRI) displaying diffuse or multifocal areas of hyperintense signal on T2-weighted, diffusion-weighted image, or fluid-attenuation inversion recovery (FLAIR) sequences, suggestive of inflammation or demyelination.

Tabe 2. Brighton Collaboration Case Definition for Encephalitis as an AEFI (see www.brightoncollaboration.org)

3. Assessment of the problem

Most of the attempts to standardize the diagnosis of encephalitis are focusing on adults whereas pediatric studies are facing specific challenges in the differential diagnosis, such as age-dependent symptoms while intellectual capabilities are still developing and the difficulty to distinguish acute neurologic impairment from consequences of perinatal asphyxia and congenital malformations, developmental delay, intoxication and other alternative possible non-infectious causes of encephalopathy.[2, 5] Due to the immaturity of the immune system and the blood-brain barrier, children under the age of two are at a particularly high risk of developing encephalitis during bacterial sepsis or systemic infection with herpesviridae, Tb and many other pathogens. At the same time the chance of recurrence of HSV meningo-encephalitis is difficult to assess and consequences of premature discontinuation of antiviral therapy can be detrimental. [94-99] Even in older children, the difficulty to identify symptoms of encephalopathy such as behavioral outbursts, decreased responsiveness, and other subtle signs may delay the diagnosis and thus, treatment. [100, 101] In other cases, the differentiation of autoimmune from viral causes of encephalitis causes problems. [100,4] Without the identification of potential causes of encephalitis, however, the treatment options and prognosis in different types of encephalitis will remain poorly understood.[1, 102]

With additional diagnostic and therapeutic options becoming available, and several types of encephalitis vaccine-preventable, the systematic surveillance of encephalitis in children has gained significance, also with respect to everyday clinical care.

As indicated above, prospective and retrospective case ascertainment both provide a number of challenges. Prospective surveillance of large cohorts using predefined case definitions is key to avoid inter-rater variability and selection bias. The installment of active surveillance systems in specialized reference centers will ultimately improve the monitoring of encephalitis as an AEFI. Children with acute CNS adverse events are most likely to present in emergency rooms and tertiary care centers rather than private pediatric practices, where the child has usually been immunized. Unless immunizations are systematically captured at the time of investigation, rates of encephalitis and other CNS adverse events following immunization - as opposed to other triggers or causes - can hardly be established. [90, 103] In addition, lumbar puncture is difficult to perform in infants and children, and even if CSF has been obtained, pathogens other than HSV and bacteria are rarely assessed in routine practice. Very little is known for example, about incidence rates of enterovirus infection in pediatric CNS disease.[104] However, effective enterovirus surveillance can also be utilized as a tool for regional polio disease surveillance, as is the case at the German National Reference Laboratory for Enteroviruses at the Robert Koch Institute in Berlin.[105, 106]

Hospital-based prospective surveillance systems have been introduced in several locations, including country-wide surveillance systems in the US[4], France[107], the UK [2] and Sweden [1], as well as smaller programs in Taiwan [108], Crete [109], and India.[110] Unfortunately, each of these programs use their own case definitions for encephalitis.

Table three provides several examples of clinical case definitions used in recent pediatric encephalitis studies:

First Author	Title	Country	Type/Category	Year(s) of Study	Clinical Case Definition for Encephalitis
Amin [67]	Acute childhood encephalitis and encephalopathy associated with influenza: a prospective 11-year review	Canada	Influenza Encephalitis	1994 - 2004	"Encephalopathy was defined as a depressed or altered level of consciousness persisting for 24 hours. Encephalitis was defined by the presence of encephalopathy plus 2 or more of the following criteria: fever (temperature 38.0°C), seizure(s), focal neurologic findings, cerebrospinal fluid (CSF) pleocytosis (WBC count 5 106 cells/L), EEG findings compatible with encephalitis, or abnormal neuroimaging"

First Author	Title	Country	Type/Category	Year(s) of Study	Clinical Case Definition for Encephalitis
Anga [111]	The aetiology, clinical presentations and outcome of febrile encephalopathy in children in Papua New Guinea	Papua New Guinea	Febrile Encephalo-pathy	ND	"Children aged between 1 month and 12 years presenting to Port Moresby General Hospital with febrile encephalopathy, defined as fever, seizures and/or altered consciousness"
Beig [110]	Etiology and clinico-epidemiological profile of acute viral encephalitis in children of western Uttar Pradesh, India	India	Acute viral encephalitis	Jul 2004-Nov 2006	"Acute encephalopathy was defined as fever with alteration of consciousness and/or with neurological deficit, secondary to central nervous system involvement lasting more than 24 hours, and not more than a oneweek history. Patients with a different final diagnosis (e.g., epilepsy, febrile convulsion, bacterial meningitis, tuberculosis, brain tumor, cerebral malaria, or metabolic disorder) were excluded from the study."
Elbers [112]	A 12-year prospective study of childhood herpes simplex encephalitis: is there a broader spectrum of disease?	USA	HSV Encephalitis	1994-2005	"Inclusion criteria for this registry are documented encephalopathy, defined as depressed or altered level of consciousness persisting for >24 hours, plus 2 of the following: fever (>38°C), seizure, focal central nervous system (CNS) findings, CSF pleocytosis (>5 x 106 cells per L), EEG abnormalities, or diagnostic imaging abnormalities (on brain computed tomography [CT]/MRI scans). Patients were excluded if they had underlying neurologic disease or were known to have immunosuppression. This study did not include cases of neonatal encephalitis and focused on children between 4 weeks and 18 years of age. For identification of a cohort of children with clinically and diagnostically definite HSE, patients in our study fulfilled stringent inclusion criteria: the aforementioned criteria of the encephalitis registry, CSF PCR and/or serologic evidence of HSV infection, and 1 of the following: CSF abnormalities, including the presence of pleocytosis, >50 x 106 red blood cells (RBCs) per L, and/or elevated protein levels (>0.4 g/L), EEG readings consistent with HSE, or CT and MRI findings suggesting HSE, such as focal signal abnormalities or hemorrhage. Patients were excluded if an alternative diagnosis accounted for their symptoms."

First Author	Title	Country	Type/Category	Year(s) of Study	Clinical Case Definition for Encephalitis
Fowler [1]	Childhood encephalitis in Sweden: etiology, clinical presentation and outcome	Sweden	Encephalitis	2000-2004	A. Age 1 month–18 years B. Signs of cerebral dysfunction either as. 1. encephalopathy defined as altered consciousness, personality or behavioral changes lasting for more than 24 hr, or 2. abnormal EEG finding compatible with encephalitis, plus at least one of the following: - Abnormal results of neuroimaging compatible with encephalitis, -Positive focal neurological findings, -Seizures. C. Signs of inflammation, defined either as pleocytosis (X6 white blood cells/mL), fever (38C) or elevated infectious parameters (CRP,WBC). Mild symptoms from eyes, nose or throat were not considered to be sufficient."
Ganerod [2]	Causes of encephalitis and differences in their clinical presentations in England: a multicentre, population-based prospective study	UK	Encephalitis	Oct 2005-Nov 2006	"The case definition included any person of any age admitted to hospital with encephalopathy (altered consciousness that persisted for longer than 24 h, including lethargy, irritability, or a change in personality and behaviour) and with two or more of the following:fever or history of fever (≥38°C) during the presenting illness; seizures and/or focal neurological fi ndings (with evidence of brain parenchyma involvement); CSF pleocytosis (more than four white blood cells per µL); electroencephalographic (EEG) fi ndings indicative of encephalitis; and abnormal results of neuroimaging (CTor MRI) suggestive of encephalitis."
Glaser [113]	In search of encephalitis etiologies: diagnostic challenges in the California Encephalitis Project, 1998-2000	USA	Encephalitis	1998-2000	"A case was defined as encephalopathy (depressed or altered level of consciousness lasting 24 h, lethargy, or change in personality) requiring hospitalization with 1 of the following symptoms: fever, seizure, focal neurological findings, CSF pleocytosis, or electroencephalography or neuroimaging findings consistent with encephalitis.", > 6 months of age
Glaser [4]	Beyond viruses: clinical profiles and etiologies associated with encephalitis.	USA	Encephalitis	1998 -2005	">= 6 months of age, and met the CEP case definition of encephalitis. A "case patient" was defined as a patient hospitalized with encephalopathy (defined by a depressed or altered sonality change) with level of consciousness lasting 24 h, lethargy, or a per 1 of the following characteristics: fever, seizure, focal neurological findings, pleocytosis, or electroencephalography or neuroimaging findings consistent with encephalitis."

First Author	Title	Country	Type/Category	Year(s) of Study	Clinical Case Definition for Encephalitis
Ward [90]	Risk of Serious Neurologic Disease After Immunization of Young Children in Britain and Ireland	Britain and Ireland	Immunization		"Case definiton of serious neurologic disease: children 2 to 35 month with suspected encephalitis and/or severe illness with fever and convulsions. Convulsion: total duration of >30 min OR followed by encephalopathy of 2-23h OR followed by paralysis or other neurological signs not previously present for ≥24h. Fever: ≥37.5°C. Encephalopathy: depressed or altered level of consciousness. Encephalitis: Encephalopathy for ≥24h and TWO of the following: fever, convulsions, focal neurological findings (≥24h), pleocystosis (>5 leucocytes per µl CSF), characteristic abnormal results of neuroimaging (CT or MRI), herpes simplex virus nucleis acid (or nucleic acid of any other virus proven to cause encephalitis) in CSF; OR postmortem histologic evidence of encephalitis. Exclusion criteria: viral meningitis without encephalopathy; the following confirmed causes: hypoxic/ischemic; vascular; toxic; metabolic, neoplastic, traumatic, pyogenic infections; uncomplicated convulsions or a series of convulsions lasting 30 min; immunocompromised children."
Hossain [48]	Hospital-based surveillance for Japanese encephalitis at four sites in Bangladesh, 2003-2005.	Bangladesh	Japanese Encephalitis	2003-2005	".. clinical case definition of acute encephalitis with indication for lumbar puncture, based on the judgment of the patient's attending physician. The clinical case definition of acute encephalitis included new onset of fever (temperature > 38°C) or history of fever during the present illness along with altered mental status, (e.g., confusion, disorientation, coma) and/or a neurological deficit (i.e., focal or diffuse neurological dysfunction or new onset of seizures) with onset of the neurological symptoms within five days prior to hospitalization. Enrollment in the study required that the patient met the clinical case definition and that he or she had cerebrospinal fluid (CSF) pleocytosis (defined as > 4 leukocytes/mm3 for patients > 6 weeks of age and > 14 leukocytes/mm3 for the patients > 6 weeks of age)..."
Huang [102]	Long-term cognitive and motor deficits after enterovirus 71 brainstem encephalitis in children	Taiwan	Enterovirus Encephalitis	1998 - 2004	"case definition for enterovirus 71 brainstem encephalitis: myoclonus, ataxia, nystagmus, oculomotor palsies, and bulbar palsy, in various combinations, with or without confirmation by neuroimaging".

First Author	Title	Country	Type/Category	Year(s) of Study	Clinical Case Definition for Encephalitis
Le [3]	Viral etiology of encephalitis in children in southern Vietnam: results of a one-year prospective descriptive study	Vietnam	Encephalitis	Jan-Dec 2004	"Children admitted [..] with suspected acute encephalitis of viral origin, based on the clinical judgment of admitting physicians, and with no preexisting neurological conditions or evidence of bacterial meningitis by microscopy or culture of cerebrospinal fluid (CSF) samples, and no febrile convulsion (defined by a single convulsion lasting less than 15 minutes with regaining of consciousness within 60 minutes in a child between 6 months and 6 years of age) were eligible for inclusion in the study after provision of written informed consent by the patient's parents or legal guardians"
Lee [108]	Encephalitis in Taiwan: a prospective hospital-based study	Taiwan	Encephalitis	2000-2001	"Encephalitis was defined as follows: acute and severe neurological dysfunction in the context of suspected encephalitis, which included signs and symptoms of acute mental dysfunction, memory impairment, LOC, pareses, abnormal behaviour, convulsions, and involuntary movement. The patient's EEG and/or CT scan and LP were also compatible with the diagnosis of encephalitis. Patients with high fever, headache, nausea and vomiting were excluded by LP, CT/MRI or EEG examination. Patients with other diseases, especially with other systemic infection (sepsis), cerebral vascular accident, neoplasm of the brain or psychiatric diseases that caused disturbed consciousness were also excluded by LP, CT/MI or EEG examination."
Mailles [107]	Infectious encephalitis in France in 2007: a national prospective study	France	Encephalitis	Jan-Dec 2007	"Inclusion criteria: age ≥ 28 days hospitalized in mainland France in 2007 AND (1) acute onset of illness, (2) at least 1 abnormality of the CSF (white blood cell count of ≥ 4 cells/mm^3 OR protein level of ≥ 40mg/dl), (3) temperature ≥ 38°C, (4) decreased consciousness OR seizures OR altered mental status OR focal neurologic signs. Exclusion criteria: hospitalization of fewer than 5 days (to avoid including patients with aseptic meningitis without brain involvement), positive HIV status, meningitis without clinical brain involvement, brain abscess, prion disease, cerebral malaria, non-infectious CNS-disease"
Morishima [114]	Encephalitis and encephalopathy associated with an influenza epidemic in Japan	Japan	Influenza Encephalitis	winter of 1998–1999	"The diagnosis of encephalitis/ encephalopathy was made on the basis of all clinical signs. All patients had altered consciousness or loss of consciousness. Patients with meningitis, myelitis, and febrile convulsions without prolonged unconsciousness were excluded. Postictal unconsciousness with prompt recovery was classified as febrile convulsion"

First Author	Title	Country	Type/Category	Year(s) of Study	Clinical Case Definition for Encephalitis
Olsen [115]	Japanese encephalitis virus remains an important cause of encephalitis in Thailand	Thailand	Encephalitis	2003-2005	"the following criteria were approached for enrollment: (1) fever or hypothermia (i.e., history of fever or documented temperature 38 8C or 35 8C); (2) evidence of acute brain dysfunction (i.e., encephalopathy, central neurological findings, or seizures) with onset 14 days prior to admission; and (3) clinical indication for lumbar puncture as determined by a staff physician."
Schubart [116]	Short report: Role of viruses in Kenyan children presenting with acute encephalopathy in a malaria-endemic area	Kenya	Cerebral Malaria	1999-2001	"Differenciation between cerebral malaria, bacterial meningitis and viral encephalitis. Cerebral malaria: WHO definition. Bacterial meningitis confirmed by the examination and culture of CSF. Viral encephalitis confirmed by looking for evidence of herpesviruses and enteroviruses."
Solomon [50]	A cohort study to assess the new WHO Japanese encephalitis surveillance standards	Viet Nam	Japanese Encephalitis	Jan-Dec 1995	"Clinically, a case of acute encephalitis syndrome (AES) is defined as a person of any age, at any time of year, with the acute onset of fever and a change in mental status (including symptoms such as confusion, disorientation, coma, or inability to talk) AND/OR new onset of seizures (excluding simple febrile seizures).[a] Other early clinical findings can include an increase in irritability, somnolence or abnormal behaviour greater than that seen with usual febrile illness."
Ward [90]	Risk of serious neurologic disease after immunization of young children in Britain and Ireland	UK and Ireland (British Pediatric Surveillance Unit)	Encephalitis and Severe Illness with Convulsions and Fever	Oct 1998 - Sept 2001	"pediatricians were requested to report all children 2 to 35 months old with suspected encephalitis and/or severe illness with fever and convulsions- -> anaöytical case definition: Fever: temperature of 37.5°C; the questionnaire asked whether there was a fever and also for the maximum temperature recorded at any site by any method. Encephalopathy: a depressed or altered level of consciousness. Case definition of serious neurologic disease: any child 2–35 mo old with a severe illness with fever and convulsions (a) and/or encephalitis (b) was included. (a) Severe illness with fever and convulsions: (i) with a total duration of 30 min; or (ii) followed by encephalopathy for 2–23 h; or (iii) followed by paralysis or other neurologic signs not previously present for 24 h. (b) Encephalitis as adapted from [117].(i) Encephalopathy for 24 h and 2 of the following:fever, convulsions, focal neurologic findings (24 h), pleocytosis (5 leukocytes per L CSF), characteristic

First Author	Title	Country	Type/Category	Year(s) of Study	Clinical Case Definition for Encephalitis
					abnormal results of neuroimaging (CT or MRI), herpes simplex virus nucleic acid (or nucleic acid of any other virus proven to cause encephalitis) in CSF; or (ii) postmortem histologic evidence of encephalitis. (c) Exclude (i) viral (aseptic) meningitis without encephalopathy (ii) the following confirmed causes were excluded: hypoxic/ischemic; vascular; toxic; metabolic, neoplastic, traumatic, and pyogenic infections (iii) uncomplicated convulsions or a series of convulsions lasting 30 min (iv) immunocompromised children"

Table 3. Examples of encephalitis surveillance systems and clinical case definitions used.

4. Summary and future perspectives

In conclusion, it may be stated that

- prospective surveillance systems for encephalitis have been developed in several sites
- universal case definitions or inclusion criteria are currently not being applied
- clinical encephalitis case definitions are usually not adjusted to age
- a large number of prospective studies are laboratory-based with clinical information added after the fact
- evidence-based information on the multiple causes of encephalitis only slowly emerging.

With the emergence of surveillance systems for encephalitis worldwide, it would be desirable to introduce the use of uniform case definitions and clinical criteria allowing meta-analysis and head-to-head comparisons between studies and sites. As a first step into this direction, a model surveillance system has been introduced in the pediatric emergency rooms at Charité University Medical Center in Berlin in collaboration with the adjacent Robert Koch Institute, as a first cohort to prospectively implement the neurologic case definitions by the Brighton Collaboration while assessing vaccine preventable neurologic disease along with neurologic adverse events following immunization in the same population.

The Charité Meningitis Surveillance at Charité (MenSCh) Cohort: Prospective Surveillance Systems for CNS inflammation and natural infection.

At Charité, a prospective surveillance system has been put in place monitoring acute presentations of children and adolescents to one of the largest pediatric ERs in Europe. The ERs are located in two different areas of Berlin representing an ethnically diverse population, including up to 40% of children with migratory background (Turkish, Kurdish, Arab/North African, Eastern European). All patients fulfilling predefined case definitions while presenting on regular screening days are automatically enrolled, tested immediately in close collaboration with epidemiologists and the adjacent Robert Koch Institute and followed-up clinically. In the absence of an HMO system in most European countries, this is a powerful method to capture a comprehensive sample of a typical pediatric urban tertiary care population with "naturally occurring infection" and adverse events. Precise immunization histories are taken at the time of presentation. Case-control and other methodology can be used to compensate for lack of randomization. The **MenSCh (Meningitis Surveillance at Charité) Cohort** is a prospective cohort of children presenting with signs and symptoms of CNS inflammation/infection to the ER. Presentations are classified according to age-adjusted clinical and disease severity scores, but also classified according to standardized case definitions for meningitis, encephalitis, myelitis, ADEM, GBS, seizure and Bell's Palsy by the Brighton Collaboration. Confirmed clinical cases according to the definitions of the Brighton Collaboration, regardless of the trigger (infection, immunization, autoimmune disease), are followed until discharge. Again, detailed immunization histories and laboratory data are captured. After case ascertainment according to standardized case definitions, patients presenting with rare autoimmune AE following immunization will be studied in detail.

Vaccines are among the most effective methodologies available to date for the prevention of infectious diseases of childhood. With declining vaccine acceptance in many parts of the world, it will become increasingly important to learn more about the causes of neurologic adverse events in children. It is hoped that the MenSch cohort will provide a useful contribution to the field while monitoring incidences of vaccine preventable disease alongside with adverse events following immunization.

5. Acknowledgements

The authors kindly thank Ewelina Türk and Jörg Seckinger for their assistance with subsections of the literature review and colleagues at the National Reference Laboratory for Enteroviruses at the Robert Koch Institute in Berlin, for their active collaboration in the development of the MenSCh Cohort.

6. References

[1] Fowler A, Stodberg T, Eriksson M, Wickstrom R. Childhood encephalitis in Sweden: etiology, clinical presentation and outcome. *Eur J Paediatr Neurol* 2008;12(6):484-90.

[2] Granerod J, Ambrose HE, Davies NW, Clewley JP, Walsh AL, Morgan D, et al. Causes of encephalitis and differences in their clinical presentations in England: a multicentre, population-based prospective study. *Lancet Infect Dis* 2010;10(12):835-44.

[3] Le VT, Phan TQ, Do QH, Nguyen BH, Lam QB, Bach VC, et al. Viral etiology of encephalitis in children in southern Vietnam: results of a one-year prospective descriptive study. *PLoS Negl Trop Dis* 2010;4(10):e854.

[4] Glaser CA, Honarmand S, Anderson LJ, Schnurr DP, Forghani B, Cossen CK, et al. Beyond viruses: clinical profiles and etiologies associated with encephalitis. *Clinical infectious diseases: an official publication of the Infectious Diseases Society of America* 2006;43(12):1565.

[5] Stahl JP, Mailles A. Infectious causes of encephalitis. *Lancet Infect Dis* 2010;10(12):814-5.

[6] Ulbert S. West nile virus: the complex biology of an emerging pathogen. *Intervirology* 2011;54(4):171-84.

[7] Salmi TT, Arstila P, Koivikko A. Central nervous system involvement in patients with rotavirus gastroenteritis. *Scand J Infect Dis* 1978;10(1):29-31.

[8] Wong CJ, Price Z, Bruckner DA. Aseptic meningitis in an infant with rotavirus gastroenteritis. *Pediatr Infect Dis* 1984;3(3):244-6.

[9] Ushijima H, Bosu K, Abe T, Shinozaki T. Suspected rotavirus encephalitis. *Archives of Disease in Childhood* 1986;61(7):692.

[10] Keidan I, Shif I, Keren G, Passwell JH. Rotavirus encephalopathy: evidence of central nervous system involvement during rotavirus infection. *Pediatr Infect Dis J* 1992;11(9):773-5.

[11] Yoshida A, Kawamitu T, Tanaka R, Okumura M, Yamakura S, Takasaki Y, et al. Rotavirus encephalitis: detection of the virus genomic RNA in the cerebrospinal fluid of a child. *Pediatr Infect Dis J* 1995;14(10):914-6.

[12] Pang XL, Joensuu J, Vesikari T. Detection of rotavirus RNA in cerebrospinal fluid in a case of rotavirus gastroenteritis with febrile seizures. *Pediatr Infect Dis J* 1996;15(6):543-545.

[13] Makino M, Tanabe Y, Shinozaki K, Matsuno S, Furuya T. Haemorrhagic shock and encephalopathy associated with rotavirus infection. *Acta Paediatr* 1996;85(5):632-4.

[14] Hongou K, Konishi T, Yagi S, Araki K, Miyawaki T. Rotavirus encephalitis mimicking afebrile benign convulsions in infants. *Pediatr Neurol* 1998;18(4):354-7.

[15] Pager C, Steele D, Gwamanda P, Driessen M. A neonatal death associated with rotavirus infection--detection of rotavirus dsRNA in the cerebrospinal fluid. *S Afr Med J* 2000;90(4):364-5.

[16] Lynch M, Lee B, Azimi P, Gentsch J, Glaser C, Gilliam S, et al. Rotavirus and Central Nervous System Symptoms: Cause or Contaminant? Case Reports and Review. *Clinical Infectious Diseases* 2001;33(7):932-938.

[17] Goldwater PN, Rowland K, Power R, Thesinger M, Abbott K, Grieve A, et al. Rotavirus encephalopathy: Pathogenesis reviewed. *Journal of Paediatrics and Child Health* 2001;37(2):206-209.

[18] Nigrovic LE, Lumeng C, Landrigan C, Chiang VW. Rotavirus Cerebellitis? *Clinical Infectious Diseases* 2002;34(1):130-130.

[19] Morrison C, Gilson T, Nuovo GJ. Histologic distribution of fatal rotaviral infection: An immunohistochemical and reverse transcriptase in situ polymerase chain reaction analysis. *Human Pathology* 2001;32(2):216-221.

[20] Kobata R, Tsukahara H, Nakai A, Tanizawa A, Ishimori Y, Kawamura Y, et al. Transient MR signal changes in the splenium of the corpus callosum in rotavirus encephalopathy: value of diffusion-weighted imaging. *J Comput Assist Tomogr* 2002;26(5):825-828.

[21] Iturriza-Gomara M, Auchterlonie IA, Zaw W, Molyneaux P, Desselberger U, Gray J. Rotavirus gastroenteritis and central nervous system (CNS) infection: characterization of the VP7 and VP4 genes of rotavirus strains isolated from paired fecal and cerebrospinal fluid samples from a child with CNS disease. *J Clin Microbiol* 2002;40(12):4797-9.

[22] Kehle J, Metzger-Boddien C, Tewald F, Wald M, Schuurmann J, Enders G. First case of confirmed rotavirus meningoencephalitis in Germany. *Pediatr Infect Dis J* 2003;22(5):468-70.

[23] Rath B, Gentsch J, Seckinger J, Ward K, Deputy S. Rotavirus encephalitis with basal ganglia involvement in an eight-month old infant. *Clinical Pediatrics* 2011;in press.

[24] Nakagomi T, Nakagomi O. Rotavirus antigenemia in children with encephalopathy accompanied by rotavirus gastroenteritis. *Archives of Virology* 2005;150(9):1927-1931.

[25] Kirton A, Busche K, Ross C, Wirrell E. Acute necrotizing encephalopathy in caucasian children: two cases and review of the literature. *J Child Neurol* 2005;20(6):527-32.

[26] Shiihara T, Watanabe M, Honma A, Kato M, Morita Y, Ichiyama T, et al. Rotavirus associated acute encephalitis/encephalopathy and concurrent cerebellitis: Report of two cases. *Brain Dev* 2007;29(10):670-673

[27] Furuya Y, Katayama T, Miyahara K, Kobayashi A, Funabiki T. Detection of the rotavirus a genome from the cerebrospinal fluid of a gastroenteritis patient: a case report. *Jpn J Infect Dis* 2007;60(2-3):148-9.

[28] Wong V. Acute gastroenteritis-related encephalopathy. *J Child Neurol* 2001;16(12):906-10.

[29] Dickey M, Jamison L, Michaud L, Care M, Bernstein DI, Staat MA. Rotavirus meningoencephalitis in a previously healthy child and a review of the literature. *The Pediatric infectious disease journal* 2009;28(4):318.

[30] Fukuda S, Kishi K, Yasuda K, Sejima H, Yamaguchi S. Rotavirus-associated encephalopathy with a reversible splenial lesion. *Pediatric Neurology* 2009;40(2):131-133.

[31] Hickey PW, DiFazio MP. Management of Neurologic Complications of Rotavirus. *The Pediatric infectious disease journal* 2009;28(10):935.

[32] Incecik F, Herguner MO, Altunbasak S, Solgun H. Acute encephalopathy associated rotavirus gastroenteritis. *Journal of Pediatric Neurosciences* 2009;4(2):141.

[33] Kato Z, Orii KE, Morimoto M, Sasai H, Funato M, Sawatari S, et al. A transient lesion in the corpus callosum during rotavirus infection. *Pediatric Neurology* 2009;41(6):467.

[34] Liu B, Fujita Y, Arakawa C, Kohira R, Fuchigami T, Mugishima H, et al. Detection of rotavirus RNA and antigens in serum and cerebrospinal fluid samples from diarrheic children with seizures. *Jpn. J. Infect. Dis* 2009;62(4):279-283.

[35] Jang YY, Lee KH. Transient splenial lesion of the corpus callosum in a case of benign convulsion associated with rotaviral gastroenteritis. *Korean Journal of Pediatrics* 2010;53(9):859-862.

[36] Kobayashi S, Negishi Y, Ando N, Ito T, Nakano M, Togari H, et al. Two patients with acute rotavirus encephalitis associated with cerebellar signs and symptoms. *European journal of pediatrics* 2010.

[37] Takanashi J, Miyamoto T, Ando N, Kubota T, Oka M, Kato Z, et al. Clinical and radiological features of rotavirus cerebellitis. *American Journal of Neuroradiology* 2010;31(9):1591.

[38] Mori T, Morii M, Kuroiwa Y, Hotsubo T, Fuse S, Tsustumi H. Rotavirus encephalitis and cerebellitis with reversible magnetic resonance signal changes. *Pediatrics international: official journal of the Japan Pediatric Society* 2011;53(2):252.

[39] Lloyd MB, Lloyd JC, Gesteland PH, Bale Jr JF. Rotavirus Gastroenteritis and Seizures in Young Children. *Pediatric Neurology* 2010;42(6):404-408.

[40] Obinata K, Okumura A, Nakazawa T, Kamata A, Niizuma T, Kinoshita K, et al. Norovirus Encephalopathy in a Previously Healthy Child. *The Pediatric infectious disease journal* 2010;29(11):1057-1059.

[41] Kato Z, Manabe T, Teramoto T, Kondo N. Adenovirus infection mimics the cerebellitis caused by rotavirus infection. *European journal of pediatrics* 2011;170(3):1-2.

[42] Grgic-Vitek M, Klavs I. High burden of tick-borne encephalitis in Slovenia-Challenge for vaccination policy. *Vaccine* 2011(May 26. [Epub ahead of print]).

[43] Czupryna P, Moniuszko A, Pancewicz SA, Grygorczuk S, Kondrusik M, Zajkowska J. Tick-borne encephalitis in Poland in years 1993-2008--epidemiology and clinical presentation. A retrospective study of 687 patients. *Eur J Neurol* 2011;18(5):673-9.

[44] Karelis G, Bormane A, Logina I, Lucenko I, Suna N, Krumina A, et al. Tick-borne encephalitis in Latvia 1973-2009: epidemiology, clinical features and sequelae. *Eur J Neurol* 2011.

[45] Ehrlich HJ, Petermann R, Barrett PN. Re: Tick-borne encephalitis (TBE) trends in epidemiology and current and future management. *Travel Med Infect Dis* 2011;9(2):83.

[46] Stefanoff P, Polkowska A, Giambi C, Levy-Bruhl D, O'Flanagan D, Dematte L, et al. Reliable surveillance of tick-borne encephalitis in European countries is necessary to improve the quality of vaccine recommendations. *Vaccine* 2011;29(6):1283-8.

[47] Witt CJ, Richards AL, Masuoka PM, Foley DH, Buczak AL, Musila LA, et al. The AFHSC-Division of GEIS Operations Predictive Surveillance Program: a multidisciplinary approach for the early detection and response to disease outbreaks. *BMC Public Health* 2011;11 Suppl 2:S10.

[48] Hossain MJ, Gurley ES, Montgomery S, Petersen L, Sejvar J, Fischer M, et al. Hospital-based surveillance for Japanese encephalitis at four sites in Bangladesh, 2003-2005. *Am J Trop Med Hyg* 2010;82(2):344-9.

[49] Bista MB, Banerjee MK, Shin SH, Tandan JB, Kim MH, Sohn YM, et al. Efficacy of single-dose SA 14-14-2 vaccine against Japanese encephalitis: a case control study. *Lancet* 2001;358(9284):791.

[50] Solomon T, Thao TT, Lewthwaite P, Ooi MH, Kneen R, Dung NM, et al. A cohort study to assess the new WHO Japanese encephalitis surveillance standards. *Bull World Health Organ* 2008;86(3):178-86.

[51] Douglas A, Harris P, Francis F, Norton R. Herpes zoster meningoencephalitis: not only a disease of the immunocompromised? *Infection* 2010;38(1):73-5.

[52] Braun-Falco M, Hoffmann M. Herpes zoster with progression to acute varicella zoster virus-meningoencephalitis. *Int J Dermatol* 2009;48(8):834-9.

[53] Ziebold C, von Kries R, Lang R, Weigl J, Schmitt HJ. Severe complications of varicella in previously healthy children in Germany: a 1-year survey. *Pediatrics* 2001;108(5):E79.

[54] Marchetto S, de Benedictis FM, de Martino M, Versace A, Chiappini E, Bertaine C, et al. Epidemiology of hospital admissions for chickenpox in children: an Italian multicentre study in the pre-vaccine era. *Acta Paediatr* 2007;96(10):1490-3.

[55] Frenos S, Galli L, Chiappini E, de Martino M. An increasing incidence of chickenpox central nervous system complications in children: what's happening in Tuscany? *J Clin Virol* 2007;38(4):358-61.

[56] Cameron JC, Allan G, Johnston F, Finn A, Heath PT, Booy R. Severe complications of chickenpox in hospitalised children in the UK and Ireland. *Arch Dis Child* 2007;92(12):1062-6.

[57] Almuneef M, Memish ZA, Balkhy HH, Alotaibi B, Helmy M. Chickenpox complications in Saudi Arabia: Is it time for routine varicella vaccination? *Int J Infect Dis* 2006;10(2):156-61.

[58] Azevedo RS, Amaku M. Modelling immunization strategies with cytomegalovirus vaccine candidates. *Epidemiol Infect* 2011:1-9.

[59] Griffiths PD, Stanton A, McCarrell E, Smith C, Osman M, Harber M, et al. Cytomegalovirus glycoprotein-B vaccine with MF59 adjuvant in transplant recipients: a phase 2 randomised placebo-controlled trial. *Lancet* 2011;377(9773): 1256-63.

[60] Heineman TC. Human cytomegalovirus vaccines. 2007.

[61] Sabbaj S, Pass RF, Goepfert PA, Pichon S. Glycoprotein B vaccine is capable of boosting both antibody and CD4 T-cell responses to cytomegalovirus in chronically infected women. *J Infect Dis* 2011;203(11):1534-41.

[62] Dollard SC, Grosse SD, Ross DS. New estimates of the prevalence of neurological and sensory sequelae and mortality associated with congenital cytomegalovirus infection. *Rev Med Virol* 2007;17(5):355-63.

[63] Berger A, Reitter A, Harter PN, Buxmann H, Allwinn R, Louwen F, et al. Problems and challenges in the diagnosis of vertical infection with human cytomegalovirus (CMV): Lessons from two accidental cases. *J Clin Virol* 2011.

[64] Montesinos P, Sanz J, Cantero S, Lorenzo I, Martin G, Saavedra S, et al. Incidence, risk factors, and outcome of cytomegalovirus infection and disease in patients receiving prophylaxis with oral valganciclovir or intravenous ganciclovir after umbilical cord blood transplantation. *Biol Blood Marrow Transplant* 2009;15(6):730-40.

[65] Kenneson A, Cannon MJ. Review and meta-analysis of the epidemiology of congenital cytomegalovirus (CMV) infection. *Rev Med Virol* 2007;17(4):253-76.

[66] Miron D, Brosilow S, Felszer K, Reich D, Halle D, Wachtel D, et al. Incidence and clinical manifestations of breast milk-acquired Cytomegalovirus infection in low birth weight infants. *J Perinatol* 2005;25(5):299-303.

[67] Amin R, Ford-Jones E, Richardson SE, MacGregor D, Tellier R, Heurter H, et al. Acute childhood encephalitis and encephalopathy associated with influenza: a prospective 11-year review. *Pediatr Infect Dis J* 2008;27(5):390-5.

[68] Maricich SM, Neul JL, Lotze TE, Cazacu AC, Uyeki TM, Demmler GJ, et al. Neurologic complications associated with influenza A in children during the 2003-2004 influenza season in Houston, Texas. *Pediatrics* 2004;114(5):e626-33.

[69] Okabe N, Yamashita K, Taniguchi K, Inouye S. Influenza surveillance system of Japan and acute encephalitis and encephalopathy in the influenza season. *Pediatr Int* 2000;42(2):187-91.

[70] Ono S, Kudo M, Aoki K, Ezaki F, Misumi J. Effect of mass immunization against influenza encephalopathy on mortality rates in children. *Pediatr Int* 2003;45(6):680-7.
[71] Steininger C, Popow-Kraupp T, Laferl H, Seiser A, Godl I, Djamshidian S, et al. Acute encephalopathy associated with influenza A virus infection. *Clin Infect Dis* 2003;36(5):567-74.
[72] Togashi T, Matsuzono Y, Narita M. Epidemiology of influenza-associated encephalitis-encephalopathy in Hokkaido, the northernmost island of Japan. *Pediatr Int* 2000;42(2):192-6.
[73] Togashi T, Matsuzono Y, Narita M, Morishima T. Influenza-associated acute encephalopathy in Japanese children in 1994-2002. *Virus Res* 2004;103(1-2):75-8.
[74] Wada T, Morishima T, Okumura A, Tashiro M, Hosoya M, Shiomi M, et al. Differences in clinical manifestations of influenza-associated encephalopathy by age. *Microbiol Immunol* 2009;53(2):83-8.
[75] Yoshikawa H, Yamazaki S, Watanabe T, Abe T. Study of influenza-associated encephalitis/encephalopathy in children during the 1997 to 2001 influenza seasons. *J Child Neurol* 2001;16(12):885-90.
[76] Citerio G, Sala F, Patruno A, Gori A, Grioni D, Rossi M, et al. Influenza A (H1N1) encephalitis with severe intracranial hypertension. *Minerva Anestesiol*;76(6):459-62.
[77] Fluss J, Ferey S, Menache-Starobinski C, Delavelle J, Van Bogaert P, Vargas MI. Mild influenza-associated encephalopathy/encephalitis with a reversible splenial lesion in a Caucasian child with additional cerebellar features. *Eur J Paediatr Neurol*;14(1):97-100.
[78] Gika AD, Rich P, Gupta S, Neilson DE, Clarke A. Recurrent acute necrotizing encephalopathy following influenza A in a genetically predisposed family. *Dev Med Child Neurol*;52(1):99-102.
[79] Goenka AH, Mukund A, Ahuja J, Kumar A. Reversible lesion in the splenium of the corpus callosum in a child with influenza-associated encephalitis-encephalopathy (IAEE). *J Clin Neurosci*;17(5):607, 678.
[80] Ichiyama T. Acute encephalopathy/encephalitis in childhood: a relatively common and potentially devastating clinical syndrome. *Brain Dev*;32(6):433-4.
[81] Kulkarni R, Kinikar A. Encephalitis in a child with H1N1 infection: First case report from India. *J Pediatr Neurosci*;5(2):157-9.
[82] Landau YE, Grisaru-Soen G, Reif S, Fattal-Valevski A. Pediatric Neurologic Complications Associated With Influenza A H1N1. *Pediatr Neurol*;44(1):47-51.
[83] Lyon JB, Remigio C, Milligan T, Deline C. Acute necrotizing encephalopathy in a child with H1N1 influenza infection. *Pediatr Radiol*;40(2):200-5.
[84] Martin A, Reade EP. Acute necrotizing encephalopathy progressing to brain death in a pediatric patient with novel influenza A (H1N1) infection. *Clin Infect Dis*;50(8):e50-2.
[85] Ormitti F, Ventura E, Summa A, Picetti E, Crisi G. Acute necrotizing encephalopathy in a child during the 2009 influenza A(H1N1) pandemia: MR imaging in diagnosis and follow-up. *AJNR Am J Neuroradiol*;31(3):396-400.
[86] Rellosa N, Bloch KC, Shane AL, Debiasi RL. Neurologic manifestations of pediatric novel h1n1 influenza infection. *Pediatr Infect Dis J*;30(2):165-7.

[87] Samuel N, Attias O, Tatour S, Brik R. Novel influenza A (H1N1) and acute encephalitis in a child. *Isr Med Assoc J*;12(7):446-7.

[88] Webster RI, Hazelton B, Suleiman J, Macartney K, Kesson A, Dale RC. Severe encephalopathy with swine origin influenza A H1N1 infection in childhood: case reports. *Neurology*;74(13):1077-8.

[89] Sejvar JJ, Kohl KS, Bilynsky R, Blumberg D, Cvetkovich T, Galama J, et al. Encephalitis, myelitis, and acute disseminated encephalomyelitis (ADEM): case definitions and guidelines for collection, analysis, and presentation of immunization safety data. *Vaccine* 2007;25(31):5771-92.

[90] Ward KN, Bryant NJ, Andrews NJ, Bowley JS, Ohrling A, Verity CM, et al. Risk of serious neurologic disease after immunization of young children in Britain and Ireland. *Pediatrics* 2007;120(2):314-21.

[91] Okais C, Gay C, Seon F, Buchaille L, Chary E, Soubeyrand B. Disease-specific adverse events following nonlive vaccines: A paradoxical placebo effect or a nocebo phenomenon? *Vaccine* 2011;May 31. [Epub ahead of print].

[92] Bonhoeffer J, Menkes J, Gold MS, de Souza-Brito G, Fisher MC, Halsey N, et al. Generalized convulsive seizure as an adverse event following immunization: case definition and guidelines for data collection, analysis, and presentation. *Vaccine* 2004;22(5-6):557-62.

[93] Rath B, Magnus M, Heininger U. Evaluating the Brighton Collaboration case definitions, aseptic meningitis, encephalitis, myelitis, and acute disseminated encephalomyelitis, by systematic analysis of 255 clinical cases. *Vaccine* 2010;28(19): 3488-95.

[94] Devrim I, Tezer H, Haliloglu G, Kara A, Secmeer G. Relapsing Herpes simplex virus encephalitis despite high-dose acyclovir therapy: a case report. *Turk J Pediatr* 2008;50(4):380-2.

[95] Jha S, Patel R, Yadav RK, Kumar V. Clinical spectrum, pitfalls in diagnosis and therapeutic implications in herpes simplex encephalitis. *J Assoc Physicians India* 2004;52:24-6.

[96] James SH, Whitley RJ. Treatment of herpes simplex virus infections in pediatric patients: current status and future needs. *Clin Pharmacol Ther* 2010;88(5):720-4.

[97] Jones CA, Walker KS, Badawi N. Antiviral agents for treatment of herpes simplex virus infection in neonates. *Cochrane Database Syst Rev* 2009(3):CD004206.

[98] Long SS, Pool TE, Vodzak J, Daskalaki I, Gould JM. Herpes simplex virus infection in young infants during 2 decades of empiric acyclovir therapy. *Pediatr Infect Dis J* 2011;30(7):556-61.

[99] Wang IJ, Lee PI, Huang LM, Chen CJ, Chen CL, Lee WT. The correlation between neurological evaluations and neurological outcome in acute encephalitis: a hospital-based study. *Eur J Paediatr Neurol* 2007;11(2):63-9.

[100] Tamma PD, Agwu AL, Hartman AL. Behavior Outbursts, Orofacial Dyskinesias, and CSF Pleocytosis in a Healthy Child. *Pediatrics* 2011;Jun 6. [Epub ahead of print].

[101] Banatvala JE. Herpes simplex encephalitis. *Lancet Infect Dis* 2011;11(2):80-1.

[102] Huang MC, Wang SM, Hsu YW, Lin HC, Chi CY, Liu CC. Long-term cognitive and motor deficits after enterovirus 71 brainstem encephalitis in children. *Pediatrics* 2006;118(6):e1785.

[103] Schessl J, Luther B, Kirschner J, Mauff G, Korinthenberg R. Infections and vaccinations preceding childhood Guillain-Barre syndrome: a prospective study. *Eur J Pediatr* 2006;165(9):605-12.

[104] Huang MC, Wang SM, Hsu YW, Lin HC, Chi CY, Liu CC. Long-term cognitive and motor deficits after enterovirus 71 brainstem encephalitis in children. *Pediatrics* 2006;118(6):e1785-8.

[105] Diedrich S, Claus H, Schreier E. Immunity status against poliomyelitis in Germany: determination of cut-off values in International Units. *BMC Infect Dis* 2002;2:2.

[106] Diedrich S, Schreier E. Aseptic meningitis in Germany associated with echovirus type 13. *BMC Infect Dis* 2001;1:14.

[107] Mailles A, Stahl JP. Infectious encephalitis in france in 2007: a national prospective study. *Clin Infect Dis* 2009;49(12):1838-47.

[108] Lee TC, Tsai CP, Yuan CL, Wei CY, Tsao WL, Lee RJ, et al. Encephalitis in Taiwan: a prospective hospital-based study. *Jpn J Infect Dis* 2003;56(5-6):193-9.

[109] Ilias A, Galanakis E, Raissaki M, Kalmanti M. Childhood encephalitis in Crete, Greece. *J Child Neurol* 2006;21(10):910-2.

[110] Beig FK, Malik A, Rizvi M, Acharya D, Khare S. Etiology and clinico-epidemiological profile of acute viral encephalitis in children of western Uttar Pradesh, India. *Int J Infect Dis* 2010;14(2):e141-6.

[111] Anga G, Barnabas R, Kaminiel O, Tefuarani N, Vince J, Ripa P, et al. The aetiology, clinical presentations and outcome of febrile encephalopathy in children in Papua New Guinea. *Ann Trop Paediatr* 2010;30(2):109-18.

[112] Elbers JM, Bitnun A, Richardson SE, Ford-Jones EL, Tellier R, Wald RM, et al. A 12-year prospective study of childhood herpes simplex encephalitis: is there a broader spectrum of disease? *Pediatrics* 2007;119(2):e399.

[113] Glaser CA, Gilliam S, Schnurr D, Forghani B, Honarmand S, Khetsuriani N, et al. In search of encephalitis etiologies: diagnostic challenges in the California Encephalitis Project, 1998-2000. *Clinical infectious diseases: an official publication of the Infectious Diseases Society of America* 2003;36(6):731.

[114] Morishima T, Togashi T, Yokota S, Okuno Y, Miyazaki C, Tashiro M, et al. Encephalitis and encephalopathy associated with an influenza epidemic in Japan. *Clinical infectious diseases: an official publication of the Infectious Diseases Society of America* 2002;35(5):512.

[115] Olsen SJ, Supawat K, Campbell AP, Anantapreecha S, Liamsuwan S, Tunlayadechanont S, et al. Japanese encephalitis virus remains an important cause of encephalitis in Thailand. *Int J Infect Dis* 2010;14(10):e888-92.

[116] Schubart CD, Mturi N, Beld MG, Wertheim PM, Newton CR. Role of viruses in Kenyan children presenting with acute encephalopathy in a malaria-endemic area. *Am J Trop Med Hyg* 2006;75(6):1148-50.

[117] Kolski H, Ford-Jones EL, Richardson S, Petric M, Nelson S, Jamieson F, et al. Etiology of acute childhood encephalitis at The Hospital for Sick Children, Toronto, 1994-1995. *Clin Infect Dis* 1998;26(2):398-409.

Part 2

Virus Infections

7

The Inflammatory Response to Viral Infection of the Central Nervous System

Nicholas Johnson[1]* and Adam F. Cunningham[2]
[1]*Animal Health and Veterinary Laboratories Agency*
[2]*University of Birmingham*
United Kingdom

1. Introduction

Encephalitis, inflammation of the brain, is a rare condition in humans characterised by a triad of clinical features that include fever, headache and an altered level of consciousness that can persist for over 24 hours. There are many causes for the condition ranging from infection with an array of pathogens to autoimmune reactions. A major cause, and the one which this review will focus on, are viral infections (Whitley and Gnann, 2002). A diverse range of viruses are capable of invading the Central Nervous System (CNS) and infecting a variety of cell types within it (Tyler, 2009a; Tyler, 2009b). Examples from a range of viral species will be used to illustrate initial infection of the CNS, early innate immune responses, viral evasion of these early responses and the development of the adaptive immune response. The majority of viral CNS infections are transient but some can lead to long- term disability or death.

Structurally, the CNS consists of the brain and spinal cord that are both encased within bone. Three membranes surround the brain, which are collectively called the meninges. These are the thick dura mater, the web-like arachnoid mater and the delicate pia mater. This structure can itself become inflamed giving rise to meningitis. Within this, the brain is divided at a gross level into the forebrain containing the frontal, parietal, occipital and temporal lobes, and the hindbrain containing specialist structures including the hippocampus, pituitary and cerebellum. Below this is the brainstem that connects the brain to the spinal cord that extends through the body of all vertebrates. Neuronal processes leave the spinal cord to innervate the organs and structures of the body through sensory and motor neurons, forming the peripheral nervous system. The cellular content of the CNS is varied. The key cell-type is the neuron although this only constitutes around 5% of the cellular total and can vary between regions of the brain. Neurons typically have a large cell body containing the nucleus, from which extensions, termed axons extend. At the termini of axons, small processes or dendrites make contact with other neurons creating an extensive network of connections enabling the brain to act as an information-processing centre for the organism. In addition to neurons are cells collectively termed glia. Glial cells support neurons through a range of functional phenotypes. Astrocytes assist in sustaining neuronal metabolism and neurotransmission. Oligodendrocytes have elongated processes that

* Corresponding Author

surround axons and produce myelin, which effectively insulates axonal processes and enables efficient electrical transmission along axons. Finally, microglia provide an immune function within the CNS, acting as the resident macrophage population removing dead cells, and are particularly important in the development of the foetal brain.

Infection of the leptomeninges (aracnoid mater and pia mater) generally does not result in serious disease. However, infection of glial cells and neurons can result in acute disease through direct cellular destruction and/or the initiation of immune pathology. The loss of non-renewable, specialized cells responsible for cognition, mobility and almost all organ function can have profound impact on the host. The immediate consequence of infection is inflammation, manifest as viral encephalitis, the outcome of which can vary from a transient episode to long term neurological deficit or in the death of the host. The pathology of disease is characterised by a cellular thickening of blood vessels or perivascular cuffing and a proliferation of astrocytes, or gliosis. Changes are also observed in the cerebro spinal fluid (CSF) including the presence of predominantly mononuclear cells (pleocytosis), increased levels of protein and antibodies. Infecting viruses can be detected in the CSF using specific molecular tests such as the polymerase chain reaction (PCR).

When considering any host-pathogen relationships within the CNS, the issue of immune-privilege must be acknowledged. The CNS is considered an immuno-privileged site, a term first coined by Peter Medawar resulting from the observation that allografts placed in certain locations, such as the eye or brain were not rejected by the immune system with the rapidity observed in other organs (Brent, 1990). The cause of this privilege has been attributed almost exclusively to the barrier separating the periphery from the CNS, which is collectively termed the blood-brain barrier (BBB). At a basic level this is formed by the endothelium found on the luminal side of blood vasculature within the brain (Bailey et al., 2006). Tight junctions between endothelial cells prevent entry of cells, large molecules and proteins. Furthermore, under normal conditions these endothelial cells express no or very low levels of adhesion molecules preventing attachment of immune cells and blocking a potential route of entry for cells involved in immune surveillance. Surrounding the endothelial cells, on the CNS side, is a thick basement membrane that is itself surrounded by processes from astrocytes termed astrocytic end feet. The BBB is present over 99% of the brain vasculature. The exceptions are those structures that are involved in hormone secretion such as the pituitary and hypothalamus where free movement of proteins is required between neural tissue and the blood. In addition there are no lymphatic vessels within the parenchyma of the brain that would provide a conduit for antigen presenting dendritic cells to move directly to lymphoid tissue. However, it would be wrong to assume that the absence of comparable cells and structures found in the periphery represents an absence of these functions. Numerous studies are now identifying the multiple mechanisms of immune surveillance that support the CNS, initiating both protective and damaging immune responses (Hickey, 2001). Likewise there are now defined routes by which immune cells can enter the CNS, particularly in response to infection (Ransohoff et al., 2003). The appropriate and timely orchestration of these events is critical in responding to viral infection particularly in the early chemokine and cytokine signals that trigger the innate immune response. Much research has been conducted in recent years on these early responses with some mediators being observed repeatedly, such as the chemokine CXCL10, in response to viral infection. This in turn has dramatic consequences for the vasculature without apparently changing the efficacy of the BBB. Adjunct to this is the activation of the adaptive response to viral infection within the CNS. In this area less is known of the mechanism that leads to antigen presentation from this site. Key questions that are raised by this include the mechanism of antigen transfer from the CNS to sites of antigen presentation, the timescale of these events and the fate of effecter cells that eventually migrate to the site of infection. The coordination of immune activation and appropriate response are poorly understood and can result in a continuum of outcomes that vary from complete resolution of the infection, latent infection by the virus, severe encephalitis and cell-mediated destruction of host cells.

This review will follow the theoretical events that occur following neuroinvasion in humans by viruses that result in encephalitis. This will include:

- A brief overview of viruses that cause encephalitis. This focuses mainly on those that infect humans although includes a number that have been used extensively in murine experimental models.
- An examination of the early innate immune response generated within the CNS to viral infection. This will also consider the cell-types that these signals target that prepare the tissue for the immune response. Also of importance will be the mechanisms that viruses use to subvert the immune response at this early stage.
- Consideration of antigen presentation from CNS, which has been traditionally been considered an immuno-privileged site. In addition, the process of antibody-secreting cell development within lymphoid tissue and then migration to the CNS will be reviewed.
- The review will conclude with the final steps of leukocyte recruitment across the BBB and discuss the variable outcomes to infection with different viruses. This appears to be determined as much by the response of the host as the virulence of the virus.

2. Viruses that cause encephalitis

Many viruses have been identified as the causative agent of encephalitis. Table 1 gives a summary of many of the virus species that are associated with human and/or animal encephalitis. It is noteworthy that most have ribonucleic acid (RNA) genomes. Many are found worldwide although some, particularly those that are associated with an arthropod vector, have a more limited distribution. Most are established causative agents of disease.

2.1 Herpesviruses that cause encephalitis

Herpes viruses are one of the few groups that preferentially infect neurons or show neurotropism. Herpes simplex virus type 1 infects trigeminal ganglia and establishes a latent infection. Periodically, the virus reactivates and returns to the site which the ganglia innervates, causing a vesicular rash. Virus is released into the exudate and can be transmitted onwards through contact. This cycle occurs repeatedly through the life of the infected individual but occasionally this can develop into encephalitis in both immunocompetent and particularly immunocompromised individuals (Kleinschmidt-DeMaster and Gilden, 2001). A recent investigation into the causes of encephalitis in England found that 42% could be attributed to infectious disease with 19% being caused by herpes simplex virus and 5% being caused by varicella zoster virus (Granerod et al., 2010). A further 30% were caused by immune-mediated encephalitis. However, the largest group (42%) were of unknown origin, some of which could have had a viral aetiology but not diagnosed. Similar findings were made from a retrospective study of encephalitis in

Australia with Herpes simplex viruses being the most common virus associated with human encephalitis (Huppatz et al., 2010), although in this study, flaviviruses such as Murray Valley encephalitis virus and Kunjin virus were also reported.

2.2 Arthropod-borne viruses that cause encephalitis

Prominent amongst the viruses that cause encephalitis are the flaviviruses (Gould and Solomon, 2008). These are transmitted by an arthropod vector (mosquitoes and ticks) and thus disease characteristically occurs in human populations in synchrony with seasonal peaks in vector abundance. In the Northern Hemisphere this is typically late summer for mosquito-borne infections. Infection with arthropod-borne viruses usually results in replication in lymphoid tissue close to the bite site that results in a transient viraemia and febrile illness. The viraemia following infection with some viruses, either through its transient nature or low titres, does not result in onward transmission to the vector such as the case of West Nile virus and humans are a dead end host. However, in other cases, human infection is critical to maintaining the infection such as in outbreaks of chikungunya virus (see below). Encephalitis usually occurs subsequent to the resolution of viraemia. The flavivirus genus includes viruses such as mosquito-borne West Nile virus, which following its introduction into the United States in 1999 resulted in a sharp increase in human cases of encephalitis as it rapidly spread west (Granwehr et al., 2004). In experimental studies, West Nile virus is highly neurovirulent in mice, spreading rapidly though the brain. Figure 1 illustrates the rapid spread of West Nile virus following intranasal infection. The morphology of infected cells indicates that they are predominantly neuronal. Another prominent member of this genus is Japanese encephalitis virus, present throughout Asia. Mortality rates can reach 30% with a further 50% having severe neurological sequelae (Tyler, 2009a). In addition to mosquito-borne viruses, the flaviviruses also include tick-borne viruses of which the most prominent is tick-borne encephalitis virus (TBEV) found in an uninterrupted belt from Western Europe to the far east of Asia (Mansfield et al., 2009). The virus is transmitted by *Ixodes* species of ticks and is currently increasing in many countries, likely through changes in human behaviour such as leisure pursuits that bring humans into areas inhabited by ticks. TBEV causes asymptomatic infection in wildlife but can result in severe encephalitis in humans. The exception to this is a variant of TBEV named louping ill virus found almost exclusively in the United Kingdom that has been rarely associated with human illness but causes fatal encephalitic disease in sheep and grouse (Sheahan et al., 2002).

Another group of mosquito-borne viruses capable of causing encephalitis is the genus Alphavirus (Zacks and Paessler, 2009). Prominent among these are the equine encephalitides of North, Central and South America Although less rarely associated with human encephalitis, infection with Eastern equine encephalitis virus can be devastating with mortality rates ranging between 50 and 75%. As the names of these virus indicates, they also cause severe encephalitis in horses with mortality rates reaching up to 90%. This group also includes emerging viruses such as chikungunya virus, that has caused explosive outbreaks of febrile disease in countries around the Indian Ocean that have sporadically been transported back to Europe by infected individuals. In one year this resulted in autochthonous transmission of chikungunya virus in Italy potentially vectored by the invasive mosquito species *Aedes albopictus* (Seyler et al., 2008).

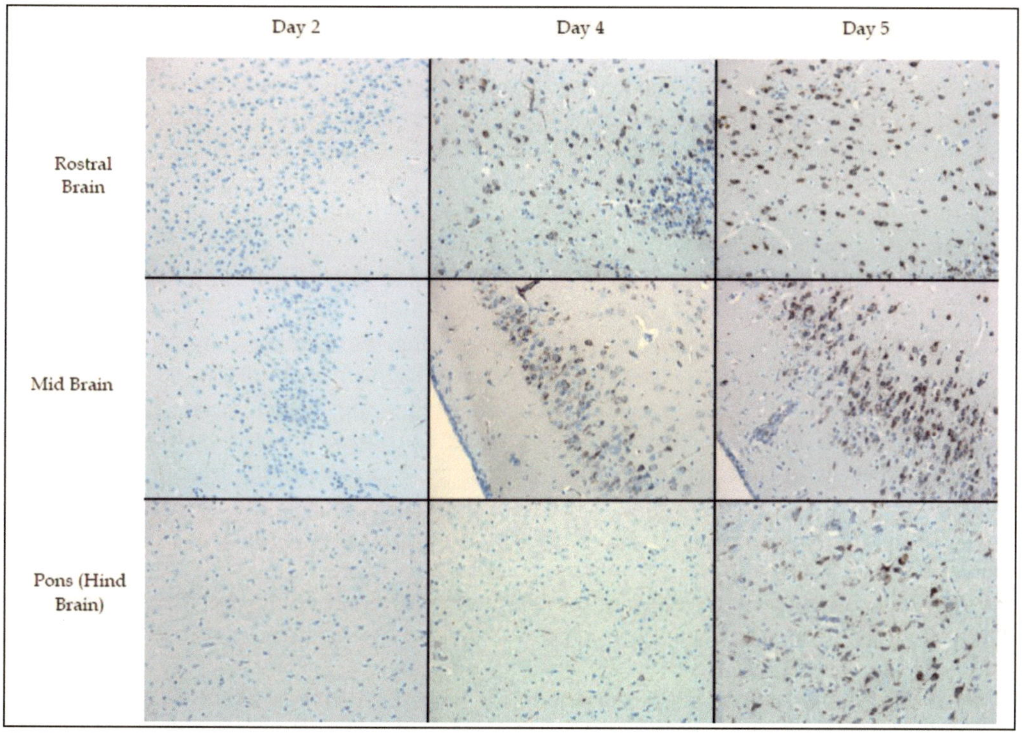

Fig. 1. Spread of West Nile virus through the murine brain following intranasal infection. Individual mice were inoculated with West Nile virus and sampled at the time points indicated. Serial 4 μm sections were cut and stained with a monoclonal antibody specific for the West Nile virus envelope protein. Brown staining indicates detection of West Nile virus within regions of the brain indicated.

2.3 Lyssaviruses that cause encephalitis

One group of viruses of special note are the lyssaviruses of which every member is believed to be neurotropic and capable of causing encephalitis. This group is dominated by the rabies virus, a virus that infects all mammals and is transmitted by animal bites that with rare exceptions cause fatal encephalitis in all those where infection reaches the brain (Rupprecht et al., 2002). Estimates are vague on the actual number of annual deaths due to rabies, particularly in regions of the world with poorly developed public health infrastructures but figures upwards of 50,000 are regularly quoted. Transmission of rabies virus occurs when virus is deposited within skin or muscle following a bite and if not treated either by wound cleansing or vaccination, infects neurons close to the wound. The virus then ascends rapidly to the CNS by retrograde axonal transport leading to replication within the spinal cord and brain (Schnell et al., 2010). Vaccination post-bite is highly effective and has virtually eliminated rabies as a human disease in the Americas and Europe. The main human burden of this disease falls in Asia and Africa where the cost of treatment or ignorance prevents its use. The lyssavirus genus also contains viruses that are associated with certain bat species and that on occasion have resulted in human fatalities following contact with an infected bat. These viruses appear to have a limited geographical distribution (Fooks et al., 2003; Johnson et al., 2010).

2.4 Emerging viruses that cause encephalitis

Others species are considered emerging viruses (Tyler, 2009a). Human immunodeficiency virus is a prime example of a virus emerging as a recognised disease in the 1970s. The virus emerged in the human population following a jump from primates into man in Africa at a much earlier point in the century (Zhu et al., 1998; Tebit and Arts, 2011). It has spread rapidly and continues to be a global public health problem. In addition to progressive immunodeficiency, up to one third of individuals infected with HIV-1 develop encephalitis (Lipton and Gendelman, 1995).

Another virus that has emerged, particularly in Italy as one of the major causes of encephalitis, is Toscana virus and the closely related virus Naples sandfly fever (Tyler, 2009a). The virus is transmitted by sandflies (*Phlebotomus perniciosus*) during the summer months causing mild febrile illness that can develop into severe encephalitis (Dionisio et al., 2001).

Further examples include the recently described Hendra and Nipah viruses (Tyler, 2009b). Hendra virus was first isolated in 1994 as a result of disease affected horses in Brisbane, Australia, that in turn lead to disease amongst veterinarians who treated the animals (Tulsiani et al., 2011). Subsequent investigation demonstrated that the virus had made the jump from its natural host, pteropid fruit bats, into an amplifying host, the horse, from which it then made the jump to humans. A similar sequence of events occurred with the emergence Nipah virus that caused an outbreak of acute encephalitis among Malaysian pig handlers in 1998, with farmed pigs acting as the amplifying host. Immunohistochemical analysis of autopsy specimens observed extensive parenchymal necrosis with widespread Nipah virus antigen staining associated with the smooth muscle of blood vessels (Wong et al., 2002). Again, fruit bats were identified as the original host of the virus and the Malaysian outbreak was controlled by mass slaughter of pigs. Repeated sporadic outbreaks of Nipah virus infections continue to occur in Asia.

2.5 Rare viral encephalopathies

Although more commonly associated with haemorrhagic fever, Lassa fever virus can cause encephalopathy during the course of infection (Cummins et al., 1992). A related virus, lymphocytic choriomeningitis virus, is used as a model for encephalitis in mice. Measles virus is a common childhood infection which usually resolves rapidly with no neural involvement. However a small number of cases develop subacute sclerosing panencephalitis (SSPE), a fatal condition in which the virus persists in the brain, spreading through the CNS causing progressive demyelination and destruction of neurons (Allen et al., 1996).

3. Innate response to viral infection of the Central Nervous System

Entry of virus into the CNS can be haematogenous, resulting from changes in the vasculature that enable virus to cross the blood-brain-barrier either directly or within infected cells crossing the endothelium. Alternatively entry can be neuronal of which rabies virus and herpes viruses are the best characterised. By the haematogenous route there is likely to have been prior virus replication in the periphery often resulting in a detectable viraemia and an opportunity for systemic immune activation and an adaptive response demonstrable by the presence of anti-virus antibodies in serum. There is usually a febrile phase that often resolves and the appearance of virus-neutralising antibodies in the blood that rapidly controls viraemia. Entry by the neuronal route may occur with minimal virus replication in the periphery and therefore the first contact between the immune response

Virus Family	Genome	Virus Species	Geographical Distribution
Adenoviridae	Double-stranded DNA	Adenovirus	Worldwide
Arenaviridae	Single-stranded RNA (negative sense, segmented)	Lassa fever virus	West Africa
		Lymphocytic choriomeningitis virus	Worldwide
Bunyaviridae	Single-stranded RNA (negative sense, segmented)	California encephalitis virus	North America
			Worldwide
		Rift Valley fever virus	Africa
		Toscana virus	Europe
		La Crosse virus	North America
Flaviviridae	Single-stranded RNA (negative sense, non-segmented)	Japanese encephalitis virus	Asia
		Kyasanur Forest virus	India
		Louping ill virus	United Kingdom
		Murray Valley encephalitis virus	Australia
		St. Louis encephalitis	North and South America
		Tick-borne encephalitis virus	Europe and Asia
		West Nile virus	Worldwide
Herpesviridae	Double-stranded DNA	Human herpes virus 1 (Herpes simplex virus)	Worldwide
		Human herpes virus 3 (Varicella zoster virus)	Worldwide
		Human herpes virus 6	Worldwide
Orthomyxoviridae	Single stranded RNA (negative sense, segmented)	Influenza A virus	Worldwide
Paramyxoviridae	Single stranded RNA, (negative sense, non-segmented)	Mumps virus	Worldwide
		Measles virus	Worldwide
		Nipah virus	Asia
		Hendra virus	Australia
Picornaviridae	Single stranded RNA (positive sense, non-segmented)	Poliovirus	Africa

Virus Family	Genome	Virus Species	Geographical Distribution
		Coxsackie virus	Worldwide
		Echovirus	Worldwide
Retroviridae	Single stranded RNA (positive sense, non-segmented). Capable of integration into the host genome through a DNA intermediate genome.	Human Immunodeficiency virus	Worldwide
Rhabdoviridae	Single-stranded RNA (negative sense, non-segmented)	Rabies virus	Worldwide
		Duvenhage virus	Africa
		European bat lyssavirus type 1	Europe
		European bat lyssavirus type 2	Europe
		Australian bat lyssavirus	Australia
Togaviridae	Single-standed RNA (negative sense, non-segmented).	Eastern equine encephalitis virus	North and South America
		Western equine encephalitis virus	North America
		Venezuelan equine encephalitis virus	North and South America
		Chikungunya virus	Africa and Asia

Table 1. Viruses that cause encephalitis

and infecting virus occurs within the CNS and can provide a direct challenge to the survival of the host. In this case, the earliest response to the appearance of virus within the CNS is the innate-immune response.

Innate immune responses are activated by recognition of pathogen-associated molecular patterns or PAMPs. For viruses, this includes surface glycoproteins and structures associated with single- or double-stranded RNA. Recognition is mediated by a number of protein families, the most prominent being the toll-like receptors (TLRs), NOD-like receptors and RIG-I helicases (Creagh and O'Neill, 2006; Rehwinkel and Reis e Sousa, 2010). These receptors are expressed in many compartments of the cell and trigger the production of type I interferons, a key element in controlling virus replication and spread (Randall and Goodbourn, 2008). Type 2 interferons are produced exclusively by lymphoid cells, which are absent early in infection but contribute to later control of pathogens. Interferons in turn activate the up-regulation of a large number of proteins that act to control infection at the cellular level and attract immune effector cells. Three mechanisms of direct inhibition of virus replication have been identified. Activation of protein kinase R (PKR) in response to double stranded RNA (e.g. virus replication intermediates) which inhibits eukaryotic translational factor 2 that in turn restricts synthesis of viral proteins. Activation of 2'5' oligoadenylate synthetase (OAS), which activates RNase L and in turn degrades viral RNA. Finally, the Mx family of proteins are activated that target nucleocapsids (viral structures that contain the genome bound to viral proteins including the nucleoprotein, a protein encoded by many viruses). Whilst the CNS has unique immunological status there is increasing evidence that there is a vigorous innate immune response to viral infection of cells within it (Savarin and Bergman, 2008). For example, TLRs are selectively up-regulated in the brain in response to infection with different viruses (McKimmie et al., 2005). Neurons can produce a range of innate immune-associated proteins including type 1 interferons in response to infection with rabies virus (Prehaud et al., 2005), Theilers virus and La Crosse virus (Delhaye et al., 2006). Microglial cells are capable of producing a wide range of inflammatory mediators in response to activation (Rock et al., 2004) or direct infection (Nakamichi et al., 2005).

Unsurprisingly, viruses have evolved a range of mechanisms to subvert the innate immune response, particularly through inhibition of the interferon system (Randall and Goodbourn, 2008). These often involve direct interaction of virally expressed proteins with signaling intermediates that would normally trigger the expression of interferon or interferon-induced proteins. Many such viral proteins have multiple roles, both in viral replication and subversion of the immune response. The influenza virus NS1 protein inhibits export of host mRNA from the nucleus during infection (Satterley et al., 2007) whereas the La Crosse virus nonstructural protein NSs targets inhibition of type 1 interferon production (Blaqori et al., 2007). The rabies virus phosphoprotein blocks interferon signaling through interaction with interferon regulatory factor 3 (Brzozka et al., 2005) and STAT proteins (Chelibi-Alix et al., 2006; Brzozka et al., 2006; Vidy et al., 2007).

Whilst innate immune inhibition occurs within the cell, neuroinvasion by viruses rapidly induces immune responses across the CNS (See Figure 2). A key family of proteins produced in response to infection are the chemokines whose primary role is to attract immune effecter cells to sites of infection. The chemokine family consists of a growing number of small proteins (<100 amino acids) that are produced at sites of pathology. They contain four conserved cysteine residues that form structurally critical disulphide bonds. The position of the first two cysteines, either adjacent (CC) or separated by a single amino acid (CXC) dictates the current naming of chemokines (Baggiolini, 1998). These in turn bind to specific receptors expressed on target cells. A summary of a number of well-characterized chemokines is shown in Table 2.

Current name	Former name	Receptors	Receptor expressed on
CCL2	MCP1	CCR2	Monocytes, activated T cells
CCL3	MIP-1α	CCR1,4,5	Activated T cells
CCL4	MIP-1β	CCR5	Monocytes, activated T cells
CCL5	RANTES	CCR1,3,4,5	Monocytes, activated T cells
CXCL10	IP-10	CXCR3	Activated T cells

Table 2. Summary of a small number of human chemokines and their receptors

Studies of *in vivo* models generally show transcriptional up-regulation of a wide range of chemokines in the CNS following viral infection. Numerous studies using murine models of infection have consistently shown up-regulation of chemokines including those on rabies virus (Wang et al., 2005) and this is associated with infiltration of mononuclear cells, particularly T cells (Johnson et al., 2008). Likewise, West Nile virus infection up-regulates a wide range of pro-inflammatory genes within the murine brain (Venter et al., 2005), prominent among these is CXCL10. Figure 2 shows the transcriptional up-regulation of a small panel of chemokines from time-points that correspond with those in Figure 1. Most show a detectable up-regulation by day 4 with CXCL10 showing the greatest increase both temporally and in magnitude. Functionally, expression of CXCL10 leads to recruitment of CD8+ T-cells and control of infections such as West Nile virus and lymphocytic choriomeningitis virus (Klein et al., 2005; Christensen et al., 2006). Conversely, the majority of T cells entering the CNS express the CXCL10 receptor CXCR3 (Stiles et al., 2006) and expression of this receptor is critical for targeting CD8+ T cells to specific regions of the CNS (Zhang et al., 2008).

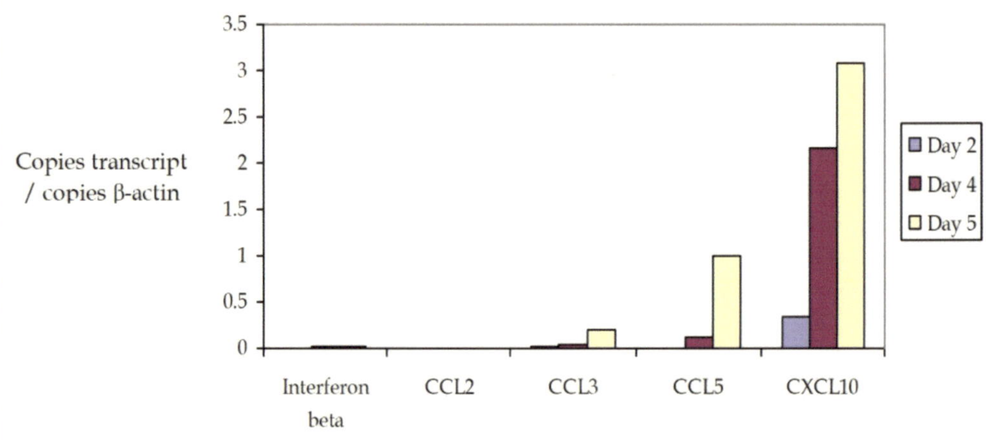

Fig. 2. Expression of interferon β and selected chemokine transcripts following intranasal infection with West Nile virus. Groups of three mice were infected with West Nile virus by the intranasal route and sampled at the time points indicated. Total RNA was extracted from whole brain and the level of transcript was measured by quantitiative real-time reverse transcription polymerase chain reaction as previously described (Johnson et al., 2008).

Many cytokines are toxic to neurons and oligodendrocytes including IL1β, TNF-α and interferon-γ. Uncontrolled cytokine expression would inevitably lead to tissue damage, a situation that occurs in auto-immune mediated encephalopathies such as multiple sclerosis and Alzheimer's disease. It is therefore not suprising to find mechanisms for controlling inflammation within the CNS. Innate immune responses are suppressed by TGF-β, produced by resting and active astrocytes (Constam et al., 1992). During inflammation, the family of suppressors of cytokine signaling (SOCS) proteins are induced by cytokine expression and block signal transduction activated by these same cytokines providing feedback inhibition of inflammation (Yoshimura et al., 2007). There is also evidence that these proteins are selectively expressed in the brain to control inflammation in response to viral infection (Mansfield et al., 2010). A delicate balance is required to ensure that inflammation, a natural response to infection and vital to initiate the process of infection resolution does not result in excessive cellular destruction. It is also clear that innate immune responses are not alone capable of controlling and eliminating the cause of infection and that an adaptive response is required.

4. Antigen presentation, lymphatic drainage and the development of the adaptive immune response

The adaptive immune response to CNS infection is presented with a unique challenge compared to other sites within the body. There appears to be limited antigen presentation capacity within the CNS and no lymphatic drainage vessels. There is no lymphoid tissue within the CNS in which antigen responses can develop and activated immune cells that develop externally to the CNS need to cross the BBB in order to reach locations where they are required. Direct viral infection can lead to disruption of the BBB such as the infection of endothelial cells by Semliki Forest virus in a murine model of disease (Soilu-Hanninen et al., 1994). However, during the early stages of most infections the BBB remains intact, indeed it is possible that failure to open the BBB may be a contributory factor in the failure to control rabies virus infection (Roy et al., 2007). The ability to detect, present and rapidly respond to the presence of virus are critical determinants in controlling infection.

Throughout the body, the principal cell-type that detects non-host antigens are plasmacytoid dendritic cells that present antigen on the cell surface to other cell-types of the adaptive immune system. They are also the main type 1 interferon producing cells. However, cells with dendritic cell morphology and phenotype are absent from the CNS (Hart and Fabre, 1981). A possible alternative within the CNS is the microglia cell component, which in some areas of the CNS form over 15% of the cellular composition (Rock et al., 2004). In their resting form, microglia express very low levels of MHC class II molecules, but this along with a range of co-stimulatory molecules are up-regulated when microglia enter an activated state enabling antigen presentation (Constam et al., 1992; Fischer and Reichmann, 2001). In addition, there appears to be a discrete population of dendritic cells associated with the vascular endothelium within the brain that could provide antigen-presenting function (Gieber et al., 2005) and could act to draw immune effectors into the CNS.

A key challenge to understanding the development of the adaptive immune response is to find appropriate means of introducing antigen or pathogen into the CNS without disruption of the BBB. It has long been recognised that direct injection of large volumes (upto 30μl) causes a dramatic increase of intra-cranial pressure leading to the expulsion of most of the inoculum into peripheral locations (Cairns, 1950; Mims 1960). One means of overcoming this has been the inoculation of laboratory animals with stereotactically guided small volumes of virus (< 2 μl). Stevenson and co-workers used this approach to study influenza virus infection in mice. Inoculation of virus into the CSF or intranasally resulted in a rapid induction of IgM (2-4 days) and IgG (3-5 days), and proliferative responses from cells prepared from cervical lymph nodes were observed 10 days after inoculation. However, direct inoculation of virus into the brain parenchyma failed to induce either antibody of cellular responses despite demonstration of virus replication within the brain (Stevenson et al., 1997). This scenario reflects the antibody responses observed in rabies patients. Infection of peripheral nerves occurs in the skin or muscle, subsequent retrograde axonal transport enables the virus to ascend directly into the CNS accompanied by a rapid increase in replication. It is possible in most infections with rabies virus that no replication occurs within the periphery and thus rabies virus bypasses normal immune surveillance and response. Hence few patients have detectable levels of antibody on admission with disease (Noah et al., 1998; Hunter et al., 2010). These observations suggest that under some circumstances, the adaptive immune response to antigen or whole virus is delayed.

A further obstacle to development of the immune response is the absence of a discrete lymphatic vasculature. This has gradually undergone revision with the recognition that this must occur. There is a net influx of fluid into the CNS that requires some form of drainage (Cserr and Knopf, 1992). Up to 50% of protein introduced into the brain of laboratory animals could be detected in the cervical lymphatics and that this can be extremely rapid with tracer being detected in deep cervical lymph nodes within six hours (Yamada et al., 1991). It is now recognised that there are discrete drainage routes from the CNS and these include passage through the arachnoid villi into the blood supplying the dural sinus. There is also drainage to the lymph system along spaces adjacent to the cranial and spinal nerves, and through the Virchow-Robin perivascular spaces surrounding brain blood vessels (Knopf et al., 1995; Kida et al., 1995). Antibody secreting cells responding to CNS antigen can be detected in cervical lymph nodes and removal of these lymph nodes in experimental animals following introduction of antigen ablates the antibody response (Knopf et al., 1995). However, it is not clear that the response to virally infected cells and thus cellular associated virus will have the same dynamics and kinetics as soluble antigen. Recent studies have shown that activated CD4+ cells can traffic from the brain parenchyma to the nasal mucosa and cervical lymph nodes, using a similar route to that of soluble antigen (Goldmann et al., 2006). This opens the possibility that classical antigen presentation is possible from within the CNS leading to development of virus specific immune cells within lymphoid tissue that are external in the presence of an intact BBB. Although this fails to explain the late emergence of antibodies to rabies virus in patients that present with disease (Noah et al., 1998).

5. Leukocyte recruitment and immune control of infection

The mechanism that directs activated immune cells from lymphoid tissue to particular organs has not been elucidated. However, some form of targeting is likely to occur in order to achieve successful resolution of infection and it is likely that chemokines play a key role in this. Activated T cells can enter the CNS in an antigen-independent manner and rates of entry do increase when inflammatory responses are triggered in the periphery. However retention and anti-viral function are dependent on MHC restricted antigen recognition. Cells can enter the CNS through a number of routes (Ransohoff et al., 2003). The first is to cross the choroid plexus stromal venules, the region of the brain where CSF is produced, and can lead to an influx of cells within the CSF. Secondly, lymphocytes can enter through the vasculature supplying the pia membrane. Finally, lymphocytes can migrate into the parenchyma across vascular endothelium throughout the brain. This leads to the common histological feature observed during encephalitis of the perivascular cuff (Figure 3). Lymphocyte entry through the vasculature is divided into a series of events controlled by the expression of a range of adhesion molecules expressed on the lymphocyte and endothelium (Ransohoff et al., 2003). The first stage is rolling or tethering as the cell becomes attached to the blood vessel. Critical amongst these are the intercellular adhesion molecules (ICAMs) that are stimulated within vascular endothelium by a range of cytokines directly or through positive feedback once adhesion has occurred between the lymphocyte and the endothelium (Dietrich, 2002). Finally the lymphocyte undergoes diapedesis, where processes extend between the endothelial cells, driven in part by chemokine-induced chemotaxis.

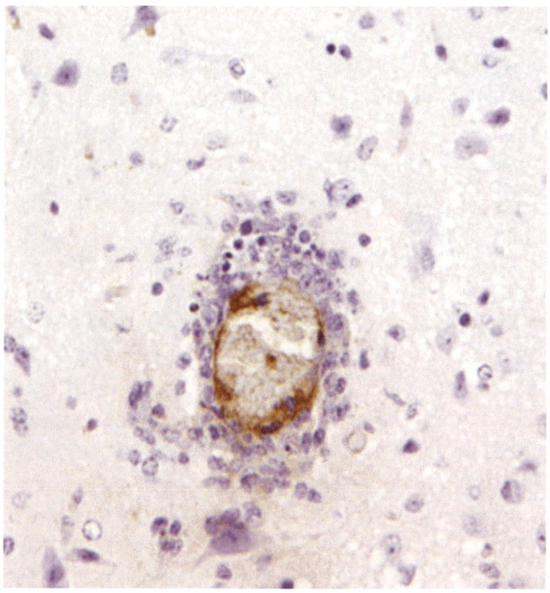

Fig. 3. Example of a perivascular cuff forming around a parenchymal blood vessel observed within the brain following infection with a lyssavirus. The fixed section of murine brain has been paraffin mounted and stained with haematoxylin and eosin. There is distinct accumulation of mononuclear cells around the vessel Further details can be found in Hicks et al. (Hicks et al., 2009).

The current understanding of effector cell infiltration of the CNS suggests that the earliest responders to viral infection are T cells, whereas B cell development takes longer and these enter the CNS later in the course of infection (Savarin and Bergmann, 2008). T cells control virally infected cells whereas antibody is critical in controlling virus spread. However, in some instances there may also be antibody-mediated control of infected host cells through antibody-dependent cellular cytotoxicity. This mechanism may be more prominent in humans than in mice.

B cells originate in the bone marrow and after development in this site, migrate as immature cells to secondary lymphoid tissues to complete the maturation process. B cells that encounter protein antigens through their B cell receptor can interact with primed T cells in a cognate-dependent manner (MacLennan et al., 2003). Productive contacts with T cells result in the B cell differentiating into antibody-secreting plasma cells in extrafollicular sites such as the splenic red pulp or medulla, in lymph nodes or entering the germinal centre reaction (MacLennan et al., 2003; Cozine et al., 2005). There are differences between these two pathways. Extrafollicular responses develop to T-dependent and T-independent antigens and produce the first wave of IgM and IgG, the latter of which is generally of modest affinity. High affinity persisting, effective life-long antibody responses and memory B cells derive from germinal centres. In germinal centres B cells undergo somatic hypermutation with subsequent competition for antigen, and require further survival signals from T cells. Plasma cells that derive from this response then usually migrate to sites such as the bone marrow and secrete antibody. Thus, these effector cells can contribute to protection from sites distal from the sites of infection. Nevertheless, cells generated through the response may also be able to migrate to sites of inflammation, possibly through mechanisms such as their expression of CXCR3 resulting in migration to sites with elevated levels of CXCL10. What is significant in the context of the current discussion is that the type of B cell response induced and the kinetics in which it develops can vary markedly between different pathogens. Fundamental work on the development of antibodies has focused on the response to bacterial infection. For instance, in responses to alum-precipitated proteins extrafollicular and germinal centre responses develop in parallel, with both detectable within the first 5 days of immunization in mice. In contrast, extrafollicular responses to *Salmonella* infection are detectable within 3 days of systemic infection yet germinal centre responses do not develop until the infection has all but resolved (Cunningham et al., 2007). Furthermore, after infection with mycobacteria antibody responses may not be detectable until weeks after infection. This means that there are likely to be host-dependent and pathogen-dependent factors that shape the type and timing of the antibody response that is induced during infection. For rabies infection of humans this is likely to be important and possibly more influenced by pathogen-intrinsic factors, since post-exposure antibody is clearly able to control the infection if present early enough.

The majority of cells undergoing migration across the CNS vasculature appear to be CD3+ T cells (Man et al., 2007). This is illustrated in Figure 4 where the average counts of T or B cells have been compared across three regions of the brain of a mouse infected with rabies virus. In each region over 90% of cells counted are T cells. Under normal conditions, low numbers of B cells can be detected in the CNS with an activated phenotype (Anthony et al., 2003). These presumably provide a low level of immune surveillance. The development of inflammation within the CNS causes this proportion to increase. The explanation for this may be in the longer development and maturation of B cells compared to other cell types prior to migration to the CNS.

The evolution of intrathecal production of antibody has been demonstrated through introduction of antigen through a permanent cannula (Knopf et al., 1998). This study demonstrated trafficking of B cells into the CNS and detection of antigen-specific intrathecal antibody 14 days after injection. It was also observed that there was localisation of mononuclear cells at the site of antigen introduction suggesting a homing process. Similar kinetics have been demonstrated for antibody secreting cell entry into the CNS following viral infection with mouse hepatitis virus (Tschen et al., 2002). Four pathways have been proposed to account for the presence of antibody secreting cells within the CNS (Meinl et al., 2006). These include migration of plasmablasts to the CNS, migration of memory B cells that subsequently differentiate into antibody-secreting cells, development of antibody secreting cells within lymphoid follicles in the meninges and antigen independent differentiation of B cells within the CNS itself. Recruitment and survival within the CNS is controlled by chemokines particularly CXCL12 / CXCL13 (Krumholz et al., 2006), and B cell promoting factors such as BAFF produced locally by astrocytes (Avery et al., 2003; Schneider, 2005).

The presence of antigen secreting cells can have both positive and negative effects within the CNS (Meinl et al., 2006). B cell secretion of cytokines such as TGF-β can down-regulate inflammation whereas expression of IL-6 and IL-12 can increase tissue destruction. Similarly, secretion of antibodies that bind to autoantigens can lead to tissue damage as observed in multiple sclerosis lesions where B cells are prominent. However, secretion of antibodies against viruses will have a direct beneficial impact by controlling virus spread. One critical observation of B cells within the CNS is that they have undergone hypersomatic mutation, confirming that they have at some stage been present within a lymphoid germinal centre (Baranzini et al., 1999). This in turn suggests that the development of mature antibody secreting B cells requires a distinct period of time before it eventually reaches the CNS and that if excessive cell death has occurred during this period permanent damage may result.

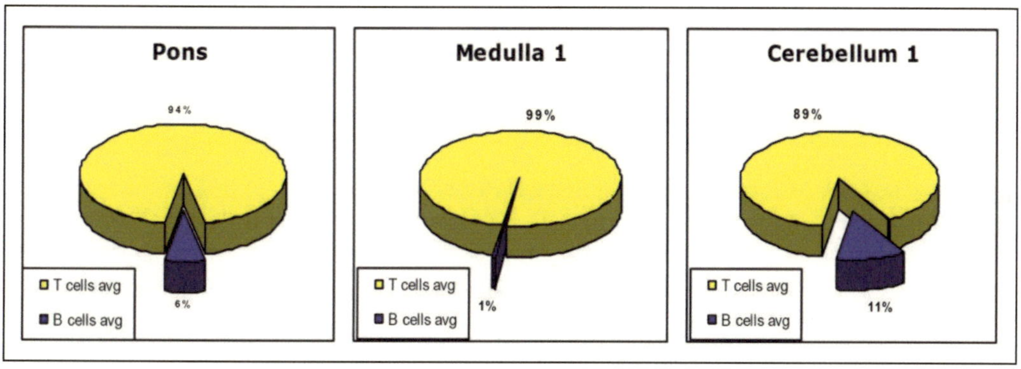

Fig. 4. Illustration of the proportion of T and B cells present with different regions of the brain following infection with rabies virus. Sections of murine brain were prepared and stained with anti-CD3 for T cells and anti-CD45R/B220 for B cells.

6. Conclusions

This review has attempted to follow the course of events that lead to the development of viral encephalitis from the viruses that cause it, through the early and late events of the host response. The proposed mechanisms that viruses use to cross the blood-brain barrier are limited and evidence for each is incomplete. The first, and one used by the most devastating viruses, is through direct infection of neurons within the periphery and effectively bypassing the BBB to infect neurons within the CNS. Examples include rabies virus and herpes viruses. Pulzova and co-workers suggested three further methods by which pathogens can cross the endothelial barrier (Pulzova et al., 2009). The first involves direct infection of endothelial cells although this appears to be rare for viruses that invade the CNS. Secondly crossing between cells, again this is likely to be rare in the absence of other factors that might lead to a breakdown of the BBB although it has been proposed for West Nile virus (Verma et al., 2009). Finally, entry may result following transit within an infected cell, the so-called Trojan horse mechanism suggested for infection with HIV. Once within the CNS, viruses can spread rapidly. The consequences of uncontrolled viral-induced damage and subsequent un-regulated inflammation within the CNS can have severe consequences to the host. The brain is enclosed within the skull and the tough dural membranes so that there can be no increase in brain-case volume. This could occur in response to increases in extracellular fluids or cellular content during inflammation with consequences for arterial influx and the possibility of ischaemia (Ransohoff et al., 2003). Furthermore, destruction of non-replaceable neurons can leave the patient with permanent disability, commonly observed following infections with Japanese encephalitis virus and West Nile virus, or death as happens following infection with rabies virus. Indeed, T cell infiltration has been associated with paralysis in experimental models of rabies virus infection (Sugamata et al., 1992).

Infection and cellular destruction triggers the innate immune response that attracts immune-effector cells with the aim of controlling virus replication. Viruses, in turn, possess mechanisms to inhibit the innate immune response, or in the case of herpesviruses are able to remain latent within infected neurons. This delays the host reponse providing a window for early rounds of virus replication. A further delay occurs through limited antigen presentation within the CNS. Early responders tend to be T cells and often appear to dominate the response when viewed at a single time-point (see Figure 4), whereas B-cells tend to enter later during the course of infection (Savarin and Bergmann, 2008). CD8 cells in particular have been shown in experimental models to be critical for clearance of some viral infections (Borrow et al., 1992) and control of others such as Herpes simplex infection (Lang and Nikolich-Zuglich, 2005). By contrast, antibody production within the CNS is considered critical to the control of rabies virus (Hooper et al., 2009).

The difficulty in identifying the aetiological agent of encephalitis presents a real challenge to treatment. Herpes simplex viruses are the most common viral cause of encephalitis and are readily treatable with nucleoside analogues such as acyclovir. However, resistance has been observed leading to the development of alternatives such as helicase inhibitors and TLR agonists (Grauer et al., 2008; Wilson et al., 2009). Nitric oxide inhibitors have been suggested as a possible therapy in HIV to inhibit BBB disruption during HIV encephalopathy (Giovannoni et al., 1998). Recently, the use of therapeutic coma has been promoted as a method for treating rabies virus infection, particularly following the survival of a teenager using this treatment (Willoughby et al., 2005). However, numerous attempts to replicate this have not met with success (Maier et al., 2010; Hunter et al., 2010). Effective prevention for rabies, as with many other virus infections is best achieved by prior vaccination. Future alternatives to treatment of viral encephalitis may focus on innate immune agonists that will assist in the early anti-viral response.

7. Acknowledgements

The authors would like to thank Dr Alejandro Nunez and Daniel Hicks for immunohistochemistry on West Nile and lyssavirus infected mouse brains. The authors were funded by Defra grant SE4107 and SE0530.

8. References

Allen, I.V., McQuaid, S., McMahon, J., Kirk, H. and McConnell, R. (1996). The significance of measles virus antigen and genome distribution in the CNS in SSPE for mechanisms of viral spread and demyelination. J. *Neuropathol. Exp. Neurol.* Vol 55, pp. 471-480.

Anthony, I.C., Crawford, D.H. and Bell, J.E. (2003). B lymphocytes in the normal brain: contrasts with HIV-associated lymphoid infiltrates and lymphomas. *Brain* Vol 126, pp. 1058-1067.

Avery, D.T., Kaled, S.L., Ellyard, J.I., et al. (2003). BAFF selectively enhances the survival of plasmablasts generated from human memory cells. *J. Clin. Invest.* 112, pp. 286-297.
Baggiolini, M. (1998). Chemokines and leukocyte traffic. *Nature* Vol 392, 565-568.
Bailey, S.L., Carpenier, P.A., McMahon, E.J., Begolka, A.S. and Miller, S. (2006). Innate and adaptive immune responses of the central nervous system. *Critical Reviews in Immunology* Vol 26, pp. 149-188.
Baranzini, S.E., Jeong, M.C., Butunoi, C., Murray, R.S., Bernard, C.C. and Oksenberg, J.R. (1999). B cell repertoire diversity and clonal expansion in multiple sclerosis brain lesions. *J. Immunol.* Vol 163, pp. 5133-5144.
Blakqori, G., Delhaye, S., Harbjan, M., Blair, C.D., Sanchez-Vargas, I., Olson, K.E., Attarzadeh-Yazdi, G., Fragkoudis, R., Kohl, A., Kalinke, U., Weiss, S., Michelis, T., Staeheli, P. and Weber, F. (2007). La Crosse bunyavirus non-structural protein NSs serves to suppress the type 1 interferon system of mammalian hosts. *J. Virol.* Vol 81, pp. 4991-4999.
Borrow, P., Tonks, P., Welsh, C.J. and Nash, A.A. (1992). The role of CD8+ T cells in the acute and chronic phases of Theiler's murine encephalomyelitis virus-induced disease in mice. *J. Gen. Virol.* Vol 73, pp. 1861-1865.
Brent, L. Immunologically privileged sites. In Pathophysiology of the Blood Brain Barrier, Eds BB Johansson, C Owmann, H Widner. Amsterdam: Elsevier, 1990: 383-402.
Brzozka, K., Finke, S. and Conzelmann, K.K. (2005). Identification of the rabies virus alpha/beta interferon antagonist: phosphoprotein P interferes with phosphorylation of interferon regulation factor 3. *J. Virol.* Vol 79, pp. 7673-7681.
Brzozka, K., Finke, S. and Conzelmann, K.K. (2006). Inhibition of interferon signalling by rabies virus phosphoprotein P: activation-dependent binding of STAT1 and STAT2. *J. Virol.* Vol 80, pp. 2675-2683.
Cairns, H.G.F. (1950). Intracerebral inoculation of mice: fate of the inoculum. *Nature,* Vol 166, pp.910-911.
Chelbi-Alix, M.K., Vidy, A., El Bougrini, J. and Blondel, D. (2006). Rabies viral mechanisms to escape IFN system: The viral protein P interferes with IRF-3, Stat1, and PML nuclear bodies. *J. Int. Cyt. Res.* Vol 26, pp 271-280.
Christensen, J.E., de Lemos, C., Moos, T., Christensen, J.P. and Thomsen, AR. (2006). CXCL10 is the key ligand for CXCR3 on CD8+ effector T cells involved in immune surveillance of the lymphocytic choriomeningitis virus-infected central nervous system. *J. Immunol.* Vol 176, pp. 4235-4243.
Constam , D.B., Philipp, J., Malipiero, U.V., ten Dijke, P., Schachner, M. and Fontana, A. (1992). Differential expression of transforming growth factor-beta 1, -beta 2, and -beta 3 by glioblastoma cells, astrocytes, and microglia. *J. Immunol.* Vol 148, pp. 1404-1410.
Cozine, C.L., Wolniak, K.L. and Waldschmidt, T.J. (2005). The primary germinal center response in mice. *Curr. Opin. Immunol.* Vol 17, pp. 298-302.
Creagh, E.M. and O'Neill, L.A. (2006). TLRs, NLRs and RLRs: a trinity of pathogen sensors that co-operate in innate immunity. *Trends Immunol.* Vol 27, pp. 352-357
Cserr, H.F. and Knopf, P.M. (1992). Cervical lymphatics, the blood-brain barrier and the immunoreactivity of the brain: a new view. *Immunology Today,* Vol 13, pp. 507-512.
Cummins, D., Bennett, D., Fisher-Hoch, S.P., Farrar, B., Machin, S.J. and McCormick, J.B. (1992). Lassa fever encephalopathy: clinical and laboratory findings. *J. Trop. Med. Hyg.* Vol 95, pp. 197-201
Cunningham, A.F., Gaspal, F., Serre, K., Mohr, E., Henderson, I.R., Scott-Tucker, A., Kenny, S.M., Khan, M., Toellner, K.M., Lane, P.J. and MacLennan, I.C. (2007). Salmonella

induces a switched antibody response without germinal centers that impedes the extracellular spread of infection. *J. Immunol.* Vol 178, pp. 6200-6207.

Delhaye, S., Paul, S., Blakqori, G., Minet, M., Weber, F., Staeheli, P. and Michiels, T. (2006). Neurons produce type 1 interferon during viral encephalitis. *Proceedings of the National Academy of Science, USA*, Vol 103, pp. 7835-7840.

Dietrich, J-B. (2002). The adhesion molecule ICAM-1 and its regulation in relation with the blood-brain barrier. *J. Neuroimmunol.* Vol 128, pp. 58-68.

Dionisio, D., Valassina, M., Ciufolini, M.G., Vivarelli, A., Esperti, F., Cusi, M.G., Marchi, A., Mazzoli, F. and Lupi, C. (2001). Encephalitis without meningitis due to sandfly fever virus serotype Toscana. *Clinical Infectious Diseases*, Vol 32, pp. 1241-1243.

Fischer, H.-G., and Reichmannm G. (2001). Brain dendritic cells and macrophages/microglia in central nervous system inflammation. *Journal of Immunology*, Vol 166, pp. 2717-2726.

Fooks, A.R., Brookes, S.M., Johnson, N., McElhinney, L.M. and Hutson, A.M. (2003). European bat lyssavirus: an emerging zoonosis. *Epidemiol. Infect.* Vol 131, pp. 1029-1039.

Giovannoni, G., Miller, R.F., Heales, S.J., Land, J.M., Harrison, M.J. and Thomson, EJ. (1998). Elevated cerebrospinal fluid and serum nitrate and nitrite levels in patients with central nervous system complications of HIV-1 infection: correlation with blood-brain-barrier dysfunction. *J. Neurol. Sci.* Vol 156, pp. 53-58

Gieber et al., (2005). Dendritic cells permit immune invasion of the CNS in an animal model of multiple sclerosis. *Nature Medicine*, Vol 11, pp.328-334.

Grauer, O.M., Molling, J.W., Bennick, E., Toonen, L.W.J., Sutmuller, R.P.M., Nierkens, S. and Adema, G.J. (2008). TLR ligands in the local treatment of established intracerebral murine gliomas. *J. Immunol.* Vol 181, pp. 6720-6729.

Gould, E.A. and Solomon, T. (2008). Pathogenic flaviviruses. *The Lancet*, Vol 371, pp.500-509.

Goldmann, J., Kwidzinski, E., Brandt, C., Mahlo, J., Richter, D. and Bechmann, I. (2006). T cells traffic from brain to cervical lymph nodes via the criboid plate and the nasal mucosa. *J. Leukoc. Biol.* Vol 80, pp. 797-801.

Granerod, J., Ambrones, H., Davies, N.W.S., Clewley, J.P., Walsh, A.L., Morgan, D., Cunningham, R., Zuckerman, M., Mutton, K.J., Solomon, T., Ward, K.N., Lunn, M.P.T., Irani, S.R., Vincent, A., Brown, D.W.G., Crowcroft, N.D.; UK Health Protection Agency (HPA) Aetiology of Encephalitis Study Group. (2010). Causes of encephalitis and differences in their clinical presentations in England: a multicentre, population-based prospective study. *Lancet Infectious Diseases*, Vol.10, pp. 835-844.

Granwehr, B.P., Lillibridge, K.M., Higgs, S., Mason, P.W., Aronson, J.F., Campbell, G.A. and Barrett, A.D.T. (2004). West Nile virus: where are we now? *Lancet Infectious Diseases*, Vol. 4, pp. 547-556.

Hart, D.N.J. and Fabre, J.W. (1981). Demonstration and characterisation of Ia-positive dendritic cells in the interstitial connective tissues of rat heart and other tissues, but no brain. *J. Exp. Med.* Vol 13, pp.347-361.

Hickey, W.F. (2001). Basic principles of immunological surveillance of the normal central nervous system. *Glia*, Vol 36, pp.118-124.

Hicks, D.J., Nunez, A., Healy, D.M., Brookes, S.M., Johnson, N. and Fooks, A.R. (2009). Comparative pathological study of the murine brain after experimental infection with classical rabies virus and European bat lyssaviruses. *J. Comp. Pathol.* Vol 140, pp. 113-126.

Hooper, D.C., Phares, T.W., Fabis, M.J. and Roy, A. (2009). The production of antibody by invading B cells is required for the clearance of rabies virus from the Central Nervous System. *PLoS Neglected Tropical Diseases* Vol 3, e535

Hunter, M., Johnson, N., Hedderwick, S., McCaughey, C., Lowry, K., McConville, J., Herron, B., McQuaid, S., Marston, D., Goddard, T., Harkess, G., Goharriz, H., Voller, K., Solomon, T., Willoughby, R.E. and Fooks, A.R. (2010). Immunological correlates in human rabies treated with therapeutic coma. *Journal of Medical Virology*, 82, 1255-1265

Huppatz, C., Gawarikar, Y., Levi, C., Kelly, P.M., Williams, D., Dalton, C., Massey, P., Givney, R. and Durrheim, D.N. (2010). Should there be a standardized approach to the diagnostic workup of suspected adult encephalitis? a case series in Australia. *BMC Infectious Diseases* Vol 10:353

Johnson, N., Mansfield, K.L., Hicks, D., Nunez, A., Healy, D.M., Brookes, S.M., McKimmie, C.S., Fazakerley, J.K. and Fooks, A.R. (2008). Inflammatory responses in the nervous system of mice infected with a street isolate of rabies virus. *Dev. Biol.* Vol 131, pp. 65-72.

Johnson, N., Vos, A., Freuling, C., Tordo, N., Fooks, A.R., and Muller, T. (2010). Human rabies de to lyssavirus infection of bat origin. *Veterinary Microbiology*, Vol 142, pp.151-159.

Kida, S., Weller, R.O., Zhang, E.-T., Phillips, M.J. and Iannotti, F. (1995). Anatomical pathways for lymphatic drainage of the brain andtheir pathological significance. *Neuropathology and Applied Neurobiology*, Vol 21, pp. 181-184.

Klein, R.S., Lin, E., Zhang, A.D., Tollett, J., Samuel, M.A., Engle, M. and Diamond, M.S. (2005). Neuronal CXCL10 direct CD8+ T-cell recruitment and control of West Nile virus encephalitis. *J. Virol.* Vol 79, pp. 11457-11466.

Kleinschmidt-DeMasters, BK. and Gilden, D.H. (2001). The expanding spectrum of herpesvirus infections of the nervous system. *Brain Pathol.* Vol 11, pp. 440-451

Knopf, P.M., Cserr, H.F., Nolan, S.C., Wu, Y-Y. and Harling-Berg, C.J. (1995). Physiology and immunology of lymphatic drainage of interstitial and cerebrospinal fluid from the brain. *Neuropathology and Applied Neurobiology*, Vol 21, pp.175-180.

Knopf, P.M., Harling-Berg, C.J., Cserr, H.F., Basu, D., Sirulnick, E.J., Nolan, S.C., Park, J.T., Keir, G., Thompson, E.J. and Hickey, S.F. (1998). Antigen-dependent intrathecal antibody synthesis in the normal rat brain: tissue entry and local retention of antigen-specific B cells. *J. Immunol.* Vol 161, pp. 692-701.

Krumbholz, M., Theil, D., Cepok, S., Hemmer, B., Kvisakk, P., Ransohoff, R.M., Hofbauer, M., Farina, C., Derfuss, T., Hartle, C., Newcombe, J., Hohlfeld, R. and Meinl, E. (2006). Chemokines in multiple sclerosis: CXCL12 and CXCL13 up-regulation is differentially linked to CNS immune cell recruitment. *Brain* Vol 129, pp. 200-211.

Lang, A. and Nikolich-Zugich, J. (2005). Development and migration of protective CD8+ T cells into the nervous system following ocular herpes simplex virus-1 infection. *J. Immunol.* 174, 2919-2925.

Lipton, S.A. and Gendelman, H.E. (1995). Seminars in medicine of the Beth Israel Hospital, Boston, Dementia associated with AIDS. New *England Journal of Medicine*, Vol 332, pp.934-940.

MacLennan, I.C.M., Toellner, K.M., Cunningham, A.F., Serre, K., Sze, D.M., Zuniga, E., Cook, M.C. and Vinuesa, C.G. (2003). Extrafollicular antibody responses. *Immunol. Rev.* Vol 198, pp. 8-18.

Maier, T., Schwarting, A., Mauer, D., Ross, R.S., Martens, A., Wahl, J., Panning, M., Baumgarte, S., Müller, T., Pfefferle, S., Ebel, H., Schmidt, J., Tenner-Racz, K., Racz,

P., Schmid, M., Strüber, M., Wolters, B., Gotthardt, D., Bitz, F., Frisch, L., Pfeiffer, N., Fickenscher, H., Sauer, P., Rupprecht, C.E., Roggendorf, M., Haverich, A., Galle, P., Hoyer, J. and Drosten, C. (2010). Management and outcomes after multiple corneal and solid organ transplants from a donor infected with rabies virus. *Clin. Infect. Dis.* Vol 50, pp. 1112-1119.

Man, S., Ubogu, E.E. and Ransohoff, R.M. (2007). Inflammatory cell migration into the central nervous system: A few new twists on an old tale. *Brain Pathology* Vol 17, pp243-250

Mansfield, K.L., Johnson, N., Stephenson, J.R., Fooks, A.R. and Solomon, T. (2009). Tick-borne encephalitis virus - a review of an emerging zoonosis. *Journal of General Virology*, Vol 90, pp. 1781-1794.

Mansfield, K.L., Johnson, N., Cosby, S.L., Solomon, T. and Fooks, A.R. (2010). Transcriptional upregulation of SOCS1 and suppressors of cytokine signalling 3 mRNA in the absence of suppressors of cytokine signalling 2 mRNA after infection with West Nile virus or tick-borne encephalitis virus. *Vector-borne and Zoonotic Diseases* Vol 7, pp. 649-653.

McKimmie, C.S., Johnson, N., Fooks, A.R. and Fazakerley, J.K. (2005). Viruses selectively upregulate Toll-like receptors in the central nervous system. *Biochemical and Biophysical Research Communications* Vol 336, pp. 925-933.

Meinl, E., Krumbholz, M. and Hohlfeld, R. (2006). B lineage cells in the inflammatory central nervous system environment: migration, maintenance, local antibody production and therapeutic modulation. *Ann. Neurol* Vol 59, pp. 880-892.

Mims, C.A. (1960). Intracerebral injections and the growth of viruses in the mouse brain. *British Journal of Experimental Pathology,* Vol 41, pp.52-59.

Nakamichi, K., Saiki, M., Sawada, M., Takayama—Ito, M., Yamamuro, Y., Morimoto, K. and Kurane, I. (2005). Rabies virus-induced activation of mitogen-activated protein kinase and NF-kappaB signalling pathways regulates expression of CXC and CC chemokine ligands in microglia. *J. Virol.* Vol 79, pp. 11801-11812.

Noah, D.L., Drenzek, C.L., Smith, J.S., Krebs, J.W., Orciari, L., Shaddock, J., Sanderlin, D., Whitfield, S., Fekadu, M., Olson, J.G., Rupprecht, C.E. and Childs, J.E. (1998). Epidemiology of human rabies in the United States, 1980 to 1996. *Annals of Internal Medicine,* Vol 128, pp. 922-930.

Prehaud, C., Megret, F., Lafage, M. and Lafon, M. (2005). Virus infection switches TLR-3-positive human neurons to become strong producers of beta interferon. *J. Virol.* Vol 79, pp. 12893-12904.

Pulzova, L., Bhide, M.R. and Andrej, K. (2009). Pathogen translocation across the blood-brain barrier. *FEMS Immunol. Med. Microbiol.* Vol 57, pp. 203-213.

Randall, R.E. and Goodbourn, S. (2008). Interferons and viruses: an interplay between induction, signalling, antiviral responses and virus countermeasures. *J. Gen. Virol.* Vol 89, pp. 1-47.

Ransohoff, R.M., Kivisakk, P. and Kidd, G. (2003). Three or more routes for leukocyte migration into the central nervous system. *Nature Reviews Immunology* Vol 3, pp. 569-581.

Rehwinkel, J. and Reis e Sousa, C. (2010). RIGorous detection: Exposing virus through RNA sensing. *Science* Vol 327, pp. 284-286.

Rock, R.B., Gekker, G., Hu, S., Sheng, W.S., Cheeran, M., Lokensgard, J.R. and Peterson, P.K. (2004). Role of microglia in central nervous system infections. *Clin. Microbiol. Rev.* Vol 17, 942-964.

Roy, A., Phares, T.W., Koprowski, H. and Hooper, D.C. (2007). Failure to open the blood-brain barrier and deliver immune effectors to central nervous system tissues leads to the lethal outcome of silver-haired bat rabies virus infection. *J. Virol.* Vol 81, pp. 1110-1118.

Rupprecht, C.E., Hanlon, C.A. and Hemachudha, T. (2002). Rabies re-examined. *Lancet Infect. Dis.* Vol 2, pp. 327-243.

Satterly, N., Tsai, P.L., van Deursen, J., Nussenzveig, D.R., Wang, Y., Faria, P.A., Levay, A., Levy, D.E. and Fontoura, B.M. (2007). Influenza virus targets the mRNA export machinery and the nuclear pore complex. *Proc. Natl. Acad. Sci. USA.* Vol 104, pp. 1853-1858.

Savarin, C. and Bergmann, C.C. (2008). Neuroimmunology of central nervous system viral infections: the cells, molecules and mechanisms involved. *Current Opinion in Pharmacology*, Vol 8, pp. 472-479.

Schneider, P. (2005). The role of APRIL and BAFF in lymphocyte activation. *Curr. Opin. Immunol.* 17, 282-289

Schnell, M.J., McGettigan, J.P., Wirblich, C. and Papaneri, A. (2010). The cell biology of rabies virus: using stealth to reach the brain. *Nat. Rev. Microbiol.* Vol 8, pp. 51-61.

Soilu-Hanninen, M., Eralinna, J.P., Hukkanen, V., Royatta, M., Salmi, A.A. and Salonen, R. (1994). Semliki Forest virus infects mouse brain endothelial cells and causes blood-brain barrier damage. *J. Virol.* Vol 68, pp. 6291-6298.

Seyler, T., Rizzo, C., Finarelli, A.C., Po, C., Alessio, P., Sambri, V., Ciofi Degli Atti, M.L. and Salmaso, S. (2008). Autochthonous chikungunya virus transmission may have occurred in Bologna, Italy, during the summer of 2007. *Euro surveill.*, Vol 13, pii=8015

Sheahan, B.J., Moore, M. and Atkins, G.J. (2002). The pathogenicity of louping ill virus for mice and lambs. *Journal of Comparative Pathology*, Vol 126, pp. 137-146

Stevenson, P.G., Hawke, S., Sloan, D.J. and Bangham, C.R.M. (1997). The immunogenicity of intracerebral virus infection depends on anatomical site. *Journal of Virology*, Vol 71, pp. 145-151.

Stiles, L.N., Hosking, M.P., Edwards, R.A., Steiter, R.M. and Lane, T.E. (2006). Differential roles for CXCR3 in CD4+ and CD8+ T cell trafficking following viral infection of the CNS. *Eur. J. Immunol.* Vol 36, pp. 613-622.

Sugamata, M., Miyazawa, M., Mori, S., Spangrude, G.J., Ewalt, L.C. and Lodmell, D.L. (1992). Paralysis of street rabies virus-infected mice is dependent on T lymphocytes. *J. Virol.* Vol 66, pp. 1252-1260.

Tebit, D.M. and Arts, E.J. (2011). Tracking a century of global expansion and evolution of HIV to drive understanding and to combat disease. *Lancet Infect. Dis.* Vol. 11, pp. 45-56.

Tschen, S-I., Bergmann, C.C., Ramakrishna, C., Morales, S., Atkinson, R. and Stolhman, S.A. (2002). Recruitment kinetics and composition of antibody-secreting cells within the central nervous system following viral encephalomyelitis. *J. Immunol.* Vol 168, pp. 2922-2929

Tulsiani, S.M., Graham, G.C., Moore, P.R., Jansen, C.C., Van Den Hurk, A.F., Moore, F.A., Simmons, R.J. and Craig, S.B. (2011). Emerging tropical diseases in Australia. Part 5. Hendra virus. *Annals of Tropical Medicine and Parasitology*, Vol 105, pp. 1-11.

Tyler, K.L. (2009a). Emerging viral infections of the Central Nervous System. Part 1. *Archives of Neurology*, Vol 66, pp. 939-948.

Tyler, K.L. (2009b). Emerging viral infections of the Central Nervous System: Part 2. *Archives of Neurology*, Vol 66, pp. 1065-1074.

Venter, M., Myers, T.G., Wilson, M.A., Kindt, T.J., Paweska, J.T., Burt, F.J., Leman, P.A. and Swanepoel, R. (2005). Gene expression in mice infected with West Nile virus strains of different neurovirulence. *Virology* Vol 342, pp. 119-140.

Verma, S., Lo, Y., Chapagain, M., Lum, S., Kumar, M., Gurjav, U., Luo, H., Nakatsuka, A. and Nerurkar, V.R. (2009). West Nile virus infection modulates human brain microvascular endothelial cells tight junction proteins and cell adhesion molecules: Transmigration across the in vitro blood-brain barrier. *Virology*. Vol 385, pp. 425-433.

Vidy, A., El Bourgrini, Chelbi-Alix, M.X. and Blondel, D. (2007). The nucleocytoplasmic rabies virus P protein counteracts interferon signalling by inhibiting both nuclear accumulation and DNA binding of STAT1. *J. Virol.* Vol 81, pp. 4255-4263.

Wang, Z.W., Sarmento, L., Wang, Y., Li, X.Q., Dhingra, V., Tseggai, T., Jiang, B. and Fu, Z.F. (2005). Attenuated rabies virus activates, while pathogenic rabies virus evades, the host innate immune responses in the central nervous system. *J. Virol.* Vol 79, pp. 12554-12565.

Whitley, R.J. and Gnann, J.W. (2002). Viral encephalitis: familiar infections and emerging pathogens. *The Lancet*, Vol 359, pp.507-514.

Willoughby, R.E., Tieves, K.S., Hoffman, G.M., Ghanayem, N.S., Amlie-Lefond, C.M., Schwabe, M.J., Chusid, M.J. and Rupprecht, C.E. (2010). Survival after treatment of rabies with induction of coma. *N. Engl. J. Med.* Vol 352, pp. 2508-2514.

Wilson, S.S., Fakioglu, E. and Herold, B.C. (2009). Novel approaches in fighting herpes simplex virus infections. *Expert Rev. Anti. Infect. Ther.* Vol 7, pp. 559-568.

Wong, K.T., Sheih, W.J., Kumar, S., Norain, K., Abdullah, W., Guarner, J., Goldsmith, C.S., Chua, K.B., Lam, S.K., Tan, C.T., Goh, K.J., Chong, H.T., Jusoh, R., Rollin, P.E., Ksiazek, T.G., Zaki, S.R.; Nipah Virus Pathology Working Group. (2002). Nipah virus infection: pathology and pathogenesis of an emerging paramyxoviral zoonosis. *American Journal of Pathology*, Vol 161, pp.2153-2167.

Yamada, S., DePasquale, M., Patlak, C.S. and Cserr, H.F. (1991). Albumin outflow into deep cervical lymph from different regions of rabbit brain. *American Journal of Physiology*, Vol 126, pp. H1197-1204.

Yoshimura, A., Naka, T. and Kubo, M. (2007). SOCS proteins, cytokine signalling and immune regulation. *Nat. Rev. Immunol.* Vol 7, pp. 454-465.

Zacks, M.A. and Paessler, S. (2010). Encephalitic alphaviruses. *Veterinary Microbiology*, Vol 140, pp.281-286.

Zhang, B., Chan, Y.K., Lu, B., Diamond, M.S. and Klein, R.S. (2008). CXCR3 mediates region-specific antiviral T cell trafficking within the central nervous system during West Nile virus encephalitis. *J. Immunol.* Vol 180, pp. 2641-2649.

Zhu, T., Korber, B.T., Nahmias, A.J., Hooper, E., Sharp, P.M. and Ho, D.D. (1998). An African HIV-1 sequence from 1959 and implications for the origin of the epidemic. *Nature*, Vol 391, pp. 594-597.

8

Chemokines and Viral Infections of the CNS

Douglas M. Durrant and Robyn S. Klein
Washington University in St. Louis
USA

1. Introduction

A critical factor in the host immune response to invading pathogens, such as viral infections, is the recruitment and infiltration of immune cells to infected tissues. Although the goal of the recruited leukocytes is to eliminate the invading pathogens, collateral tissue damage may be induced in the process, and, in certain circumstances, may pose a serious threat to the survival of the host. The central nervous system (CNS) is a unique site with limited regenerative potential and therefore a low threshold for inflammation-induced tissue damage. However, as the CNS may become the target of life-threatening viral infections, it is imperative that immunological surveillance and efficient effector responses occur in this organ to aid in pathogen clearance. Although traditionally characterized as a site of "immune privilege," evidence suggests that immune surveillance and antiviral immunity does occur in the CNS (Carson *et al.*, 2006). Understanding how the local inflammatory response within the CNS is regulated is a key to understanding the pathogenesis of viral infections in the CNS and developing therapies that promote protective and limit pathogenic responses.

Leukocyte recruitment to any organ site is generally a complex, multistep process. Under normal conditions, leukocyte migration into the CNS is maintained at low levels (Hickey, 2001). During virus-induced inflammation, however, the extravasation of leukocytes is increased and targeted to specific compartments of the CNS depending on the inflammatory stimulus and the infected region. Chemokines and chemokine receptors have been identified as pivotal players in regulating immune cell trafficking into the CNS. Chemokines consist of a large family of small, structurally related, chemotactic cytokines that are involved in regulating the normal lymphocytic traffic to both the lymphoid and nonlymphoid organs and leukocyte emigration into sites of injury and infection (Rossi & Zlotnik, 2000). Chemokines select leukocytes for tissue entry based on their expression of chemokine receptors, G-protein-coupled cell surface receptors, which have a characteristic seven transmembrane structure (Premack & Schall, 1996). In addition to targeting distinct leukocyte populations during inflammation, chemokines and their receptors have emerged as crucial mediators of a variety of biological processes including development and tissue homeostasis. With regard to virus-induced inflammation in the CNS, chemokines and chemokine receptors are in a strategic position to coordinate immune responses through both the regulation of leukocyte extravasation and also in the final positioning and activation of infiltrating cells.

Immune surveillance of the CNS and the effector function of infiltrating leukocytes into the CNS dictate the host-pathogen relationship during viral pathogenesis of the CNS. The challenge of viral pathogenesis research in the CNS has been to define how immune cells traffic in and out of the CNS to recognize foreign antigen and their effect on the biology of the CNS. In this chapter, clinically relevant viral infections of the CNS that cause meningitis or encephalitis in humans and the murine models used to study these infections will be discussed as well as the current understanding of the role of chemokines and chemokine receptors in host protection and/or in neuropathology. Because many viral infections of the CNS are rare and without animal models, we have chosen to discuss those for which chemokine studies exist and have shed light on important aspects of antiviral and immunopathologic responses. A clearer understanding of how chemokines and chemokine receptors impact the inflammatory response to viral infections within the CNS will lead to the identity of targets that can potentially be manipulated for either host defense or recovery.

2. Flaviviruses

2.1 WNV

Viruses of the family *Flaviviridae* consist of approximately 70 members, of which four, West Nile virus (WNV), St. Louis encephalitis virus (SLE), Japanese encephalitis virus (JEV) and Murray Valley encephalitis virus (MVE) comprise the neurotropic Japanese encephalitis (JE) serogroup (Mukhopadhyay *et al.*, 2005). These viruses are primarily spread through arthropod vectors. For instance, West Nile Virus (WNV) is a neurotropic virus that exists in nature as a zoonosis and is transmitted by the *Culex* mosquito to humans and other vertebrates (Hayes & Gubler, 2006). Most humans infected with WNV are asymptomatic, yet approximately 20% may develop a minor flu-like illness, known as West Nile Fever (Mostashari *et al.*, 2001). Less than 1% of these patients develop severe neurological complications, such as encephalitis, that may potentially be lethal (Petersen & Roehrig, 2001). Increased age and defects in cell-mediated immunity are risk factors for developing WNV neuroinvasive disease (Campbell *et al.*, 2002; Murray *et al.*, 2008), which provides clues to mechanisms of viral clearance within the CNS.

A mouse model of WNV has contributed to the understanding of the pathogenesis of WNV encephalitis. Typically, mice are infected intra-dermally with WNV where it is taken up by Langerhans dendritic cells and brought to draining lymph nodes where replication results in primary viremia (Johnston *et al.*, 2000). The virus continues to replicate in the spleen, kidney, and epithelial tissues before it enters the CNS (Chung *et al.*, 2007). After entering the CNS, through both retrograde axonal transport and hematogenous dissemination (Samuel & Diamond, 2005; Hunsperger & Roehrig, 2006), WNV typically infects the brain stem, hippocampal, and spinal cord neurons (Eldadah & Nathanson, 1967; Omalu *et al.*, 2003; Shrestha *et al.*, 2003; Fratkin *et al.*, 2004). Following infection of the CNS, $CD4^+$ and $CD8^+$ T cells, as well as NK cells and infiltrating monocytes/macrophages accumulate in the CNS and localize primarily in the vicinity of WNV-infected neurons. To clear virus from infected brain tissues, T cells, particularly virus-specific $CD8^+$ T cells, monocytes, macrophages and $\gamma\delta$ T cells as well as key cytokines, IFN-γ and TNF-α, are necessary and aid in the immune response during WNV infection of the brain. The murine model of WNV encephalitis exploits age-related differences in virologic control. While eight week-old mice exhibit 50-70% survival due to both peripheral and CNS control of viral replication, five week-old animals exhibit only a 10-20% survival rate due to inadequate virologic control within the CNS (Diamond *et al.*, 2003).

2.2 Role of chemokines in WNV-induced encephalitis

The recruitment of effector cells into the infected regions of the CNS is crucial for host defense against WNV and successful viral clearance within this compartment. Increased expression of inflammatory chemokines and their receptors (including CCR1, CCR2, CCR5, CXCR3 and CX3CR1) have been detected in the WNV-infected brain of 8 week-old mice (Glass *et al.*, 2005). One of the first chemokine receptors identified to have a clear functional role in the mouse model of WNV is CCR5. WNV infection of mice with targeted deletion of CCR5 results in a fatal outcome due to the loss of virologic control in the CNS. In addition, loss of CCR5 was associated with reduced infiltration of $CD4^+$ and $CD8^+$ T cells, NK cells and macrophages in the CNS of WNV-infected mice (Glass *et al.*, 2005). Thus, CCR5-depedent influx of leukocytes into the virally infected CNS is fundamental to viral clearance and recovery from WNV encephalitis.

One of the most highly expressed chemokines in the CNS in response to WNV infection is CXCL10, which is known to recruit NK and activated T cells (Muller *et al.*, 2010). CXCL10 is expressed relatively early in the course of neuroinvasion of WNV, primarily because WNV-infected neurons are the source of this chemokine (Klein *et al.*, 2005). In the mouse, CXCL10 expression exhibits a caudal-to-rostral pattern of expression, first found within Purkinje and granule cell neurons of the cerebellum and then detected within neurons of the hippocampus, frontal cortex and olfactory bulb. In mice with targeted deletion of CXCL10, the ability to control viral replication within the CNS is lost and mortality is enhanced (Klein *et al.*, 2005). The receptor for CXCL10, CXCR3, is also strongly upregulated by WNV in the mouse model and CXCR3 knockout mice demonstrate a similar increased susceptibility to the virus (Zhang *et al.*, 2008). The loss of the ability of neurons to express CXCL10 or the loss of CXCR3 resulted in decreased leukocyte trafficking, specifically $CD4^+$ and $CD8^+$ T cells, particularly within the cerebellum. Thus, WNV differentially induces CXCL10 within the brain, which results in the recruitment of effector T cells via the chemokine receptor CXCR3. These studies demonstrate the ability of resident cells of the CNS to generate antiviral immune responses in a region-specific manner.

Of interest, CXCL10 has also been shown to induce apoptosis of CXCR3-expressing neurons (Sui *et al.*, 2006). During WNV, elevated levels of CXCL10, however, promote lymphocyte entry and do not appear to simultaneously enhance neuronal death (Zhang *et al.*, 2010). Using in vivo and in vitro systems, it was determined that WNV-infected neurons also express TNF-α, which leads to down-regulation of CXCR3 mRNA levels and loss of surface expression of CXCR3 on neurons. Neuronal loss of CXCR3 in the context of WNV-infection promoted bystander survival of uninfected neurons, suggesting an adaptive mechanism to prevent CXCL10-mediated neuronal damage in the face of viral infections that require the entry of antiviral lymphocytes.

Monocytes also play an important role during CNS injury and infection as precursors to macrophages and microglial cells (Getts *et al.*, 2008). The accumulation of monocytes in the CNS occurred following a lethal intranasal inoculation with a non-neurotropic strain of WNV. Following treatment with an anti-CCL2 antibody, infiltration of these cells was delayed and survival was prolonged, suggesting a CCR2-dependent, pathogenic role for monocytes in the brain in this model (Getts *et al.*, 2008). In contrast, monocyte depletion in mice challenged intraperitoneally with a neurotropic strain of WNV resulted in increased mortality (Ben-Nathan *et al.*, 1996), suggesting a protective role for these cells. The ligands for CCR2, CCL2 and CCL7, are induced following WNV infection in the CNS (Glass *et al.*, 2005; Lim *et al.*, 2010) and in mice with targeted deletion of CCR2, increased mortality and increased viral burden occurs (Lim *et al.,* 2010). Monocytosis occurs following WNV infection in WT mice and peaks just before monocytes begin to traffic into the brain (Lim & Murphy, 2011). This appears to be dependent on CCR2 since the numbers of recruited $CD4^+$ and $CD8^+$ T cells and NK cells in the brain of CCR2 knockout mice following WNV infection are similar to wild-type mice, whereas, the accumulation of inflammatory monocytes in the CNS is severely deficient. Thus, monocytes may be beneficial or harmful depending on the infection model.

Studies of WNV infection in five week-old WT mice, which exhibit a 10-20% survival rate, indicated that impaired viral clearance and survival may be partially due to lack of migration of antiviral $CD8^+$ T cells into the CNS parenchyma. Normally, infiltrating T cells are retained in perivascular spaces through the interaction of CXCR4 with its ligand CXCL12, which is found along abluminal surfaces of the entire CNS vasculature (McCandless *et al.,* 2006; McCandless *et al.,* 2008). Following WNV infection in eight week-old mice, CXCL12 levels decline by day two post-infection, allowing egress of antiviral T cells (Durrant, unpublished data). In contrast, five week-old mice do not exhibit down-regulation of CXCL12 until eight days post-infection, which is associated with perivascular accumulation of CXCR4-expressing T cells and increasing numbers of WNV-infected neurons. These data suggest that developmental changes in regulation of CXCL12 expression at the blood-brain barrier may contribute to antiviral immune responses. In support of a critical role for CXCL12 in limiting egress of virus-specific $CD8^+$ T cells, administration of the specific CXCR4 antagonist, AMD3100, was associated with increased migration of effector T cells into the CNS and enhanced viral clearance (McCandless *et al.,* 2008). CXCR4 antagonism was also associated with a rapid decrease in immune cell trafficking as virologic control ensued, suggesting that an early increase in virus-specific immune cell trafficking that controls viral infection ultimately leads to a rapid dampening of inflammation that would otherwise have pathologic consequences.

Taken altogether, these studies support a role for chemokines in the final positioning of effector cells that dictates outcome of immune responses in response to viral invasion within the CNS. Since resolution of CNS infection is often a balance between immune-mediated pathogen clearance and the deleterious effects of inflammation, studies utilizing the murine WNV encephalitis model suggest that if the appropriate cells reach critical regions at the appropriate time, virologic control may be accomplished and less severe disease occur.

2.3 CCR5 in human WNV disease

Studies of patients that carry a 32 base-pair deletion within the coding sequence of CCR5 (*CCR5Δ32*) indicate that human CCR5 is important in WNV pathogenesis. A genotype-phenotype association study of patients carrying *CCR5Δ32*, who lack functional CCR5, suggested that WNV-infected *CCR5Δ32* homozygous individuals exhibit higher incidences of symptomatic infection. Ultimately, CCR5 deficiency resulted in 100% susceptibility to severe symptomatic disease (Glass *et al.,* 2006). This genetic deficiency supports the observations in the WNV mouse model that functional CCR5 is critical for viral control and disease progression.

2.4 JEV

Japanese encephalitis virus (JEV) is a mosquito borne pathogen that occurs throughout most of Asia. JEV causes infection of the CNS with a high mortality rate (Parida *et al.,* 2006).

Clinical manifestation of JEV include fever, headache, vomiting, altered consciousness, and severe meningo-encephalitis (Kumar *et al.*, 1990). Children appear to be at greatest risk of infection in endemic areas for unknown reasons. Following entry into the host, JEV generates a rapid inflammatory response, which results in infiltration of neutrophils into the CNS. JEV is highly neurotropic, infecting neuronal rather than non-neuronal tissues in humans (Vaughn & Hoke, 1992) with neuronal precursors as the major target cells for infection (Kimura-Kuroda *et al.*, 1993). The course of disease for JEV in humans is faithfully replicated in murine models. Following extraneural inoculation with JEV, young mice are highly susceptible to neuroinvasion and rapidly die soon after virus is detected within the CNS (Johnson *et al.*, 1985; Hase *et al.*, 1990). Thus, viral titers of JEV in the brain generally peak at five days post-infection with death occurring between five and six days post-infection.

2.5 Chemokines and JEV-associated encephalitis

Expression of the chemokines CXCL10 and CXCL1 is upregulated in neuroblastoma cells infected with JEV (Gupta *et al.*, 2010). In a JEV-infected mouse model, similar chemokines were significantly upregulated including CXCL9, CXCL10 and CXCL12 (Gupta *et al.*, 2010). In addition to the robust expression of proinflammatory chemokines there was also increased numbers of infiltrating inflammatory cells into the brain at day five post-infection. Similar to WNV, JEV-infected neurons were found to be the source of CXCL10. CCL5 was also detected in JEV-infected neuroblastoma cells, indicating a possible role for this chemokine in the early stages of infection. Interestingly, neuronal death and mortality rate increases in patients with elevated levels of proinflammatory cytokines and chemokines, including CCL5, in the serum and cerebrospinal fluid (Winter *et al.*, 2004). Whether this is simply correlative data or whether these chemokines actually contribute to pathogenesis is currently unknown. An improved understanding of the proinflammatory effects responsible for immune-mediated control of viral infection and neuronal injury during JEV infections is essential to determine the viral pathogenesis of JEV in the CNS.

2.6 TBEV

Tickborne encephalitis virus (TBEV) is an additional member of the *Flaviviridae* family that causes Tickborne encephalitis (TBE), a severe infection of the CNS. TBEV is usually transmitted to patients by infected *Ixodes ricinus* ticks (Gunther & Haglund, 2005). Infection with TBEV is characterized by a biphasic clinical course with early nonspecific influenza-like symptoms and subsequent development of neurological symptoms or meningoencephalitis (Haglund & Gunther, 2003; Holzmann, 2003). In most fatal cases, TBEV can be found in the brain tissue (Gelpi *et al.*, 2005). An animal model for TBEV has not been established to date.
The pro-inflammatory cytokines CCL2, CCL5, CXCL10 and CXCL11 have been detected in the CSF of TBE patients (Grygorczuk *et al.*, 2006; Lepej *et al.*, 2006; Michalowska-Wender *et al.*, 2006). Although these chemokines exhibit known anti-viral roles in WNV encephalitis, their specific role in TBE is yet to be fully determined. One significant study, however, demonstrated an association between carriage of the *CCR5Δ32* allele and TBE (Kindberg *et al.*, 2008). Similar to WNV, an association between severe TBE and *CCR5Δ32* homozygosity was observed. Therefore, loss of CCR5 function in humans is a risk factor for TBE in patients exposed to TBEV. Increased expression of CCL5 in the CSF of patients with TBE suggests it may indeed play a role in leukocyte trafficking within TBEV-infected patients. Thus, CCR5

may be essential for limiting viral replication within the CNS through effective antiviral immune responses that shorten the course and limit the lethality of encephalitis.

3. HSV

Herpes simplex virus (HSV) types 1 and 2 establish latent infection in dorsal root ganglia for the entire life of the host. From this reservoir they can reactivate to cause human morbidity and mortality. HSV-1 is the causative agent of encephalitis and several disorders of the peripheral nervous system. HSV-2 is responsible for meningitis in neonates and in adults (Steiner *et al.*, 2007). HSV encephalitis is considered the most frequent cause of sporadic encephalitis in North America (Whitley, 1981). In a murine model of HSV-1 infection, the intracranial inoculation of a neurotropic HSV-1 strain causes encephalitis and death by day six after infection (Vilela *et al.*, 2008). In a murine model of HSV-2 infection, intraperitoneal inoculation with a neurovirulent HSV-2 strain causes meningoencephalitis (Kristensson *et al.*, 1978) and death occurs 10-14 days after infection. Pathology of HSV-2 infection has been shown to be T-cell mediated, due specifically to the actions of Th2 cells (Ikemoto *et al.*, 1995).

3.1 Chemokines and HSV

Following intracranial inoculation of HSV-1, early chemokine expression is dominated by CCL2, CCL3, CCL5, CXCL9 and CXCL10 (Wickham *et al.*, 2005; Carr *et al.*, 2006). CCL2, in particular, exhibits an important role in the early immune response to CNS infection with HSV-1 as monocyte recruitment to the CNS is significantly diminished in mice with targeted deletion of CCL2, thus hindering viral clearance (Kodukula *et al.*, 1999). CXCR3-deficient mice similarly exhibit elevated CNS viral titers of HSV-1, but only on day seven post-infection. Interestingly, survival was enhanced in CXCR3-deficient mice compared with wild-type mice following HSV-1 infection (Wickham *et al.*, 2005), suggesting a more complex role for CXCR3. Coinciding with increased viral titer, protein levels of CCL5, CXCL9, CXCL10 and IFN-γ were increased in the CNS as well as $CD8^+$ lymphocytes, suggesting a role for this receptor in antiviral adaptive immunity. In the absence of CXCR3, a transient increase in viral burden facilitates an elevated protective immune response.

In HSV-1-infected, CCR5-deficient mice, viral load was decreased in the CNS but associated with greater neuropathology and increased lethality (Teixeira *et al.*, 2010). Following infection, CCR5-deficient mice exhibited increased chemokine levels, including CCL5 and CCL2; enhanced expression of cytokines, such as TNF-α; and a significant increase in leukocyte migration into the brain (Teixeira *et al.*, 2010). Thus, in the absence of CCR5, greater control of viral replication was achieved, but at the cost of enhanced neuropathology and ultimately death. Generally, CCR5 deficiency would lead to decreased leukocyte infiltration; therefore, these results are surprising and may be unique to HSV-1 encephalitis. Treatment with anti-CCL5 antibodies or with small molecule antagonists of CCR1 and CCR5, both CCL5 receptors, had no effect on viral titers but led to significant reduction of the number of leukocytes infiltrating into the brain (Vilela *et al.*, 2009). Therefore, blocking CCR1 and CCR5 did not affect HSV-1 replication, suggesting that other immune mechanisms are involved in the process of viral control.

CCL2 has been identified as an initiator of Th2 responses and has a pathogenic role in the development of disease in HSV-2-infected mice (Karpus *et al.*, 1997; Hogaboam *et al.*, 1998). In the absence of CCL2 the severity of disease decreased dramatically, and the amount of Th2 cytokine production also decreased (Nakajima *et al.*, 2001). It appears that a population of macrophages in mouse CSF is the primary producers of CCL2, which are postulated to increase severity of disease through induction of Th2 responses. Of note, CCL2 has been detected in the CSF from patients with herpes simplex encephalitis and has been correlated with clinical severity of herpes simplex encephalitis (Rosler *et al.*, 1998).

4. LCMV

Lymphocytic choriomeningitis virus (LCMV) is spread by the common house mouse and can cause aseptic meningitis in children and adults, neurological dysfunction in newborns and may induce spontaneous abortion in pregnant women (Enders *et al.*, 1999). Infection with LCMV can present with two separate clinical phases. Symptoms of the first phase include fever, malaise, headache and nausea, which resolve after several days and are then followed by the second phase of illness, which is characterized by symptoms of meningitis (Bonthius, 2009) with an abundant number of lymphocytes within the CSF (Chesney *et al.*, 1979). Although recovery from CNS disease is common, severe neurological disease as well as death, although rare, may occur. Congenital infection with LCMV is often fatal for the fetus or newborn (Biggar *et al.*, 1975). Survivors of congenital LCMV infection usually experience severe visual and cognitive impairment (Barton *et al.*, 1995). LCMV infection of the brain parenchyma may extend specifically to neuronal precursor cells, especially in prenatal or neonatal infections (Bonthius *et al.*, 2007).

LCMV is essentially a noncytolytic virus (Hotchin & Weigand, 1961) and in murine models of LCMV-induced meningoencephalitis (LCM), intracranial infection of LCMV into healthy adult mice results in fatal meningitis between seven and ten days after viral infection (Cole *et al.*, 1972; Allan *et al.*, 1987). Symptoms of disease are accompanied by a massive infiltration of mononuclear cells into the meninges, choroid plexus, CSF, and ependymal membranes (Doherty & Zinkernagel, 1974; Buchmeier *et al.*, 1980; Ceredig *et al.*, 1987; Doherty *et al.*, 1990). $CD8^+$ T cells and macrophages dominate the cellular infiltrate (Allan *et al.*, 1987; Ceredig *et al.*, 1987), whereas $CD4^+$ T cells and polymorphonuclear leukocytes are present in limited numbers (Ceredig *et al.*, 1987; Dixon *et al.*, 1987; Christensen *et al.*, 1995). It appears that the T cell response is a critical component for LCM because lethal meningitis does not occur in immunodeficient (irradiated or T-cell-depleted) mice following intracranial infection (Doherty *et al.*, 1974; Christoffersen *et al.*, 1976). Moreover, in the absence of $CD8^+$ T cells, mice will invariably survive intracranial LCMV infection (Christoffersen *et al.*, 1976; Leist *et al.*, 1987), suggesting that virus-specific $CD8^+$ cytotoxic T lymphocytes mediate fatal tissue damage (Buchmeier *et al.*, 1980; Doherty *et al.*, 1990). The role of virus-specific $CD8^+$ T cells during lethal LCM appears to be dependent on the strain of virus. Mice infected with the Armstrong strain of LCMV leads to killing of virus-infected cells in the meninges via a perforin-dependent mechanism (Kagi *et al.*, 1994), which leads to increased immunopathology. Whereas, mice infected with the Traub strain of LCMV exhibit lymphocytic infiltration of the neuroparenchyma rather than meningeal inflammation, which leads to a more fatal outcome (Christensen *et al.*, 2004). Overall, pathogenesis and death may be directly related to the influx of virus-specific T cells into critical regions of the CNS.

4.1 Chemokines and Lymphocytic choriomeningitis

During the mouse model of LCMV infection, expression of the T cell chemoattractants CCL2, CCL4, CCL5 and CCL7 as well as CXCL9, CXCL10 and CXCL11 is detected in the virus-infected tissues, as well as in the meninges, as early as day three post-infection

(Asensio & Campbell, 1997; Nansen *et al.*, 2000; Nansen *et al.*, 2002; Lindow *et al.*, 2003). On days six to seven post-infection, expression of these chemokines is significantly increased and accompanied by increased expression of granulocyte chemoattractants including XCL1 and CXCL2, CXCL6, CXCL16, and CCL3 (Asensio & Campbell, 1997; Nansen *et al.*, 2000). The main chemokine-producing cell types are resident cells of the CNS, particularly the meninges and choroid plexus together with astrocytes (Loetscher *et al.*, 2001). This surge of chemokine activity coincides with immune cell infiltration into the infected tissue. An analysis of chemokine receptor expression revealed local expression of receptors for these chemokines including CCR1, CCR2 and CCR5 as well as CXCR3 around day six to seven post-infection. (Nansen *et al.*, 2000; Lindow *et al.*, 2003). The analyses of cells from the inflammatory exudate of LCMV-infected mice indicate that T cells express CCR2, CCR5, and CXCR3, whereas macrophages are the predominant cell type expressing CCR1 (Nansen *et al.*, 2000; Lindow *et al.*, 2003; Christensen *et al.*, 2004). Thus, the elevated expression of these chemokines and chemokine receptors is likely to result in T lymphocytic and macrophage infiltration to the inflammatory site.

The chemokines CXCL9, CXCL10 and CXCL11 are the three known ligands for the receptor CXCR3 (Loetscher *et al.*, 2001). CXCL10 is rapidly upregulated in the virus-infected CNS (Asensio *et al.*, 1999; Nansen *et al.*, 2000), which results in the recruitment of $CXCR3^+$ cells into critical regions of the CNS. CXCL9 and CXCL11 are also expressed, but their role appears to be redundant (Christensen *et al.*, 2006). The majority of cells found to be expressing CXCR3 were activated IFN-γ-producing $CD8^+$ T cells (Homann *et al.*, 2001; Christensen *et al.*, 2004). A strong positive feedback loop is established through the local production of IFN-γ, which brings about further, marked upregulation of CXCL10 expression and therefore continued recruitment of $CXCR3^+$ effector cells. This robust recruitment positions CXCL10 as a key mediator of severe LCMV-induced CNS disease. In the absence of CXCL10, approximately half of LCMV (Traub) intracranially infected mice are protected from a lethal viral dose (Christensen *et al.*, 2006). CXCL10-deficient mice show no impairment of effector T cell generation or of immune cell infiltration, except for reduced $CD8^+$ T cell accumulation in parenchymal regions such as the corpus callosum (Christensen *et al.*, 2006). On the other hand, CXCL10 appears to be dispensable for the development of fatal neuroinflammation following infection with LCMV (Armstrong) (Hofer *et al.*, 2008). This highlights that there are underlying differences in viral strains and chemokine utilization with regards to disease outcome.

The chemokine receptor CXCR3 is upregulated in LCMV-infected CNS (Lindow *et al.*, 2003), and is predominately expressed on activated $CD8^+$ T cells (Christensen *et al.*, 2004). During intracranial infection with LCMV (Traub), CXCR3 deficiency leads to partial protection from immunopathology and death (Christensen *et al.*, 2004). In immunocompetent mice infected with LCMV (Traub), $CD8^+$ T cells preferentially traffic to the leptomeninges and choroid plexus and are also found in some parenchymal regions, such as the corpus callosum (Christensen *et al.*, 2004). However, in the absence of CXCR3, trafficking of these cells to specific regions was significantly delayed (Christensen *et al.*, 2004). This suggests that during LCMV infection, the expression of certain chemokines is necessary to target effector cells into infected CNS regions. However, this targeting, while important for viral control, may cause neuropathology. In addition, it is apparent that not only the recruitment of effector cells but the over-accumulation of the cells in infected regions of the CNS through the establishment of a CXCL10-mediated positive feedback loop may lead to immunopathology in these critical regions.

In addition to CXCR3, other chemokine receptors may also contribute to effector T cell recruitment, since in the absence of CXCR3 only partial protection is achieved. The expression of CCR1, CCR2, and CCR5, has also been associated with meningeal inflammation (Nansen *et al.*, 2000). A subpopulation of activated $CD8^+$ T cells expresses high levels of CCR2 and CCR5 (Andersson *et al.*, 1995). Yet, when CCR5 expression is absent there is no impairment of the LCMV-induced inflammation (Nansen *et al.*, 2002), supporting the notion that other chemokine receptors contribute to T cell recruitment. Overall, in addition to CXCR3, virus-activated $CD8^+$ T cells were found to express CCR2 and CCR5, whereas activated macrophages expressed CCR1 (Nansen *et al.*, 2000).

LCM is essentially the result of anti-viral effector T cells unable to control rapid replication of LCMV in the brain. Following viral infection, a highly potent T cell response is induced. There is a rapid and robust infiltration of effector T cells into the meninges of the CNS, which leads to increased local expression of IFN-γ, which leads to increased chemokine production and amplification of effector T cell infiltration. Lack of effective viral clearance contributes to persistent chemokine expression, which promotes excessive inflammation within the meninges and eventually the brain parenchyma, leading to a fatal outcome.

4.2 CXCL10/CXCR3 in human LCMV infection

One characteristic of LCMV infection in immunocompetent adults and children is the abundance of lymphocytes in the CSF (Bonthius, 2009). $CD8^+$ T cells are thought to infiltrate into the CSF to primarily clear the virus, which subsequently leads to the symptoms of aseptic meningitis during LCMV infection (Buchmeier & Lane, 1999). A predominant chemokine found in the CSF of patients with viral meningoencephalitis is CXCL10 (Lahrtz *et al.*, 1997). CXCL10 and its receptor CXCR3 have integral roles in the development of neuropathology in the mouse model of LCMV infection and may also have similar roles in the LCMV-infected CNS of certain patients. The infiltration of effector T cells into the CSF, CXCL10 expression and the resulting neuropathy are reminiscent of the mouse model, however the host factors that contribute to disease severity and, in some cases, lethality are not currently understood. Overall, chemokines appear to be important in viral control but, as seen with murine models of LCMV, also contribute to neuropathology.

5. HIV

Human immunodeficiency virus-1 (HIV) targets $CD4^+$ cells and macrophages. Infection of the CNS by HIV-1 occurs in about 80% of infected individuals. HIV-1 arrives in the CNS via infected macrophages that cross the blood-brain barrier. Neurological symptoms include meningitis, encephalitis, neuropathies, and HIV-1-associated dementia (HAD), with cognitive, motor, and behavioral dysfunctions (Marcotte *et al.*, 2003). Chemokine involvement in HIV-1 neuropathogenesis is well recognized because of their roles in the recruitment of HIV-1 infected immune cells, inflammatory responses, and as ligands for the HIV-1 coreceptors, CXCR4 and CCR5, which are expressed by neurons and directly mediate neurotoxicity and cell death (Hesselgesser *et al.*, 1998; Klein *et al.*, 1999; Hosking & Lane, 2010).

Chemokines that recruit monocytes/macrophages and lymphocytes into the brain, such as CCL2, have been detected in the CSF of individuals with HIV-1 infection (Kolb *et al.*, 1999). CCL2 levels are significantly increased during HIV-1-induced encephalitis (HIVE) and the chemokine accumulates in the CSF and brains of patients with HAD and HIVE, as well as in macaques with Simian immunodeficiency virus (SIV)-induced encephalitis (SIVE) (Mankowski *et al.*, 2004; Monteiro de Almeida *et al.*, 2005; Monteiro de Almeida *et al.*, 2006). The expression of CCL2 in the CNS is associated with enhanced progression of HIV encephalitis, due to its ability to recruit monocytes and lymphocytes (Dhillon *et al.*, 2008). In addition to CCL2, CXCL10 also can attract inflammatory cells and has been detected in the CSF of HIV-1-infected patients (Kolb *et al.*, 1999). CXCL10 is chronically expressed within the brains of patients suffering from HIV-associated neurological disorders (Christo *et al.*, 2009). In addition, HIV-1 envelope glycoprotein gp120 can induce CXCL10 gene expression in astrocytes independent of IFN-γ (Asensio *et al.*, 2001). The encephalitic brain from SIV-infected animals exhibits elevated immunohistochemical expression of CCL3, CCL4, CCL5, CCL7 and CXCL10 (Sasseville *et al.*, 1996), suggesting a role for one or multiple chemokines in the pathogenesis of acquired immune deficiency syndrome encephalitis. Elevated levels of CCL7, another ligand for CCR2, are also detected within activated astrocytes in the brains of SIV-infected macaques, and are increased further in response to TNF-α, which thus initiates neuroinvasion by SIV/HIV-infected monocytes (Renner *et al.*, 2011). The prevention of monocyte infiltration into the brains of HIV-infected patients is therefore a critical step in limiting the ability of the CNS to act as a viral reservoir.

Chemokines may also act as neuromodulators within the HIV-infected CNS. The HIV glycoprotein gp120 may induce neuronal death via excitotoxicity during activation of CXCR4 receptors (Ohagen *et al.*, 1999; Chen *et al.*, 2002) and the CXCR4 ligand, CXCL12 may be converted into a neurotoxic agent via proteolytic cleavage with the resulting peptide capable of inducing neurotoxicity and apoptosis through engagement of the chemokine receptor CXCR3 (Vergote *et al.*, 2006). Thus, in addition to attracting inflammatory cells that contribute to neuropathology, CXCL10 can also synergize with CXCL12 cleavage products to induce neuronal cell death (van Marle *et al.*, 2004).

6. Concluding remarks

An effective anti-viral immune response is vital to maintain a balance between pathogen control and immunopathology during viral infection resolution within the CNS. While chemokines may contribute to viral clearance through focused amplification of inflammatory responses, they may also contribute to immune-mediated damage that depends on the type of virus and affected CNS compartment or region. However, targeting chemokines to abrogate all CNS infiltration may lead to untoward effects on immunosurveillance, as evidenced by the recent increase in opportunistic CNS viral infection with JC virus in patients treated with the anti-α4-integrin monoclonal antibody, natalizumab. Natalizumab treats multiple sclerosis, a chronic, inflammatory demyelinating disease, by preventing leukocyte entry at CNS endothelial barriers (Kleinschmidt-DeMasters & Tyler, 2005). A side effect of this treatment is the occurrence of progressive multifocal leukoencephalopathy (PML), a fatal opportunistic viral infection of the CNS caused by the reactivation of latent JC virus infection (Havrdova *et al.*, 2009). Thus, blockade of immune cell trafficking into the CNS interferes with essential components of immune surveillance that prevent opportunistic infections. PML underscores how vital immune cell trafficking in the CNS is for monitoring and regulating immune responses.

In summary, chemokines are integrally involved in recruiting targeted leukocyte populations to critical regions of the CNS that contribute both to host defense and the pathogenesis of disease. It is clear that these proinflammatory molecules exert nonredundant roles in contributing to neuroinflammation following viral infection of the CNS thus meriting further studies on chemokines with regards to viral-induced disease. Finally, it is clear that chemokines and their receptors may represent viable targets in modulating the severity of human neuroinflammatory diseases.

7. References

Allan, J.E., Dixon, J.E. & Doherty, P.C. (1987) Nature of the inflammatory process in the central nervous system of mice infected with lymphocytic choriomeningitis virus. *Curr Top Microbiol Immunol*, 134, 131-143.

Andersson, E.C., Christensen, J.P., Scheynius, A., Marker, O. & Thomsen, A.R. (1995) Lymphocytic choriomeningitis virus infection is associated with long-standing perturbation of LFA-1 expression on CD8+ T cells. *Scand J Immunol*, 42, 110-118.

Asensio, V.C. & Campbell, I.L. (1997) Chemokine gene expression in the brains of mice with lymphocytic choriomeningitis. *J Virol*, 71, 7832-7840.

Asensio, V.C., Kincaid, C. & Campbell, I.L. (1999) Chemokines and the inflammatory response to viral infection in the central nervous system with a focus on lymphocytic choriomeningitis virus. *J Neurovirol*, 5, 65-75.

Asensio, V.C., Maier, J., Milner, R., Boztug, K., Kincaid, C., Moulard, M., Phillipson, C., Lindsley, K., Krucker, T., Fox, H.S. & Campbell, I.L. (2001) Interferon-independent, human immunodeficiency virus type 1 gp120-mediated induction of CXCL10/IP-10 gene expression by astrocytes in vivo and in vitro. *J Virol*, 75, 7067-7077.

Barton, L.L., Peters, C.J. & Ksiazek, T.G. (1995) Lymphocytic choriomeningitis virus: an unrecognized teratogenic pathogen. *Emerg Infect Dis*, 1, 152-153.

Ben-Nathan, D., Huitinga, I., Lustig, S., van Rooijen, N. & Kobiler, D. (1996) West Nile virus neuroinvasion and encephalitis induced by macrophage depletion in mice. *Arch Virol*, 141, 459-469.

Biggar, R.J., Woodall, J.P., Walter, P.D. & Haughie, G.E. (1975) Lymphocytic choriomeningitis outbreak associated with pet hamsters. Fifty-seven cases from New York State. *Jama*, 232, 494-500.

Bonthius, D.J. (2009) Lymphocytic choriomeningitis virus: a prenatal and postnatal threat. *Adv Pediatr*, 56, 75-86.

Bonthius, D.J., Nichols, B., Harb, H., Mahoney, J. & Karacay, B. (2007) Lymphocytic choriomeningitis virus infection of the developing brain: critical role of host age. *Ann Neurol*, 62, 356-374.

Buchmeier, M.J. & Lane, T.E. (1999) Viral-induced neurodegenerative disease. *Curr Opin Microbiol*, 2, 398-402.

Buchmeier, M.J., Welsh, R.M., Dutko, F.J. & Oldstone, M.B. (1980) The virology and immunobiology of lymphocytic choriomeningitis virus infection. *Adv Immunol*, 30, 275-331.

Campbell, G.L., Marfin, A.A., Lanciotti, R.S. & Gubler, D.J. (2002) West Nile virus. *Lancet Infect Dis*, 2, 519-529.

Carr, D.J., Ash, J., Lane, T.E. & Kuziel, W.A. (2006) Abnormal immune response of CCR5-deficient mice to ocular infection with herpes simplex virus type 1. *J Gen Virol*, 87, 489-499.

Carson, M.J., Doose, J.M., Melchior, B., Schmid, C.D. & Ploix, C.C. (2006) CNS immune privilege: hiding in plain sight. *Immunol Rev*, 213, 48-65.

Ceredig, R., Allan, J.E., Tabi, Z., Lynch, F. & Doherty, P.C. (1987) Phenotypic analysis of the inflammatory exudate in murine lymphocytic choriomeningitis. *J Exp Med*, 165, 1539-1551.

Chen, W., Sulcove, J., Frank, I., Jaffer, S., Ozdener, H. & Kolson, D.L. (2002) Development of a human neuronal cell model for human immunodeficiency virus (HIV)-infected macrophage-induced neurotoxicity: apoptosis induced by HIV type 1 primary isolates and evidence for involvement of the Bcl-2/Bcl-xL-sensitive intrinsic apoptosis pathway. *J Virol*, 76, 9407-9419.

Chesney, P.J., Katcher, M.L., Nelson, D.B. & Horowitz, S.D. (1979) CSF eosinophilia and chronic lymphocytic choriomeningitis virus meningitis. *J Pediatr*, 94, 750-752.

Christensen, J.E., de Lemos, C., Moos, T., Christensen, J.P. & Thomsen, A.R. (2006) CXCL10 is the key ligand for CXCR3 on CD8+ effector T cells involved in immune surveillance of the lymphocytic choriomeningitis virus-infected central nervous system. *J Immunol*, 176, 4235-4243.

Christensen, J.E., Nansen, A., Moos, T., Lu, B., Gerard, C., Christensen, J.P. & Thomsen, A.R. (2004) Efficient T-cell surveillance of the CNS requires expression of the CXC chemokine receptor 3. *J Neurosci*, 24, 4849-4858.

Christensen, J.P., Andersson, E.C., Scheynius, A., Marker, O. & Thomsen, A.R. (1995) Alpha 4 integrin directs virus-activated CD8+ T cells to sites of infection. *J Immunol*, 154, 5293-5301.

Christo, P.P., Vilela Mde, C., Bretas, T.L., Domingues, R.B., Greco, D.B., Livramento, J.A. & Teixeira, A.L. (2009) Cerebrospinal fluid levels of chemokines in HIV infected patients with and without opportunistic infection of the central nervous system. *J Neurol Sci*, 287, 79-83.

Christoffersen, P.J., Volkert, M. & Rygaard, J. (1976) Immunological unresponsiveness of nude mice to LCM virus infection. *Acta Pathol Microbiol Scand C*, 84C, 520-523.

Chung, K.M., Thompson, B.S., Fremont, D.H. & Diamond, M.S. (2007) Antibody recognition of cell surface-associated NS1 triggers Fc-gamma receptor-mediated phagocytosis and clearance of West Nile Virus-infected cells. *J Virol*, 81, 9551-9555.

Cole, G.A., Nathanson, N. & Prendergast, R.A. (1972) Requirement for theta-bearing cells in lymphocytic choriomeningitis virus-induced central nervous system disease. *Nature*, 238, 335-337.

Dhillon, N.K., Williams, R., Callen, S., Zien, C., Narayan, O. & Buch, S. (2008) Roles of MCP-1 in development of HIV-dementia. *Front Biosci*, 13, 3913-3918.

Diamond, M.S., Shrestha, B., Mehlhop, E., Sitati, E. & Engle, M. (2003) Innate and adaptive immune responses determine protection against disseminated infection by West Nile encephalitis virus. *Viral Immunol*, 16, 259-278.

Dixon, J.E., Allan, J.E. & Doherty, P.C. (1987) The acute inflammatory process in murine lymphocytic choriomeningitis is dependent on Lyt-2+ immune T cells. *Cell Immunol*, 107, 8-14.

Doherty, P.C., Allan, J.E., Lynch, F. & Ceredig, R. (1990) Dissection of an inflammatory process induced by CD8+ T cells. *Immunol Today*, 11, 55-59.

Doherty, P.C. & Zinkernagel, R.M. (1974) T-cell-mediated immunopathology in viral infections. *Transplant Rev*, 19, 89-120.

Doherty, P.C., Zinkernagel, R.M. & Ramshaw, I.A. (1974) Specificity and development of cytotoxic thymus-derived lymphocytes in lymphocytic choriomeningitis. *J Immunol*, 112, 1548-1552.

Eldadah, A.H. & Nathanson, N. (1967) Pathogenesis of West Nile Virus encepahlitis in mice and rats. II. Virus multiplication, evolution of immunofluorescence, and development of histological lesions in the brain. *Am J Epidemiol*, 86, 776-790.

Enders, G., Varho-Gobel, M., Lohler, J., Terletskaia-Ladwig, E. & Eggers, M. (1999) Congenital lymphocytic choriomeningitis virus infection: an underdiagnosed disease. *Pediatr Infect Dis J*, 18, 652-655.

Fratkin, J.D., Leis, A.A., Stokic, D.S., Slavinski, S.A. & Geiss, R.W. (2004) Spinal cord neuropathology in human West Nile virus infection. *Arch Pathol Lab Med*, 128, 533-537.

Gelpi, E., Preusser, M., Garzuly, F., Holzmann, H., Heinz, F.X. & Budka, H. (2005) Visualization of Central European tick-borne encephalitis infection in fatal human cases. *J Neuropathol Exp Neurol*, 64, 506-512.

Getts, D.R., Terry, R.L., Getts, M.T., Muller, M., Rana, S., Shrestha, B., Radford, J., Van Rooijen, N., Campbell, I.L. & King, N.J. (2008) Ly6c+ "inflammatory monocytes" are microglial precursors recruited in a pathogenic manner in West Nile virus encephalitis. *J Exp Med*, 205, 2319-2337.

Glass, W.G., Lim, J.K., Cholera, R., Pletnev, A.G., Gao, J.L. & Murphy, P.M. (2005) Chemokine receptor CCR5 promotes leukocyte trafficking to the brain and survival in West Nile virus infection. *J Exp Med*, 202, 1087-1098.

Glass, W.G., McDermott, D.H., Lim, J.K., Lekhong, S., Yu, S.F., Frank, W.A., Pape, J., Cheshier, R.C. & Murphy, P.M. (2006) CCR5 deficiency increases risk of symptomatic West Nile virus infection. *J Exp Med*, 203, 35-40.

Grygorczuk, S., Zajkowska, J., Swierzbinska, R., Pancewicz, S., Kondrusik, M. & Hermanowska-Szpakowicz, T. (2006) [Concentration of the beta-chemokine CCL5 (RANTES) in cerebrospinal fluid in patients with tick-borne encephalitis]. *Neurol Neurochir Pol*, 40, 106-111.

Gunther, G. & Haglund, M. (2005) Tick-borne encephalopathies : epidemiology, diagnosis, treatment and prevention. *CNS Drugs*, 19, 1009-1032.

Gupta, N., Santhosh, S.R., Babu, J.P., Parida, M.M. & Rao, P.V. (2010) Chemokine profiling of Japanese encephalitis virus-infected mouse neuroblastoma cells by microarray and real-time RT-PCR: implication in neuropathogenesis. *Virus Res*, 147, 107-112.

Haglund, M. & Gunther, G. (2003) Tick-borne encephalitis--pathogenesis, clinical course and long-term follow-up. *Vaccine*, 21 Suppl 1, S11-18.

Hase, T., Dubois, D.R. & Summers, P.L. (1990) Comparative study of mouse brains infected with Japanese encephalitis virus by intracerebral or intraperitoneal inoculation. *Int J Exp Pathol*, 71, 857-869.

Havrdova, E., Galetta, S., Hutchinson, M., Stefoski, D., Bates, D., Polman, C.H., O'Connor, P.W., Giovannoni, G., Phillips, J.T., Lublin, F.D., Pace, A., Kim, R. & Hyde, R. (2009) Effect of natalizumab on clinical and radiological disease activity in multiple sclerosis: a retrospective analysis of the Natalizumab Safety and Efficacy in Relapsing-Remitting Multiple Sclerosis (AFFIRM) study. *Lancet Neurol*, 8, 254-260.

Hayes, E.B. & Gubler, D.J. (2006) West Nile virus: epidemiology and clinical features of an emerging epidemic in the United States. *Annu Rev Med*, 57, 181-194.

Hesselgesser, J., Liang, M., Hoxie, J., Greenberg, M., Brass, L.F., Orsini, M.J., Taub, D. & Horuk, R. (1998) Identification and characterization of the CXCR4 chemokine receptor in human T cell lines: ligand binding, biological activity, and HIV-1 infectivity. *J Immunol*, 160, 877-883.

Hickey, W.F. (2001) Basic principles of immunological surveillance of the normal central nervous system. *Glia*, 36, 118-124.

Hofer, M.J., Carter, S.L., Muller, M. & Campbell, I.L. (2008) Unaltered neurological disease and mortality in CXCR3-deficient mice infected intracranially with lymphocytic choriomeningitis virus-Armstrong. *Viral Immunol*, 21, 425-433.

Hogaboam, C.M., Lukacs, N.W., Chensue, S.W., Strieter, R.M. & Kunkel, S.L. (1998) Monocyte chemoattractant protein-1 synthesis by murine lung fibroblasts modulates CD4+ T cell activation. *J Immunol*, 160, 4606-4614.

Holzmann, H. (2003) Diagnosis of tick-borne encephalitis. *Vaccine*, 21 Suppl 1, S36-40.

Homann, D., Teyton, L. & Oldstone, M.B. (2001) Differential regulation of antiviral T-cell immunity results in stable CD8+ but declining CD4+ T-cell memory. *Nat Med*, 7, 913-919.

Hosking, M.P. & Lane, T.E. (2010) The role of chemokines during viral infection of the CNS. *PLoS Pathog*, 6, e1000937.

Hotchin, J. & Weigand, H. (1961) Studies of lymphocytic choriomeningitis in mice. I. The relationship between age at inoculation and outcome of infection. *J Immunol*, 86, 392-400.

Hunsperger, E.A. & Roehrig, J.T. (2006) Temporal analyses of the neuropathogenesis of a West Nile virus infection in mice. *J Neurovirol*, 12, 129-139.

Ikemoto, K., Pollard, R.B., Fukumoto, T., Morimatsu, M. & Suzuki, F. (1995) Small amounts of exogenous IL-4 increase the severity of encephalitis induced in mice by the intranasal infection of herpes simplex virus type 1. *J Immunol*, 155, 1326-1333.

Johnson, R.T., Burke, D.S., Elwell, M., Leake, C.J., Nisalak, A., Hoke, C.H. & Lorsomrudee, W. (1985) Japanese encephalitis: immunocytochemical studies of viral antigen and inflammatory cells in fatal cases. *Ann Neurol*, 18, 567-573.

Johnston, L.J., Halliday, G.M. & King, N.J. (2000) Langerhans cells migrate to local lymph nodes following cutaneous infection with an arbovirus. *J Invest Dermatol*, 114, 560-568.

Kagi, D., Vignaux, F., Ledermann, B., Burki, K., Depraetere, V., Nagata, S., Hengartner, H. & Golstein, P. (1994) Fas and perforin pathways as major mechanisms of T cell-mediated cytotoxicity. *Science*, 265, 528-530.

Karpus, W.J., Lukacs, N.W., Kennedy, K.J., Smith, W.S., Hurst, S.D. & Barrett, T.A. (1997) Differential CC chemokine-induced enhancement of T helper cell cytokine production. *J Immunol*, 158, 4129-4136.

Kimura-Kuroda, J., Ichikawa, M., Ogata, A., Nagashima, K. & Yasui, K. (1993) Specific tropism of Japanese encephalitis virus for developing neurons in primary rat brain culture. *Arch Virol*, 130, 477-484.

Kinberg, E., Mickiene, A., Ax, C., Akerlind, B., Vene, S., Lindquist, L., Lundkvist, A. & Svensson, L. (2008) A deletion in the chemokine receptor 5 (CCR5) gene is associated with tickborne encephalitis. *J Infect Dis*, 197, 266-269.

Klein, R.S., Lin, E., Zhang, B., Luster, A.D., Tollett, J., Samuel, M.A., Engle, M. & Diamond, M.S. (2005) Neuronal CXCL10 directs CD8+ T-cell recruitment and control of West Nile virus encephalitis. *J Virol*, 79, 11457-11466.

Klein, R.S., Williams, K.C., Alvarez-Hernandez, X., Westmoreland, S., Force, T., Lackner, A.A. & Luster, A.D. (1999) Chemokine receptor expression and signaling in macaque and human fetal neurons and astrocytes: implications for the neuropathogenesis of AIDS. *J Immunol*, 163, 1636-1646.

Kleinschmidt-DeMasters, B.K. & Tyler, K.L. (2005) Progressive multifocal leukoencephalopathy complicating treatment with natalizumab and interferon beta-1a for multiple sclerosis. *N Engl J Med*, 353, 369-374.

Kodukula, P., Liu, T., Rooijen, N.V., Jager, M.J. & Hendricks, R.L. (1999) Macrophage control of herpes simplex virus type 1 replication in the peripheral nervous system. *J Immunol*, 162, 2895-2905.

Kolb, S.A., Sporer, B., Lahrtz, F., Koedel, U., Pfister, H.W. & Fontana, A. (1999) Identification of a T cell chemotactic factor in the cerebrospinal fluid of HIV-1-infected individuals as interferon-gamma inducible protein 10. *J Neuroimmunol*, 93, 172-181.

Kristensson, K., Vahlne, A., Persson, L.A. & Lycke, E. (1978) Neural spread of herpes simplex virus types 1 and 2 in mice after corneal or subcutaneous (footpad) inoculation. *J Neurol Sci*, 35, 331-340.

Kumar, R., Mathur, A., Kumar, A., Sethi, G.D., Sharma, S. & Chaturvedi, U.C. (1990) Virological investigations of acute encephalopathy in India. *Arch Dis Child*, 65, 1227-1230.

Lahrtz, F., Piali, L., Nadal, D., Pfister, H.W., Spanaus, K.S., Baggiolini, M. & Fontana, A. (1997) Chemotactic activity on mononuclear cells in the cerebrospinal fluid of patients with viral meningitis is mediated by interferon-gamma inducible protein-10 and monocyte chemotactic protein-1. *Eur J Immunol*, 27, 2484-2489.

Leist, T.P., Cobbold, S.P., Waldmann, H., Aguet, M. & Zinkernagel, R.M. (1987) Functional analysis of T lymphocyte subsets in antiviral host defense. *J Immunol*, 138, 2278-2281.

Lepej, S.Z., Begovac, J. & Vince, A. (2006) Changes in T-cell subpopulations during four years of suppression of HIV-1 replication in patients with advanced disease. *FEMS Immunol Med Microbiol*, 46, 351-359.

Lim, J.K., McDermott, D.H., Lisco, A., Foster, G.A., Krysztof, D., Follmann, D., Stramer, S.L. & Murphy, P.M. (2010) CCR5 deficiency is a risk factor for early clinical manifestations of West Nile virus infection but not for viral transmission. *J Infect Dis*, 201, 178-185.

Lim, J.K. & Murphy, P.M. (2011) Chemokine control of West Nile virus infection. *Exp Cell Res*, 317, 569-574.

Lindow, M., Nansen, A., Bartholdy, C., Stryhn, A., Hansen, N.J., Boesen, T.P., Wells, T.N., Schwartz, T.W. & Thomsen, A.R. (2003) The virus-encoded chemokine vMIP-II inhibits virus-induced Tc1-driven inflammation. *J Virol*, 77, 7393-7400.

Loetscher, P., Pellegrino, A., Gong, J.H., Mattioli, I., Loetscher, M., Bardi, G., Baggiolini, M. & Clark-Lewis, I. (2001) The ligands of CXC chemokine receptor 3, I-TAC, Mig, and IP10, are natural antagonists for CCR3. *J Biol Chem*, 276, 2986-2991.

Mankowski, J.L., Queen, S.E., Clements, J.E. & Zink, M.C. (2004) Cerebrospinal fluid markers that predict SIV CNS disease. *J Neuroimmunol*, 157, 66-70.

Marcotte, T.D., Deutsch, R., McCutchan, J.A., Moore, D.J., Letendre, S., Ellis, R.J., Wallace, M.R., Heaton, R.K. & Grant, I. (2003) Prediction of incident neurocognitive impairment by plasma HIV RNA and CD4 levels early after HIV seroconversion. *Arch Neurol*, 60, 1406-1412.

McCandless, E.E., Wang, Q., Woerner, B.M., Harper, J.M. & Klein, R.S. (2006) CXCL12 limits inflammation by localizing mononuclear infiltrates to the perivascular space during experimental autoimmune encephalomyelitis. *J Immunol*, 177, 8053-8064.

McCandless, E.E., Zhang, B., Diamond, M.S. & Klein, R.S. (2008) CXCR4 antagonism increases T cell trafficking in the central nervous system and improves survival from West Nile virus encephalitis. *Proc Natl Acad Sci U S A*, 105, 11270-11275.

Michalowska-Wender, G., Losy, J., Kondrusik, M., Zajkowska, J., Pancewicz, S., Grygorczuk, S. & Wender, M. (2006) [Evaluation of soluble platelet cell adhesion molecule sPECAM-1 and chemokine MCP-1 (CCL2) concentration in CSF of patients with tick-borne encephalitis]. *Pol Merkur Lekarski*, 20, 46-48.

Monteiro de Almeida, S., Letendre, S., Zimmerman, J., Kolakowski, S., Lazzaretto, D., McCutchan, J.A. & Ellis, R. (2006) Relationship of CSF leukocytosis to compartmentalized changes in MCP-1/CCL2 in the CSF of HIV-infected patients undergoing interruption of antiretroviral therapy. *J Neuroimmunol*, 179, 180-185.

Monteiro de Almeida, S., Letendre, S., Zimmerman, J., Lazzaretto, D., McCutchan, A. & Ellis, R. (2005) Dynamics of monocyte chemoattractant protein type one (MCP-1) and HIV viral load in human cerebrospinal fluid and plasma. *J Neuroimmunol*, 169, 144-152.

Mostashari, F., Bunning, M.L., Kitsutani, P.T., Singer, D.A., Nash, D., Cooper, M.J., Katz, N., Liljebjelke, K.A., Biggerstaff, B.J., Fine, A.D., Layton, M.C., Mullin, S.M., Johnson, A.J., Martin, D.A., Hayes, E.B. & Campbell, G.L. (2001) Epidemic West Nile encephalitis, New York, 1999: results of a household-based seroepidemiological survey. *Lancet*, 358, 261-264.

Mukhopadhyay, S., Kuhn, R.J. & Rossmann, M.G. (2005) A structural perspective of the flavivirus life cycle. *Nat Rev Microbiol*, 3, 13-22.

Muller, M., Carter, S., Hofer, M.J. & Campbell, I.L. (2010) Review: The chemokine receptor CXCR3 and its ligands CXCL9, CXCL10 and CXCL11 in neuroimmunity--a tale of conflict and conundrum. *Neuropathol Appl Neurobiol*, 36, 368-387.

Murray, K.O., Baraniuk, S., Resnick, M., Arafat, R., Kilborn, C., Shallenberger, R., York, T.L., Martinez, D., Malkoff, M., Elgawley, N., McNeely, W. & Khuwaja, S.A. (2008) Clinical investigation of hospitalized human cases of West Nile virus infection in Houston, Texas, 2002-2004. *Vector Borne Zoonotic Dis*, 8, 167-174.

Nakajima, H., Kobayashi, M., Pollard, R.B. & Suzuki, F. (2001) Monocyte chemoattractant protein-1 enhances HSV-induced encephalomyelitis by stimulating Th2 responses. *J Leukoc Biol*, 70, 374-380.

Nansen, A., Christensen, J.P., Andreasen, S.O., Bartholdy, C., Christensen, J.E. & Thomsen, A.R. (2002) The role of CC chemokine receptor 5 in antiviral immunity. *Blood*, 99, 1237-1245.

Nansen, A., Marker, O., Bartholdy, C. & Thomsen, A.R. (2000) CCR2+ and CCR5+ CD8+ T cells increase during viral infection and migrate to sites of infection. *Eur J Immunol*, 30, 1797-1806.

Ohagen, A., Ghosh, S., He, J., Huang, K., Chen, Y., Yuan, M., Osathanondh, R., Gartner, S., Shi, B., Shaw, G. & Gabuzda, D. (1999) Apoptosis induced by infection of primary brain cultures with diverse human immunodeficiency virus type 1 isolates: evidence for a role of the envelope. *J Virol*, 73, 897-906.

Omalu, B.I., Shakir, A.A., Wang, G., Lipkin, W.I. & Wiley, C.A. (2003) Fatal fulminant pan-meningo-polioencephalitis due to West Nile virus. *Brain Pathol*, 13, 465-472.

Parida, M., Dash, P.K., Tripathi, N.K., Ambuj, Sannarangaiah, S., Saxena, P., Agarwal, S., Sahni, A.K., Singh, S.P., Rathi, A.K., Bhargava, R., Abhyankar, A., Verma, S.K., Rao, P.V. & Sekhar, K. (2006) Japanese Encephalitis Outbreak, India, 2005. *Emerg Infect Dis*, 12, 1427-1430.

Petersen, L.R. & Roehrig, J.T. (2001) West Nile virus: a reemerging global pathogen. *Emerg Infect Dis*, 7, 611-614.

Premack, B.A. & Schall, T.J. (1996) Chemokine receptors: gateways to inflammation and infection. *Nat Med*, 2, 1174-1178.

Renner, N.A., Ivey, N.S., Redmann, R.K., Lackner, A.A. & Maclean, A.G. (2011) MCP-3/CCL7 production by astrocytes: implications for SIV neuroinvasion and AIDS encephalitis. *J Neurovirol*.

Rosler, A., Pohl, M., Braune, H.J., Oertel, W.H., Gemsa, D. & Sprenger, H. (1998) Time course of chemokines in the cerebrospinal fluid and serum during herpes simplex type 1 encephalitis. *J Neurol Sci*, 157, 82-89.

Rossi, D. & Zlotnik, A. (2000) The biology of chemokines and their receptors. *Annu Rev Immunol*, 18, 217-242.

Samuel, M.A. & Diamond, M.S. (2005) Alpha/beta interferon protects against lethal West Nile virus infection by restricting cellular tropism and enhancing neuronal survival. *J Virol*, 79, 13350-13361.

Sasseville, V.G., Smith, M.M., Mackay, C.R., Pauley, D.R., Mansfield, K.G., Ringler, D.J. & Lackner, A.A. (1996) Chemokine expression in simian immunodeficiency virus-induced AIDS encephalitis. *Am J Pathol*, 149, 1459-1467.

Shrestha, B., Gottlieb, D. & Diamond, M.S. (2003) Infection and injury of neurons by West Nile encephalitis virus. *J Virol*, 77, 13203-13213.

Steiner, I., Kennedy, P.G. & Pachner, A.R. (2007) The neurotropic herpes viruses: herpes simplex and varicella-zoster. *Lancet Neurol*, 6, 1015-1028.

Sui, Y., Stehno-Bittel, L., Li, S., Loganathan, R., Dhillon, N.K., Pinson, D., Nath, A., Kolson, D., Narayan, O. & Buch, S. (2006) CXCL10-induced cell death in neurons: role of calcium dysregulation. *Eur J Neurosci*, 23, 957-964.

Teixeira, M.M., Vilela, M.C., Soriani, F.M., Rodrigues, D.H. & Teixeira, A.L. (2010) Using intravital microscopy to study the role of chemokines during infection and inflammation in the central nervous system. *J Neuroimmunol*, 224, 62-65.

van Marle, G., Henry, S., Todoruk, T., Sullivan, A., Silva, C., Rourke, S.B., Holden, J., McArthur, J.C., Gill, M.J. & Power, C. (2004) Human immunodeficiency virus type 1 Nef protein mediates neural cell death: a neurotoxic role for IP-10. *Virology*, 329, 302-318.

Vaughn, D.W. & Hoke, C.H., Jr. (1992) The epidemiology of Japanese encephalitis: prospects for prevention. *Epidemiol Rev*, 14, 197-221.

Vergote, D., Butler, G.S., Ooms, M., Cox, J.H., Silva, C., Hollenberg, M.D., Jhamandas, J.H., Overall, C.M. & Power, C. (2006) Proteolytic processing of SDF-1alpha reveals a change in receptor specificity mediating HIV-associated neurodegeneration. *Proc Natl Acad Sci U S A*, 103, 19182-19187.

Vilela, M.C., Mansur, D.S., Lacerda-Queiroz, N., Rodrigues, D.H., Arantes, R.M., Kroon, E.G., Campos, M.A., Teixeira, M.M. & Teixeira, A.L. (2008) Traffic of leukocytes in the central nervous system is associated with chemokine up-regulation in a severe model of herpes simplex encephalitis: an intravital microscopy study. *Neurosci Lett*, 445, 18-22.

Vilela, M.C., Mansur, D.S., Lacerda-Queiroz, N., Rodrigues, D.H., Lima, G.K., Arantes, R.M., Kroon, E.G., da Silva Campos, M.A., Teixeira, M.M. & Teixeira, A.L. (2009) The chemokine CCL5 is essential for leukocyte recruitment in a model of severe Herpes simplex encephalitis. *Ann N Y Acad Sci*, 1153, 256-263.

Whitley, R. (1981) Diagnosis and treatment of herpes simplex encephalitis. *Annu Rev Med*, 32, 335-340.

Wickham, S., Lu, B., Ash, J. & Carr, D.J. (2005) Chemokine receptor deficiency is associated with increased chemokine expression in the peripheral and central nervous systems and increased resistance to herpetic encephalitis. *J Neuroimmunol*, 162, 51-59.

Winter, P.M., Dung, N.M., Loan, H.T., Kneen, R., Wills, B., Thu le, T., House, D., White, N.J., Farrar, J.J., Hart, C.A. & Solomon, T. (2004) Proinflammatory cytokines and chemokines in humans with Japanese encephalitis. *J Infect Dis*, 190, 1618-1626.

Zhang, B., Chan, Y.K., Lu, B., Diamond, M.S. & Klein, R.S. (2008) CXCR3 mediates region-specific antiviral T cell trafficking within the central nervous system during West Nile virus encephalitis. *J Immunol*, 180, 2641-2649.

Zhang, B., Patel, J., Croyle, M., Diamond, M.S. & Klein, R.S. (2010) TNF-alpha-dependent regulation of CXCR3 expression modulates neuronal survival during West Nile virus encephalitis. *J Neuroimmunol*, 224, 28-38.

9

Subacute Sclerosing Pan-Encephalitis (SSPE) – Past and Present

Natan Gadoth
Department of Neurology, Maynei Hyeshuah Medical Center, Bnei Barak, and The Sackler Faculty of Medicine, Tel-Aviv University
Israel

1. Introduction

Subacute Scerosing Pan Encephalitis (SSPE), a devastating brain disease of young children was frequently taken into account in the differential diagnosis of the so-called "neurodegenerative diseases of childhood" by paediatricians, child neurologist and psychiatrists during the second half of the last century. Fortunately, this diagnosis is considered very rarely today in well developed countries, mainly in the western hemisphere. This does not mean that the disease "vanished" although its incidence dramatically declined.

One of the reasons to include SSPE in a book dedicated to "encephalitis " is not only for historical purposes, but also to remind the young generation of physicians dealing with neuro-psychiatric disorders of children and young adults, that SSPE still exists.

Another goal of this chapter is to point out the reasons why SSPE is one of several disorders which fulfil the concept of "slow virus infection", a term brought up by Bjorn Sigurdsson in 1954, after he and his co-workers discovered that three sheep diseases, *scrapie, visna,* and *sheep pulmonary adenomathosis* are all caused by the same retrovirus. This revolutionary concept was later utilized by D. Carleton Gajdusek to study "infections of unknown origin" such as Kuru and Creuzfeldt-Jacob disease. The new generation of paediatricians and child neurologists who most probably have never seen a case of SSPE, will quite naturally skip the paragraph in the text-book which is dedicated to this disease. For those young colleagues this chapter may be more than "interesting" or "informative". It is written for them and hopefully may help them to diagnose correctly their first case and offer the present available palliative drug treatment. Regarding the readers in the field of public health, it may enhance their drive to achieve widespread and complete coverage of measles immunization of populations at risk.

2. History

The suggestion that SSPE may be a viral infection was raised by Dawson who published 2 consecutive papers in 1933 and 1934 in which he described 2 children from Tennessee who died after a progressive course characterized by involuntary jerking of the limbs and mental deterioration. In their brains he noted encephalitic changes with intracellular eosinophilic inclusion bodies in numerous cortical neurons which reminded him of viral inclusions.

(Dawson, 1933; 1934). In 1939, an additional case was described in Germany. This was a 17 year old boy who died after 2 years of progressive neurological deterioration.In his brain nodular changes in the white and gray matter resembling "encephalomyelitis with characteristics of Japanese Encephalitis", were observed. (Pette & Döring, 1939, Case 3). In 1945, Van Bogaert described a clinically similar case in whom the dominant neuropathological features consisted of demyelination and glial proliferation in the white matter which were summarized by him as "subacute sclerosing leukoencephalitis" (Van Bogaert, 1945). Thus, at this stage, 4 children with similar clinical features of progressive fatal neuro- behavioural deterioration and "jerks", have been described. However, in their brains variable and non uniform pathological findings including inflammatory changes, intraneuronal inclusion bodies, nodular "sclerotic" changes both in the white and gray matter were reported and demyelination with glial proliferation in the white matter.

During the next few years children with diverse clinical features resembling progressive encephalitis have been described. However, only in 1957, Poser and Radermecker reached the conclusion that all those patients suffer from a similar disorder which they called Subacute Sclerosing Leucoencephalitis. (Poser & Radermecker, 1957). They based their conclusion on a study of 7 cases including 3 post- mortem examinations. Finally, the term SSPE was coined by Greenfield in 1950 (Greenfield, 1950). Boutellie should be credited for his significant contribution to the understanding of the true nature of SSPE. With the aid of the electron- microscope he identified structures which resembled nucleocapsids of paramyxovirus in SSPE (Boutellie et al., 1965). This finding was soon followed by a search for antibodies to paramyxovirus in the blood and CSF of patients with SSPE which yielded very high titers of anti- measles antibodies in the blood and CSF of all patients studied (Connolly et al., 1967). These pivotal findings led to the crucial conclusion that SSPE is related to infection with measles virus (MV). Later, the mechanisms by which this virus is able to persists in nerve cells for long periods of time in a dormant form were elucidated and shed light on the processes involved in "slow virus infection". The conclusion reached by epidemiological observations that there is a relation between early measles infection and SSPE led to a world-wide measles immunization program followed by a dramatic decline in the incidence of SSPE, up to the present situation where in most of the western developed countries, SSPE was almost completely eradicated.

3. The clinical spectrum of SSPE

There are 2 forms of encephalitis following measles infection. The first is the relatively common acute post infections measles encephalitis which develops in about 0.1 percent of immunocompetent patients and carries a 20 percent mortality rate. This form of encephalitis is not caused by direct invasion of the brain by MV. Indeed, only with highly sensitive methods could MV specific nucleic acids be detected in the brains of patients with this form of encephalitis. Those findings are in line with the assumption that this is a true example of measles virus induced pathological immune mediated "post-infectious" encephalitis. In contras, MV is present in the brains of the immunocompetent patients and causes SSPE while in immunocompromized patients it causes Measles Inclusion Body Encephalitis. Both conditions are fatal and present clinically months or years after the initial measles infection.

The clinical presentation of SSPE is often insidious and frequently attributed to psychological or behavioural problems. The exception to this are those cases who present acutely with focal neurological signs and progress rapidly to coma and death.

The following case report is a classical example of the fulminant form of SSPE which affects about 10% of all patients (PeBenito et al., 1997).

3.1 Case report 1

This 7 year old, previously healthy boy was born in 1970 to healthy unrelated parents of Jewish -Yemenite origin. He was brought to the emergency room (ER), at the Beilinson Medical Center in the state of semi- coma.Past medical and family history were non-contributory. He was well until 2 days prior to admission when mild fever was followed by complains of right sided difficulties in using his hand and leg. He was previously seen by a local physician who diagnosed " common cold ". In the ER his Glasgow Coma Scale Score was 6/15 (eye opening 1, best verbal response 1, best motor response 4). The abnormal neurological findings were lack of withdrawal from deep pain with brisk DTR's and extensor plantar response on the right side. There were no involuntary movements. Immediate brain CT followed by 4 vessel cerebral angiography were normal. An EEG disclosed rhythmic periodic delta generalized discharges with flat electrical background. A lumbar puncture disclosed normal opening pressure, crystal clear sterile CSF with slightly increased protein, normal glucose and negative Gram stain. Serum measles antibody titer by complement fixation was 1:256 and that of the CSF 1:16. There were no clinical signs of measles. The boy died on the 3rd hospital day and the autopsy confirmed the clinical diagnosis of SSPE. He had measles at the age of 2 years and did not receive measles vaccination.

The following case report represents the protracted and peculiar clinical course of SSPE

3.2 Case report 2

This 16 year old girl was born in 1963 to healthy Jewish parents who immigrated to Israel from Morocco in 1949. Her past medical and developmental history was unremarkable. There was no history of clinical measles or an exanthematous early febrile illness. She received measles immunization soon after it was initiated in Israel during 1967. At the age of 7 years, during the second elementary school year, an unexplained decline in her school performance was noted. A paediatric neurological assessment was summarized as Attention Deficit Disorder for which supplementary teaching and Methylphenidate (Ritalin^{R}) 10 mg daily was prescribed. An EEG showed right sides periodic delta wave discharges and for that brain CT with contract enhancement was done and read normal. The EEG findings were attributed to "sweating artefact".The clinical course was stable for 18 months during which a slow deterioration was noticed in her general alertness and vigilance according to the mother. This was however denied by her school teachers who thought that she did quite well in school and received excellent school reports. The anxious mother consulted several child neurologists and psychiatrists who failed to find any abnormalities. A repeated EEG showed generalized periodic slow delta bursts with slow background activity. Serum and CSF measles antibody titers by complement fixation were 1: 256 and 1:32 respectively. A diagnosis of SSPE was considered for which daily Isoprinosine and several courses of intravenous "Thymic Humoral Factor" (THF), were given as part of 2 experimental treatment trials which were at that time done in Israel. That was followed by clinical improvement in her vigilance. She enjoyed the routine daily life of a young girl until the age of 11 years when frequent falls, schoolwork deterioration and sudden brief neck and back flexion movements associated with the falls were noted. She started to behave "strangely",

and had difficulties in recognition of familiar faces and objects. When examined by me for the first time she had marked visual agnosia and neck and axial myoclonus. Her EEG showed additional background slowing with "metronomic" delta bursts resembling "Burst Suppression" pattern. Clonazepam (clonex^R) was helpful only for a short period of time. Both serum and CSF measles antibody titers, and brain CT were almost unchanged.
Her condition gradually deteriorated. She spent her last 2 years of life in a nursing home during which continuous very high fever unresponsive to a variety of antipyretics, bouts of sweating accompanied by brady-tachy arrhythmia, and generalized rigidity were present. Her EEG was almost isoelectirc without evidence of periodic bursts during the last weeks of her life. She died of aspiration pneumonia. Autopsy was not permitted for religious reasons.
Those 2 cases represent the wide spectrum of the clinical features and course of SSPE and also the difficulties of considering SSPE in the differential diagnosis at the early stags of the disease, a fact which explains the delay in the diagnosis in some cases.
The classical clinical diagnostic features of SSPE are shown in Table 1, and the clinical staging of the disease is shown in table 2.

Childhood onset of mental and behavioral regression with :

- Myoclonic Jerks
- EEG- Generalized bilateral rhythmic synchronous bursts of spike-wave or slow wave complexes
- Elevated measles antibody titers in serum and CSF without concomitant evidence of clinical measles
- Elevated CSF IgG, presence of oligoclonal IgG bands

In the brain, presence of perivascular inflammatory cuffing, cortical and subcortical white matter astro-microgliosis, neurophagia and Cowdry type A, eosinophilic intaranuclear inclusion bodies

Table 1. SSPE - Clinical and laboratory diagnostic criteria

i. Personality changes accompanied by school failure and bizarre behavior
ii. Axial (Especially characteristic rapid neck flexion) massive myoclonus causing frequent and violent falls
iii. Generalized rigidity with extarapyramidal features and progressive unresponsiveness
iv. Minimal conscious state progressing to akinetic mutism with severe progressive autonomic failure

Table 2. Clinical staging of SSPE

4. Characteristic clinical features

The majority of the patients the initial symptoms are noted between the ages of 8-11 years, about 6-7 years after measles infection. Zilber et al. initiated a country survey of SSPE in Israel by obtaining information from the Israeli National Neurological Diseases Register (INNDR), the Central Virus Laboratory which at that time tested sera and CSF for measles antibodies throughout the country and the medical records of patients diagnosed with SSPE from all hospitals in the country between the years 1960-1973 (Zilebr at al., 1983). Hundred and eight such patients were detected, 40 of them were followed by the author of this chapter. The onset of SSPE accrued during 1968-1979. The mean age of onset was almost identical to that reported for children in USA (9.5 y.) and UK (9.8 y.). The interval (in years) between clinical measles and onset of SSPE in the Israeli children (7.4 y.), was also similar to that of USA and UK children (7.0 and 6.8 y. respectively). However, the interval (in years) between the time of measles vaccination and SSPE varied between 6.5 years in Israel, and 3.3 and 3.0 in the USA and UK respectively.

All Israeli children with SSPE had progressive neurobehavioral deterioration, myoclonic jerks and characteristic EEG. Sixty eight percent had elevated serum measles antibodies and 89% had increased titer of those antibodies in the CSF. A quite surprising finding was the low percentage of patients (13%) with brain pathology characteristic of SSPE.

True epileptic seizures were a rarity. We have seen only 6 out of our cohort of 40 patients who had true epileptic seizures. Those were 5 boys and 1 girl who had a similar age of onset and disease features. The mean interval between SSPE onset and the first seizure was 15 months (3 - 24). The EEG was mostly focal and the response to Anti Convulsive Drugs (ACD) varied from excellent in 2 patients, good in one and poor in 2. One patient who failed to respond to ACD was given a ketogenic diet which was beneficial. The common denominator of these patients was antecedent neurological impairment. Four suffered from viral encephalitis at one year of age, one had severe learning problems diagnosed prior to the onset of SSPE and the sixth had severe congenital sensory-neural deafness. Two similar cases have been recently reported (Demir et al., 2009). In few patients focal seizures in the form of epilepsia partialis continua and an EEG showing Periodic Lateralizing Epileptic Discharges (PLED) were reported. This pattern was associated with a fulminant course (Santoshkumar & Radhakrishnan 1996, Cherian et al., 2009). As mentioned above, earlier publications indicated that epileptic seizures are rare and appear at late stages of the disease. More recent publications such as the paper by Kissani (Kissani et al., 2001), indicate that epilepsy is rather frequent. In a series of 70 patients with SSPE from Morocco, 30 had

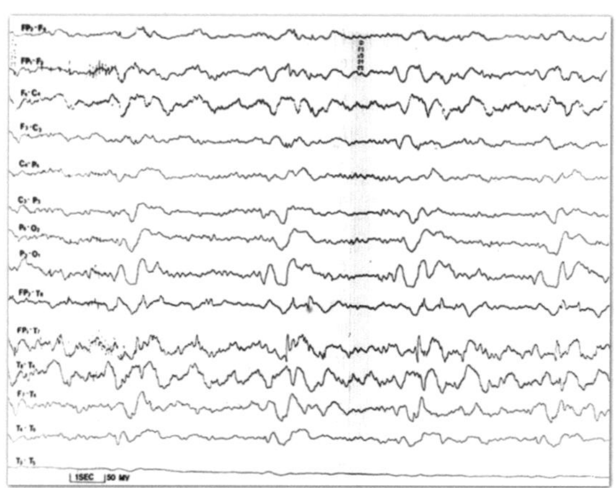

Fig. 1. Patients with SSPE and partial seizures. Note the slow background activity, continuous fronto-central delta activity, periodic non-rhytmic delta bursts and left anterior temporal spikes.

true epileptic seizures.In two-thirds of them the seizures started during the first year of the disease and in 23%, were the presenting symptom. Partial seizures with secondary generalization were most common in the very early stages of the disease and frequently led to the correct diagnosis. When seizures appeared late in the course of the disease (43%), they were mainly generalized tonic-clonic (GTCS). The "heralding" partial seizures are most probably indicators of focal onset of encephalitis with generalized spread later on.

The diagnosis of SSPE is quite straight forward and easily reached in children if the attending paediatricians and child neurologists are familiar with the disease. This is quite different when the disease affects adults. The occurrence of SSPE in subjects older than 18 years is quite rare, comprising 1-12.7% of all patients (Prashanth et al., 2006). Adult onset SSPE presents at an average age of 25 years and rarely follows the classical clinical stages mentioned above. Visual symptoms at presentation are frequent (Singer et al., 1997), while myoclonus may be absent. About 30 % of 52 such patients lacked a history of measles (Fabian et al., 2010).

5. Electroencephalographic and neuroimaging features

The most characteristic EEG feature is the periodic, stereotyped, high voltage discharges which appear concomitantly with the appearance of the myoclonic jerks. At early stages of the disease, the EEG may be normal or show moderate non-specific generalized slowing. As the diseases progresses, the periodic discharge pattern emerges, at first only during sleep, before myoclonic jerks are evident. In early stages, administration of IV diazepam can bring out the typical bursts. Somewhat later in the course and concomitantly with the appearance of typical myoclonus, the characteristic periodic discharge pattern can be seen also during wakefulness. This pattern consists of bilateral synchronous symmetrical bursts with an amplitude of 200-500 mV. Each burst consists of polyphasic, monomorphic delta waves. The bursts appear every 4-10 seconds with an identical morphology in any recording lead and are rhythmic ("metronomic"). The bursts are "time locked" with the myoclonic jerks. The interval between the bursts becomes shorter with disease progression. In advanced stages this pattern is replaced by disorganized slow delta rhythm. The voltage of the recording gets smaller and at stage IV it may became almost iso- electric (Figure.2)

In a relatively recent study from India (Praveen-Kumar et al., 2007), the EEG features of 58 patients with SSPE (stage I: 10.2%; II: 64%; III: 25.8%), were analyzed and related to the stage of disease and neuroimaging findings. Bursts as defined above were found in 98% of the patients. Those were periodic in 55%, "quasi-periodic" in 36% and non-periodic in 6%. The periodic bursts were asymmetrical in 33%. The burst morphology, frequency and inter-burst interval were not influenced by hyperventilation, photic or sensory stimulation. Normal background was recorded in all patients in stage I, and slow background in all other stages. Spike and sharp wave epileptiform discharges were present in 72.4% of the patients. Those were mostly generalized and only in 10 patients epileptiform activity was lateralized or multifocal. The focal discharges were mostly fronto-parietal. Periodic Lateralizing Epileptic Discharges (PLED's), were present in 10 recordings. Asymmetry of background activity or bursts were associated with lateralizing neurological deficits. However, there was no correlation between the EEG asymmetry and CT or MRI findings. Brain neuroimaging was performed in 44 patients and both CT and MRI in 11 patients only. The main neuro-imaging findings consisted of brain oedema and atrophy seen in all stages of the disease while signal intensity changes were present in stages II-III. Parieto-occipital white matter was affected in

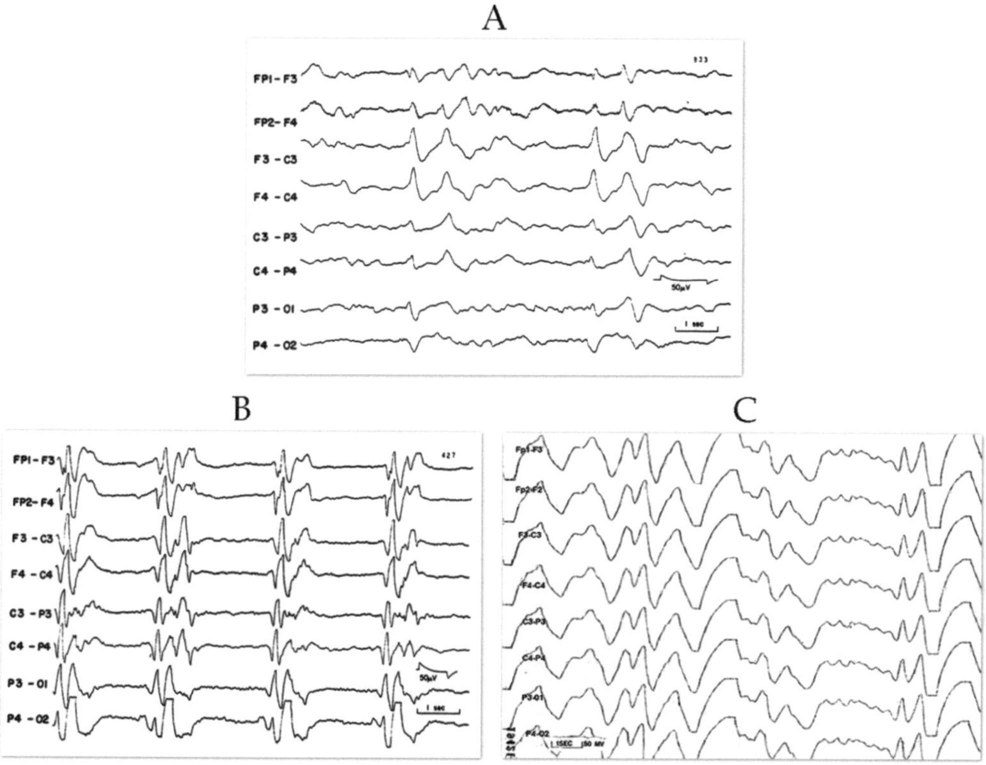

Fig. 2. EEG in various stages of SSPE. A: The background activity is disorganized with few repetitive high voltage delta bursts with fronto-central amplitude accentuation in the early stages of the disease. B: Typical "metronomic" delta burst pattern with almost flat amplitude during burst intervals recorded during the advanced stages of SSPE C: A uniform pattern of monomorphic slow waves at a very advanced stage of SSPE.

stage II while diffuse fronto-parteital changes were more common in stage II-III. There was no contrast enhancement by Iodine or Gadolinium. Although there was no correlation between the imaging features and focal EEG changes or the abnormal neurological findings, a significant association between visual deficits and parieto-occipital signal changes on MRI was found. In a more recent study (Aydin et al., 2009), 17 patients with SSPE who had a routine normal MRI and 30 healthy matched controls underwent T1-weighted magnetization-prepared rapid acquisition gradient echo images. When optimized method of voxel-based morphometry performed across-sectional analysis were applied to search for gray matter volume differences between the patients and controls, a fronto-temporal reduction of the cortical gray matter was found in the patients,regardless of the duration of symptoms or the presence and nature of neurological deficits.

6. Neuropathology

In the early phase of the disease brain oedema with DNA and RNA oxidative damage within infected cells are the typical findings. There is evidence of lipid peroxidation in areas of early demyelination (Hayashi et al., 2002). The main histopathological findings in the acute phase are inflammatory and consist of the classical cortical and subcortical "perivascular cuffing", spongiosis and demyelination, sparing the cerebellum (Figure 3).

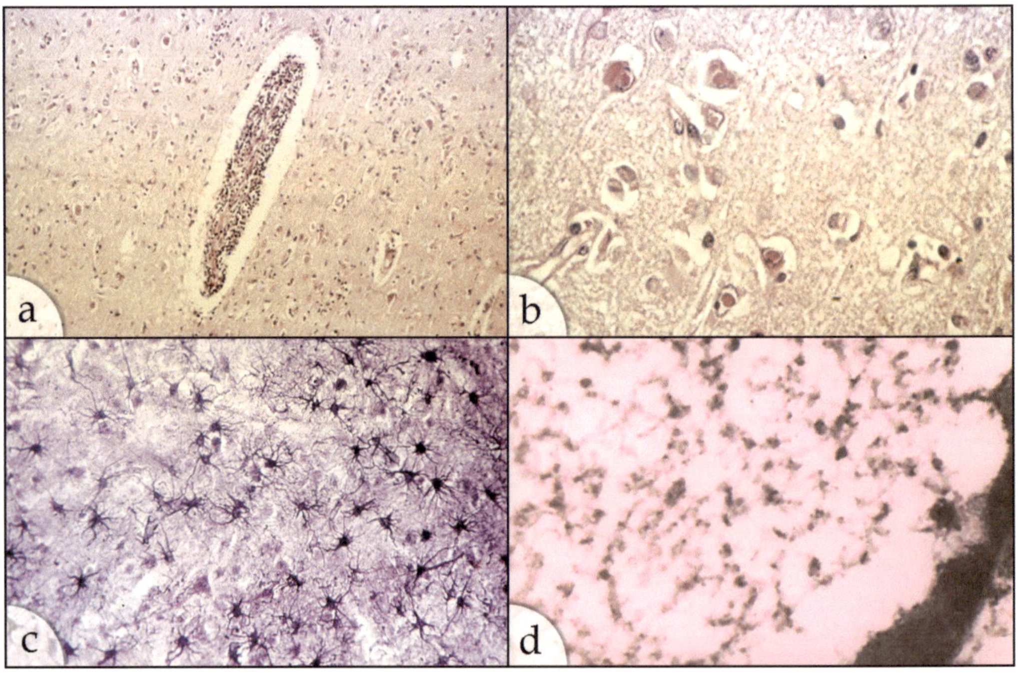

Fig. 3. Postmortem brain microscopy of SSPE. **(a).** Typical lymphocytic perivascular cuffing within brain parenchyma (H&E, X100) **(b).** Cortical neurons with the characteristic intranuclear eosinophilic Cowdry type-A inclusions surrounded by a clear hallo (H&E X400). **(c).** Profound astrocytic proliferation (PAS X190). **(d).** Elecromicrograph of an inclusion body showing curvilinear structures which are most probably viral nucleocapsids (X 20000).

Initially, posterior brain regions are the most affected. Pronounced changes are seen in the medial thalamus and the deep structures. With disease progression more anterior areas, brain stem and spinal cord are also affected. The inflammatory cellular response consists of focal and/or diffuse perivascular infiltrates of lymphocytes, plasma cells and phagocytes which are present within brain parenchyma as well as in the menings. The astrocytes, oligodendrocytes and microvascular endothelium are the mostly infected cell types (Allen et al., 1996).The nuclear and cytoplasmic inclusion bodies seen in neurons and oligodendrocytes are Cowdry type-A inclusions which contain homogeneous eosinophilic material. They are diffusely distributed mostly in the fulminant cases while the small multiple Cowdry type-B inclusion bodies, are almost always present in the brainstem. The nuclear inclusions correspond to measles viral particles and contain viral antigens. Neurofibrillary tangles may be present within neurons and oligodendrocytes. The tangles contain viral genome as shown by in-situ hybridization. Those findings suggest that the tangles are the result of the viral infection. (McQuaid et al., 1994). The inflammatory reaction and even the inclusion bodies are typical for the early stages of the disease and are hard to find at the later stages. Typically for SSPE as a model for slow virus infection, it is very difficult to isolate even a small amount of infectious virus from the brain while viral antigens can be quite easily identified.

7. Immunopathology

A large number of major histocompatibility complex (MHC) class I-II positive cells were seen by immunohistochemical methods in SSPE brains, especially in a perivascular distribution. By morphological criteria, HLA -DR positive microglia and reactive astrocytes were also identified. (Hofman et al., 1991). Although cell mediated immunity was found to be abnormal in a small series of patients such as our own where 11/15 patients had some evidence of such an impairment (Handzel et al.,1983), no specific immune defect was found in SSPE (Schneider-Schaulies et al., 2003). The inflammatory perivascular cell infiltrates are predominantly CD4+ T cells, while B cells are seen more frequently in parenchymal inflammatory infiltrates. We have shown in 11 patients with SSPE, that similar to matched controls, they had no detectable plasma interferon (INF) activity. However, their PBMC failed to produce INF following stimulation with polyinosinic:polycytidilic acid (poly I:C and Phytohemagglutinin (PHA) (Gadoth et al., 1989)

8. Pathophysiology

One of the prevailing theories suggests that in spite of the lack of evidence for a specific immune defect causing SSPE, impaired immune response plays an important role in its pathophysiology. The observation that early infection with MV virus at the time when the immune system is relatively immature, is associated with increased risk for SSPE (Tuxhorn, 2004), was a pivotal step in understanding the disease. Normally, during the incubation phase of measles, the invading virus induces a cell mediated immune response with activation of T-Helper 1 (Th1) lymphocytes, release of INF- α, and interleukin 2 (IL-2), which is capable of eradicating the invading virus particles from the infected cells. Following the characteristic measles papulo-macular skin rash, a humoral antibody mediated long term immunity against future infection is established via the production of Th2 lymphocytes, release of mainly IL- 4 and to a lesser extent INF-α and IL-2. (Griffin et al., 1994). Due to genetic polymorphism, patients with SSPE have an inadequate cellular immune responses to common antigens and produce markedly decreased amounts of IFN (Handzel et al., 1983), and IL - 2,10,12, while producing increased amounts of IL -4 and IL-1b. (Yentür et al., 2005). The induction of this set of humoral immune responses in patients with SSPE rather than producing a cellular immune response which is capable of completely eradicate the MV from the infected cells, is believed to play a major role in the pathogenesis of the disease and contributes to the ability of the mutated measles virus to persist in a dormant form within the brain. (Inoue et al., 2002).

The variable incidence rates of SSPE in different populations and ethnic groups can be partially attributed to genetic polymorphism in addition to a number of epidemiological variables which will be discussed below.

Measles virus uses the cluster of differentiation (CD) protein 46 and fusion protein (protein F), to invade the neuron. The fact that high antibody titers to CD9 were detected in CSF of patients with SSPE who had severe brain atrophy, indicates that this protein plays also a role in neuronal invasion of the virus (Shimizu et al., 2002). After entering the cell the viral matrix protein undergoes mutations and cannot be recognized by the immune system. This is followed by virus replication and persistence within the infected cell without being eradicated by the immune system (Makhortova et al., 2007). In addition, a truncated protein F receptor may also play a causative role. Neurokinin-1 is implicated in the spread of the mutated virus to adjacent cells. After a variable period when the virus is dormant, it induces an inflammatory immune mediated reaction directed against the infected cells, which results in widespread CNS damage. Those mentioned immune mechanisms may also play a role in other chronic demyelinating CNS disorders.

9. Treatment

SPEE is always fatal. A relative beneficial effect was achieved with either daily oral Isoprinosine or in combination with weekly intrathecal INF -α. Although this combination is considered the most beneficial, approximately 22% of the treated patients suffered from complications related to the intrathecal reservoir. Isoprinosine (Inosiplex^R), is a derivative of Inosine and p-acetamidobenzoic acid salt of N,N-dimethylamydo-2- propanol. This drug is considered as an immunomodulator agent capable of impairing viral replication. It is quite safe when given for extended periods of time. The positive immunomodulation effect of Isoprinosine was demonstrated by an experiment during which PBMC of patients with SSPE failed to produce INF after stimulation with poly I:C and PHA. The patients were then given oral Isoprinosine for several days which resulted in significant elevation of serum INF and corrected the failure of INF production by the similarly stimulated PBMC. Moreover, 10 days after discontinuation of the drug, the INF system returned to its inactive state. Several patients were treated for extended periods of time with a 20% remission rate and or 4 year survival. (Gadoth et al., 1989). Other investigators have shown a beneficial effect of the drug in up to 30-35% of the patients which is significantly higher than the reported 5% spontaneous remission rate (Dyken et al., 1982).
Other agents such as Ribavirin, which blocks RNA polymerase without and in combination with INF, Anti CD2O antibodies, THF, Amantadine, Steroids and plasmapehresis showed some beneficial effect in selected non-randomized trials.
Several patients have been treated with intraventricular INF-α alone or in combination with oral Isoprinosine but with no advantage over the intrathecal route (Yalaz et al., 1992).

10. Epidemiology

The dramatic changes in the epidemiology of SSPE in relation to the world-wide immunization project against measles are fascinating. The reduction in measles incidence especially in immunized infants was followed by a dramatic fall in the rate of SSPE in the developed countries of the western hemisphere and in other world regions where measles immunization became mandatory. In addition, some changes occurred in the previously described "classical" characteristics of the disease such as the age of onset and a number of clinical features. In a relatively recent world wide review of the rate of measles and SSPE before and after the institution of measles immunization, the dramatic drop in the incidence of SSPE due to immunization was clearly shown (Campbell et al., 2007).
Israel served and still serves as a good site for classical epidemiological studies because of its heterogenic ethnic population, high standard of medical care and a well organized medical and health system which enables the particular researcher to obtain well

documented data throughout the country. For this reason data from Israel can provide an excellent example of the role of mass measles immunization on the rate of SSPE. The country has a wide-spread network of Mother and Child health clinics which serve the entire county's population. The individual clinics keep careful records of each child's immunization program, and the medical staff is alert to those who fail to show for their clinic visits or to the immunization schedule, established by the Israeli Ministry of health. Due to the nominal cost of those services, it can be assumed that the diagnosis and reports of patients with SSPE are accurate and most probably complete. Population studies of SSPE were carried out in Israel since 1960, while mass measles vaccination was introduced in 1967. Thus, most of the children born after February 1965 were immunized. Considering the standard of medical care in Israel and the size of its population in 1975 (3.5 million), it can be assumed that a rare disease such as SSPE was reported in sufficient numbers during those years when the local and world wide SSPE "epidemic" suddenly emerged. All those factors enabled an accurate analysis of SSPE incidence in regard to a number of variables including the role of mass immunization against measles. Zilber (Zilber et al., 1983), obtained data on SSPE rates from the Israeli National Neurological Disease Register which received notification on all neurological disorders recorded in all hospitalized patients around the country. Death certifications with a code for any neurological disorder were also retrieved. Assuming that the varied and dramatic symptoms of SSPE will eventually lead to hospitalization of the affected child, it is highly likely that the register was notified of almost all patients with SSPE during the period of this study which covered the period of 1968-1979. The medical records of all detected cases were obtained. As the register was notified also on cases of measles encephalitis, non-specific encephalitis, and degenerative progressive neurological diseases in children, the charts of such cases were also obtained and reviewed for possible SSPE. The records from the central virology laboratory which performed serum and CSF measles antibody titers for the entire country since 1968 until the publication of the mentioned study were searched for tests with increased measles antibody titers and the patients details and medical records were obtained. In a previous study by the same group (Soffer et al., 1975) the medical records of patients with the diagnosis of SSPE from all Israeli hospitals for the period of 1960-1973 were reviewed. In addition, the departments of paediatrics, neurology and the EEG laboratories across the country were asked to provide information on additional patients. The multi-source information thus gathered enabled to exclude multiple reports of the same patient and provided a high level of ascertainment of the data obtained. The main findings of this study confirmed the presence of a steep drop in incidence of SSPE in vaccinated Israeli children noted mainly in 1977, 10 years after the initiation of mass immunization. The rate of SSPE remained low at the completion of this study in 1979. The calculated rate of SSPE (per 10^6 live births) during the period of 1965-1971 was 246 in non vaccinated patients compared to 27 in vaccinated subjects. The rate of 27 included patients who developed measles after immunization. When those patients were excluded the rate dropped to 17. The relation between the rate of measles infection and SSPE in Israel is shown in Figure 4. The rates of SSPE for Israeli Jews and Arabs were compared to rates for Arabs living in Gaza and the west bank where measles immunization was not compulsory but available. The rates dropped steeply for both Israeli Jews and Arabs in 1977 with a significant delay in Gaza and the west bank. However, even in this particular population the decline in the number of new cases was dramatic to the point that no new cases were reported in both populations after 1986 (Figure 5).

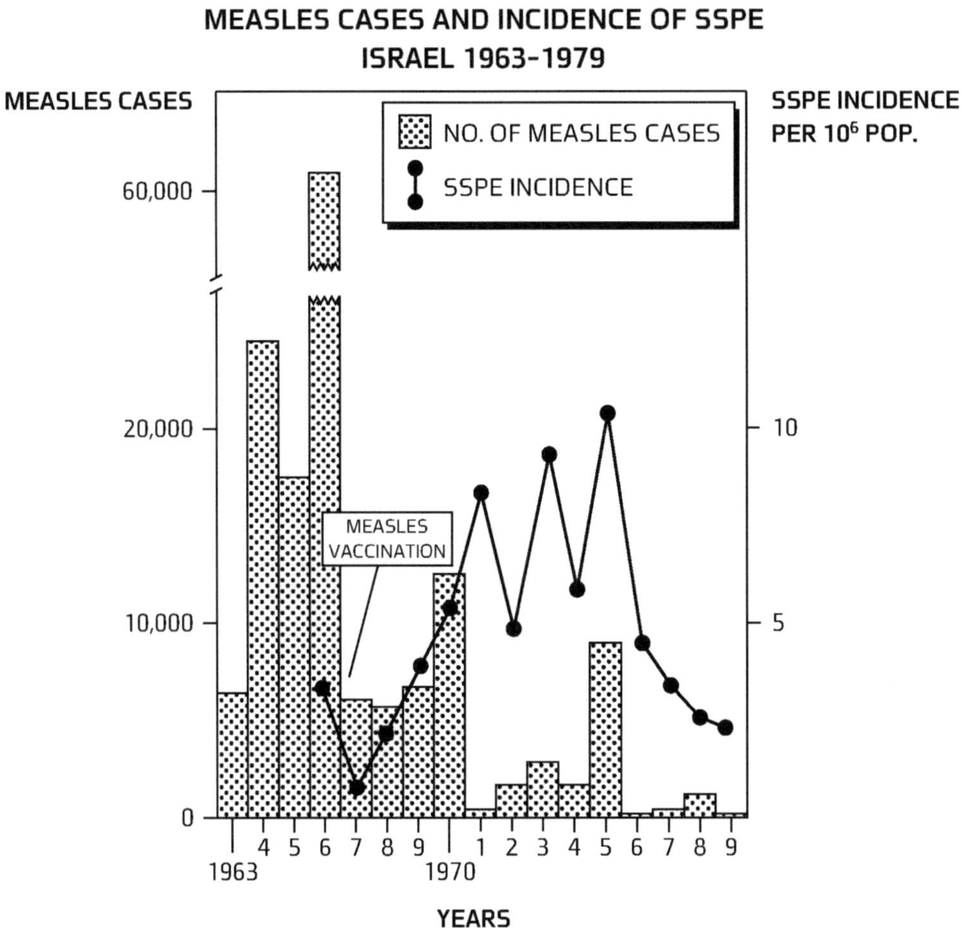

Fig. 4. The incidence of SSPE in relation to the rate of measles infection in Israel during the epidemic years of SSPE.

Similar to data from other countries, the age of onset in Israeli patients increased parallel to the decrease in the rate of measles and SSPE, although in Arabs it remained around 10 years of age. (Figure 6).

While new cases are a rarity today in counties with good measles control such as USA where the rate is very low ($0.01/10^6$), it is still quite high in counties with poor measles control (India; $21/10^6$, Japan; $11/10^6$, and Turkey; $0.461/10^6$,(Gutierrez et al., 2010). One of the highest rates of SSPE was found and is still present in Papua- New Guinea (PNG). This rate is only partially related to poor immunization control. During the years 1988-1999, a rate of $13\text{-}98/10^6$ was found in individuals younger than 20 years of age. The rate of measles immunization in this particular population was stable at a level between 50-60 % of the population at risk during 1997-2008. A recent study from the referral hospital of the Madang Province in PNG mentioned a rate of $54/10^6$ in individuals younger than 20 years, during 2007–2009. The rate was much higher in 4 sub-districts with an annual incidence of $> 100/10^6$ among the same age group. Those rates are the highest ever reported. The patients in this study contracted measles during their first year of life in 2002 and presented with SSPE 6-7 years later. A possible explanation for that very high rate in spite of a 60% rate of measles immunization in this region is the observation that only 36% of young Melanesian children respond well to measles vaccine and develop immunity to measles.(Manning et al., 2011).

From the above mentioned epidemiological data it is evident that SSPE is a "vanishing" disease in well developed countries while the disease is still taking the life of children in underdeveloped world regions. The variable incidence of SSPE can be explained not only in relation to the variability in measles morbidity, the degree of immunization coverage, the age of immunization, the different rates of virus mutations, male gender preponderance and ethnic origin, but it is also related to genetic polymorphism which determines the individual immune system reaction to measles vaccine as it happened in PNG.

The different ethnic susceptibility to SSPE was studied in the multiethnic Israeli population. It was found that SSPE was more frequent among Sephardic than Ashkenazi Jews (3.4 vs. $0.5/10^6$, respectively) (Zilber et al., 1998).

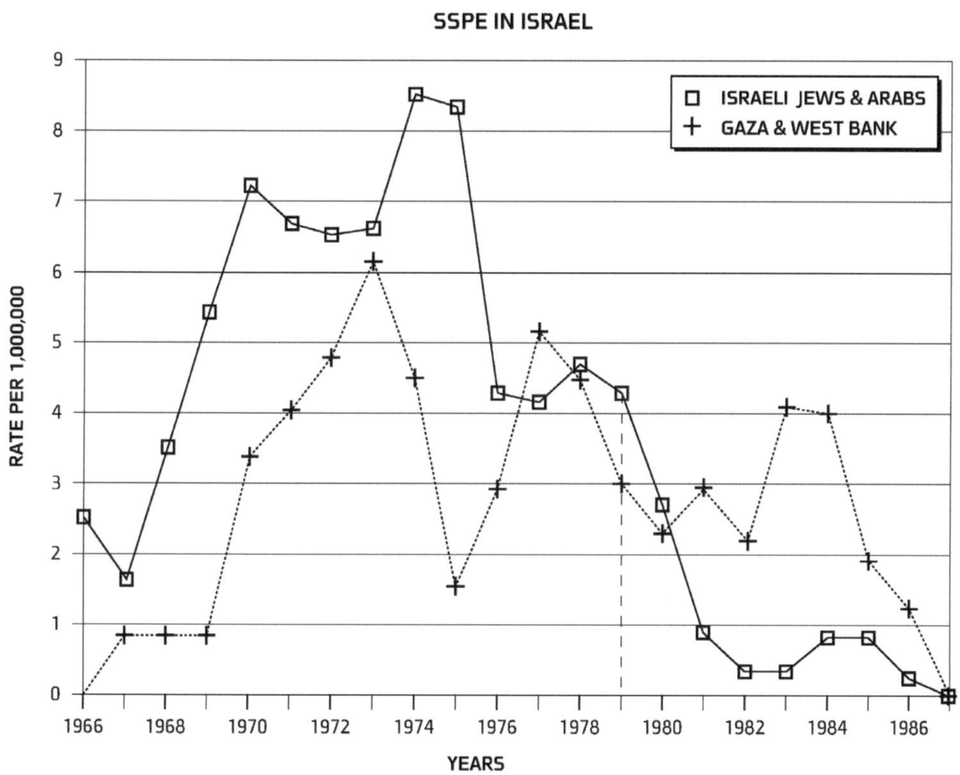

Fig. 5. Differences in incidence of SSPE between Israel and Gaza -West bank. Note the dramatic drop in the incidence in both populations (Vertical broken line).

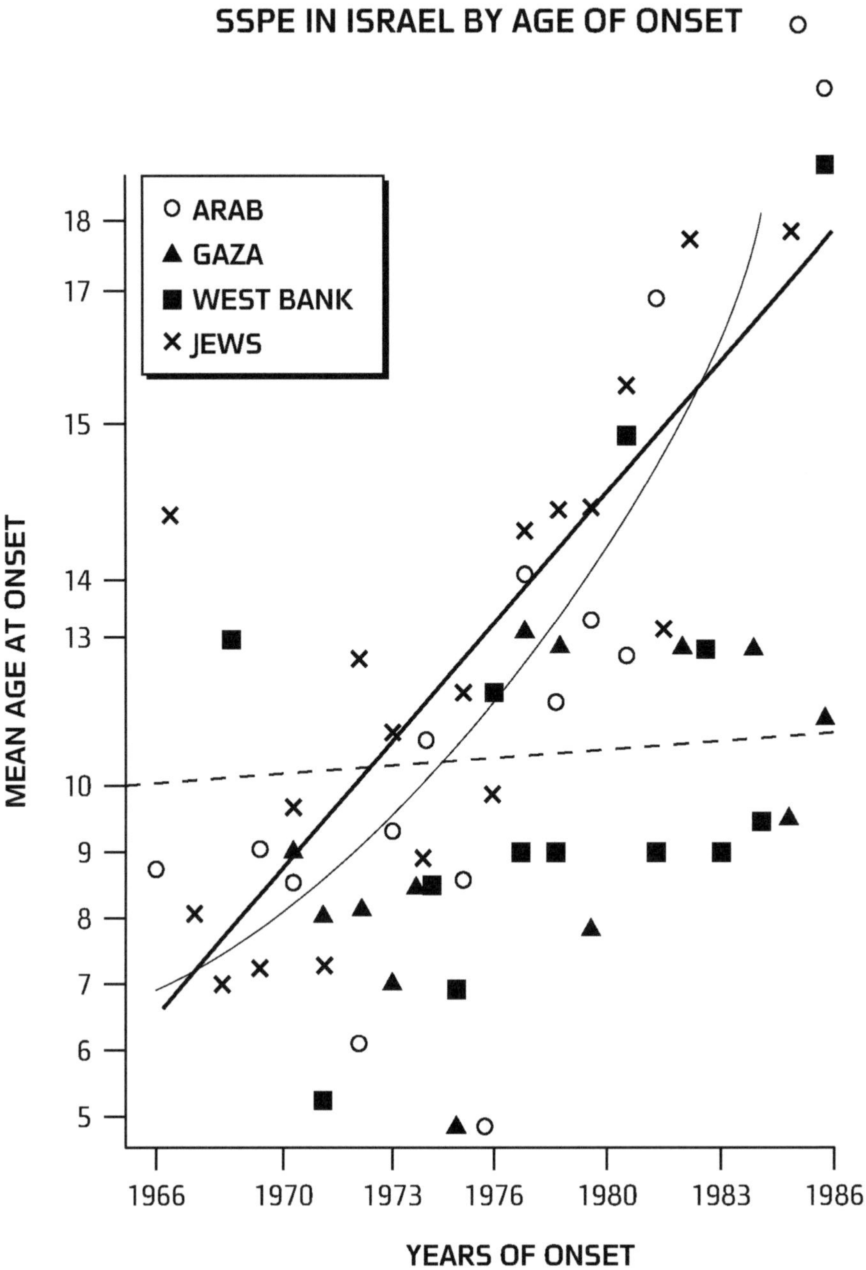

Fig. 6. The increase in age of onset in Jewish Israeli patients with SSPE which followed the steep decline in the incidence of SSPE.

11. Conclusion

SSPE can be added to the past pandemics such as small pox and poliomyelitis which were eradicated due to mass vaccination creating a world wide and an almost complete immunity to those devastating diseases. Although SSPE is not an acute infection "per se " like those mentioned above, this horrible disease was also eradicated due to mass immunization initiated when the "old" traditional methods of keen clinical judgment, basic epidemiology and the progress made by understanding the mechanisms involved in persistent viral infections made it clear that early infection with measles can cause SSPE.
There is still an urgent need to lower the rate of SSPE in areas with poor measles immunization coverage. Although we are at present unable to offer efficient treatment and cure to patients with a variety of degenerative progressive neurological disorders there are some hints to suggest that some of them might be the result of yet unknown "slow virus" infections.

12. Acknowledgment

I would like to thank Professor E. Kahana MD, one of the most enthusiastic pioneers of neuro-epidemiological research, who studied the epidemiology of degenerative progressive neurological disorders in Israel, among them, multiple sclerosis, Creutzfeldt- Jacob disease and SSPE. She has willingly provided some of the diagrams shown in this chapter which have not been published before.

13. References

Allen, IV. McQuaid, S. McMahon, J. Kirk, J. & McConnell, R. (1996). The significance of measles virus antigen and genome distribution in the CNS in SSPE for mechanism of viral spread and demyelination, *Journal of Neuropathology and Experimental Neurology*, Vol.55, No 4, (April 1996), pp. 471-480, ISSN 0022-3069

Aydin, K. Okur, O. Tatli, B. Sarwar, SG, Ozturk, C. & Dilber, C. (2009), Reduced Gray Matter Volume in the Frontotemporal Cortex of Patients with Early Subacute Sclerosing Panencephalitis., *American Journal of Neuroradiology*, Vol. 30, No. 2, (February 2009), pp. 271-275, ISSN 0195-6108

Boutellie, M. Fontaine, C. & Vedrenne, CL. (1965). Sur un cas d'encephalite subaigue a inclusions. Etude Anatomoclinique et ultrastructurale. *Revue neurologique,* Vol. 113, No. 4, (October 1965), pp. 454-458, ISSN 0035-3787

Cherian, A. Sreedharan, S. Raghavendra, S. Nayak, D. & Radhakrishnan,A.(2009).Periodic lateralized epileptiform discharges in fulminant form of SSPE. *The Canadian Journal of Neurological Sciences,* Vol. 36, No. 4, (July 2009), pp. 524-526, ISSN 0317-1671

Connolly, JH. Allen, IV. Hurwitz, LI. & Millar, JH. (1967). Measles virus antibody and antigen in subacute sclerosing panencephalitis. *Lancet,* Vol. 1, No. 7489, (March 1967), pp. 542-544, ISSN 0140-6736

Dawson, JR. (1933). Cellular inclusions in cerebral lesions of lethargic encephalitis. *American Journal of Pathology* , Vol. 9, No 1. (January 1933), pp. 7-15, ISSN 0002-9440

Dawson, JR. (1934). Cellular inclusions in cerebral lesions of epidemic encephalitis. *Archives of Neurology and Psychiatry,* Vol. 31, No. 4, (April 1934) , pp. 685-700, ISSN 0096-6754

Demir, E. Ozcelik, A. Arhan, E. Serdaroglu, A. & Gucuyener, K. (2009). Atypical presentations of subacute sclerosing panencephalitis in two neurologically handicapped cases. *Neuropediatrics,* Vol. 40, No. 4, (August 2009) , pp. 195-198,ISSN 0174-304X

Dyken, PR. Swift, A. & DuRant, RH. (1982). Long-term follow-up of patients with subacute sclerosing panencephalitis treated with inosiplex. *Annals of Neurology* Vol. 11, No. 4, (April 1982), pp. 359-364, ISSN 0364-5134

Fabian, VA. Yee Lee, H. Keith-Rokosh, JL. de Souza, JL. & Stewart-Wynne, E. (2010). A 22-year-old Australian woman with atypical subacute sclerosing panencephalitis diagnosed at postmortem. *Journal of Clinical Neuroscience,* Vol. 17, No. 9, (September 2010), pp. 1192-1194, ISSN 0967-5868

Gadoth, N. Kott, E. Levin, S. & Hahn, T. (1989). The interferon system in subacute sclerosing panencephalitis and its response to Isoprinosine. *Brain and Development* Vol. 11, No. 5, (May 1989), pp. 308-312, ISSN 0387-7604

Greenfield, JG. (1950). Encephalitis and encephalomyelitis in England and Wales during the last decade. *Brain.* Vol. 73, No. 2,(June 1950), pp. 141-166, ISSN 0006-8950

Griffin, DE. Ward, BJ. & Esolen, LM. (1994). Pathogenesis of measles virus infection: a hypothesis for altered immune responses. *Journal of Infectious Diseases,* Vol. 170, Suppl. 1, (November 1994), pp. S24-S31, ISSN 1344-6304

Gutierrez, J. Issacson, RS. & Koppel, BS. (2010). Subacute sclerosing panencephalitis: an update. *Developmental Medicine and Child Neurology,* Vol. 52, No.10, (October 2010), pp. 901-907, ISSN 1469- 8749

Handzel, Z. Gadoth, N. Idar, D. Schlesinger, M. Kahana, E. Dagan, R. Levin, S. & Trainin N. (1983). Cell mediated immunity and effect of "thymic humoral factor " in 15 patients with SSPE. *Brain and Development,* Vol. 5, No. 1,(January 1983) , pp. 29-35, ISSN 0387-7604

Hayashi, M. Arai, N. Satoh, J. Suzuki, H. Katayama, K. Tamagawa, K. & Morimatsu, Y. (2002). Neurodegenerative mechanisms in subacute sclerosing panencephalitis. *Journal of Child Neurology,* Vol. 17, No. 10, (October 2002), pp. 725-730, ISSN 0883-0738

Hofman, FM. Hinton, DR. Baemayr, J. Weil, M. & Merrill, JE. (1991). Lymphokines and immunoregulatory molecules in subacute sclerosing panencephalitis. *Clinical Immunology and Immunopathology.* Vol. 58, No. 3, (March 1991), pp. 331-342, ISSN 0090-1229

Inoue, T. Kira, R. Nakao, F. Ihara, K. Bassuny, WM. Kusuhara, K. Nihei, K. Takeshita, K. & Hara, T. (2002). Contribution of the interleukin 4 gene to susceptibility to subacute sclerosing panencephalitis. *Archives of Neurology,* Vol. 59, No. 5, (May 2002), pp. 822-827, ISSN 0003-9942

Kissani, N. Ouazzani, R. Belaidi, H. Ouahabi, H. & Chkili, T. (2001).Crises épileptiques et épilepsie dans le cadre d'une panencéphalite sclérosante subaiguë (à propos de 30 cas). *Neurophysiologie Clinique,* Vol. 31, No. 6, (December 2001), pp. 398-405, ISSN 0987-7053

Makhortova, NR. Askovich, P. Patterson, CE. Gechman, LA. Gerard, NP. & Rall, GF. (2007). Neurokinin-1 enables measles virus trans-synaptic spread in neurons. *Virology,* Vol. 362, No. 1, (May 2007), pp. 35–44, ISSN 0042-6822

Manning, L. Laman, M. Edoni, H. Mueller, I. Karunajeewa, HA. Smith, D. Hwaiwhanje, I. Siba, PM. & Davis, TME. (2011). Subacute Sclerosing Panencephalitis in Papua New Guinean Children: The Cost of Continuing Inadequate Measles Vaccine Coverage. *Public Library of Science (PLoS) Neglected Tropical Diseases*, Vol. 5, No. 1, (January 2001), pp. e932 (1-8). ISSN 1935-2735

McQuaid, S. Allen, IV. McMahon, J. & Kirk, J. (1994). Association of measles virus with neurofibrillary tangles in subacute sclerosing panencephalitis: a combined in situ hybridization and immunocytochemical investigation. *Neuropathology and Applied Neurobiology*, Vol. 20, No. 2, (April 1994), pp. 103–110, ISSN 0305-1846

Pette, H, & Döring, G.(1939). Über einheimische panencephalomyelitis vom charaker der encephalitis japonica. *Deutsche Zeitschrift fur Nervenheilkunde*, Vol. 149, No. 1-2, (June 1939), pp. 7-44, ISSN 0340-5354

PeBenito, R. Naqvi, SH. Arca, MM. & Schubert, R. (1997). Fulminating subacute sclerosing panencephalitis: case report and literature review. *Clinical Pediatrics (Phila)*, Vol. 36, No. 3, (March 1997), pp.-149–154, ISSN 0009-9228

Poser, CM. & Radermecker, J. (1957). Subacute Scelorsing leucoencephalitis. *Journal of Pediatrics*, Vol. 50, No. 4, (April 1957), pp. 408-425, ISSN 0022-3476

Prashanth, LK. Taly, AB. Ravi, V. Sinha, S. & Arunodaya, GR. (2006). Adult onset subacute sclerosing panencephalitis: clinical profile of 39 patients from a tertiary care centre. *Journal of Neurology Neurosurgery and Psychiatry*, Vol. 77, No. 5, (May 2006), pp. 630-633, ISSN 0022-3050

Praveen- kumar, S. Sinha, S. Taly, AB. Jayasree, S. Ravi, V. Vijayan, J. & Ravishankar, S. (2007). Electroencephalographic and imaging profile in a subacute sclerosing panencephalitis (SSPE) cohort: A correlative study. *Clinical Neurophysiology*, Vol. 118, No. 9, (September 2007), pp. 1947-1954, ISSN 1388-2457

Santoshkumar, B. & Radhakrishnan, K. (1996). Periodic electroencephalographic pattern in subacute sclerosing panencephalitis modified by preexisting damaged cerebral hemisphere. *Electroencephalogry and Clinical Neurophysiology*, Vol. 99, No 5, (November 1996), pp. 440-443, ISSN 0013-4694

Schneider-Schaulies, J. Meulen, V. & Schneider-Schaulies, S. (2003). Measles infection of the central nervous system. *Journal of Neurovirology*, Vol. 9, No. 2, (April 2003), pp. 247-252, ISSN 1355-0284

Shimizu, T. Matsuishi, T. Iwamoto, R. Handa, K. Yoshioka, H. Kato, H. Ueda, S. Hara, H. Tabira, T. & Mekada, E. (2002). Elevated levels of anti-CD9 antibodies in the cerebrospinal fluid of patients with subacute sclerosing panencephalitis. *Journal of Infectious Diseases*, Vol. 185, No. 9, (May 2002), pp- 1346–1350, ISSN 1344-6304

Singer, C. Lang, AE. & Suchowersky, O. (1997). Adult-onset subacute sclerosing panencephalitis: case reports and review of the literature. *Movement Disorders*. Vol. 12, No. 3, (May 1997), pp. 342-353, ISSN 0885-3185

Soffer, D. Rannon, L. Alter, M. Kahana, E. & Feldman, S.(1975). Subacute scerosing panencephalitis: incidence among ethnic groups in Israel. *Israel Journal of Medical Sciences*, Vol. 11, No. 1, (January 1975), pp. 1-4, ISSN 0021-2180

Tuxhorn, IE. (2004). Familial subacute sclerosing panencephalitis in two siblings. *Pediatric Neurology* Vol. 31, No. 4, (October 2004), pp. 291–294, ISSN 0887-8994

Van Bogaert, L. (1945). Une leocoencephalite sclerosante subaigue. *Jouranl of Neurolorgy, Neurosurgery & Psychiatry*, Vol. 8, No. 3-4, (July 1945), pp. 101-120, ISSN 0022-3050

Yalaz, K. Anlar, B. Oktem, F. Aysun, S. Ustacelebi, S. Gurcay, O. Gucuyener, K. & Renda, Y. (1992). Intraventricular interferon and oral inosiplex in the treatment of subacute sclerosing panencephalitis. *Neurology*, Vol. 42, No. 3, (March 1992), pp-488-491, 0028-3878

Yentür, SP. Gürses, C. Demirbilek, V. Yilmaz, G. Onal, AE. Yapici, Z. Yalçinkaya, C. Cokar, O. Gökyiğit, A. & Saruhan-Direskeneli, G. (2005). Alterations in cell-mediated immune response in subacute sclerosing panencephalitis. *Journal of Neuroimmunology*, Vol. 170, No. 1-2, (December 2005), pp. 179–185,ISSN 0165-5728

Zilber, N. Rannon, L. Alter, M. & Kahana, E. (1983). Measles, measles Vaccination and risk of subacute sclerosing panencephalitis (SSPE). *Neurology* Vol. 33, No. 12, (December 1983), pp. 1558-1564,ISSN 0028-3878

Zilber, N. & Kahana, E. (1998). Environmental risk factors of subacute scleroisng panenecephalitis (SSPE). *Acta Neurologica Scandinavica*, Vol. 98, No. 1, (July 1998), pp. 49-54, ISSN 0001-6314

10

Herpes Simplex Myelitis: Differences in Clinical Manifestations Between Herpes Simplex Virus Type 1 and Type 2

Hideto Nakajima[1,2] and Hiroshi Shoji[3]
[1]*Department of Internal Medicine, Seikeikai Hospital*
[2]*Division of Neurology, Department of Internal Medicine, Osaka Medical College*
[3]*Division of Neurology, St.Mary's Hospital*
Japan

1. Introduction

Various clinical types of central nerve infection caused by herpes simplex virus (HSV) have been identified, and the clinical features of not only encephalitis and meningitis, but also Mollaret meningitis and Elsberg syndrome, have been clarified (Tyler, 2004; Eberhardt et al., 2004). Myelitis is rare, and it has been mostly reported as ascending myelitis, necrotizing myelitis or myeloradiculitis (Klastersky et al, 1972; Koskiniemi et al., 1982; Britton et al., 1985; Tucker et al., 1985; Wiley et al., 1987; Ahmed,1988; Nakagawa et al., 1991; Iwamasa et al., 1991). The initial symptoms of herpes simplex myelitis (HSM) are sensory-motor disturbance of lower limbs and urinary disturbance. Then, transverse myelopathy ascends from level of the lumbosacral spinal cord to level of the cervicothoracic spinal cord. As ascending necrotizing form of HSM often accompanied encephalitis, quadriplegia, or respiratory muscle paralysis, the prognosis of this condition is poor (Table 1). In terms of pathological features, necrotic changes are common, and hemorrhagic lesions are occasionally seen. As a result of technical advances in the 1990s, including diagnostic imaging using MRI and virological diagnosis using PCR, HSM is now more frequently identified. Consequently, in addition to acute ascending myelitis, patients with transverse

Clinical symptoms:	
(initially)	Sensorimotor disturbances of lower limbs, Urinary disturbance
	Ascending progression of myelopathy (1-2 weeks)
Complication:	Genital herpes
Associated condition:	HIV, Malignancy, Diabetes mellitus
	(immunocompromised)
HSV typing:	HSV-2
Diagnosis:	Autopsy
Prognosis:	Fatal

Table 1. Characteristic of acute ascending necrotizing myelitis

myelitis that arises in the cervicothoracic spinal cord and does not ascend, mild myelitis, and recurrent myelitis, have been reported. The present article summarizes the clinical features of HSM and discusses diagnosis and therapy.

2. Case presentation

2.1 Case 1: Acute ascending myelitis by HSV-2

A 44-year-old man with diabetes mellitus presented with urinary retention and weakness in both legs following scrotal numbness. He had genital herpes, and sensory-motor disturbance of his lower limbs ascended to the level of thoracic spinal cord in 5 days. Neurological examination revealed paraparesis and sensory disturbances below the T6 level. The urodynamic study showed atonic contraction. Analysis of his CSF showed 105 WBC (all mononuclear cells), protein of 68 mg/dl, and the test for serum antibody to human T lymphotropic virus type I (HTLV-I) antibody and results of collagen vascular screening test were both negative. He was treated with acyclovir (1,500 mg/day) and betamethasone (8mg/day) for 4 weeks. He showed some improvement in urinary retention, but the paraparesis persisted as sequelae. The anti-HSV antibody (neutralizing test) in his serum antibody was 1:4, and did not change in paired samples. On admission, the test for anti-HSV antibody (ELISA) in the CSF showed positive IgM-HSV 2.000 (4+) and negative IgG-HSV IgG 0.076 (-). Following CSF tests showed the decrease of the IgM-HSV level 0.234(+) and the increase of the IgG-HSV 0.366(+). HSV-2 DNA was detected in his CSF sample by PCR.

2.2 Case 2: Recurrent HSM by HSV-2

A 49-year-old female presented with urinary retention, back pain, numbness and a sudden onset of weakness in both legs. Neurological examination showed paraparesis, positive Babinski sign, and sensory disturbances below the T5 level on the right and below the T7 level on the left. The urodynamic study showed atonic contraction. Analysis of her CSF showed 30 WBC (all mononuclear cells), protein of 79 mg/dl, IgG index of 0.32, myelin basic protein of 3.1 µg/ml, and an absence of oligoclonal IgG bands. A myelogram revealed cord enlargement at the levels of T3 to T7 segments. Anti-HSV antibody by EIA was positive in her CSF. After treatment with intravenous acyclovir (1,500 mg/day) and betamethasone (8 mg/day) for 4 weeks, she recovered significantly. One year and 10 months later, she again developed myelopathy at the T6 level, and she showed Romberg's sign. CSF analysis showed 196 WBC (100% mononuclear cells), protein of 90 mg/dl, IgG index of 0.51, and myelin basic protein of 6.7 µg/ml. MRI of her thoracic cord indicated an increased signal intensity in the posterior portion of spinal cord at the 2nd thoracic vertebra Tl-weighted image with Gd-DTPA enhancement. Brain MRI was normal. In her CSF, anti-HSV antibody using EIA remained positive. No herpetic vesicles were observed in either episode. The test for serum antibody to HTLV-I antibody and results of collagen vascular screening test were both negative. Flow cytometry showed no abnormality in lymphocyte subset. She was treated with acyclovir (1,500 mg/day) and betamethasone (8mg/day) for 3 weeks and again showed complete recovery. HSV-2 DNA was detected at both first and second episode.

2.3 Case 3: Chronic myelitis by HSV-2

A 38-year-old male presented with progressive weakness in both legs, urinary retention, and numbness, for one month. Neurological examination revealed paraparesis and sensory disturbances below the T6 level. Babinski's sign was negative. His bladder was distended.

Analysis of his CSF showed 11 WBC (all mononuclear cells), protein of 75 mg/dl, IgG index of 0.44, and a positive oligoclonal IgG band. The myelogram revealed the cord enlargement at the T2 to T6 segments. The anti-HSV-1 antibody in his CSF determined by immunofluorescence (IF) was 1:4, and in serum it was 1:640. After administration of intravenous acyclovir (750 mg/day for 4 weeks) and prednisolone (60 mg/day for 2 weeks), his paraparesis improved. The anti-HSV-1 antibody in his CSF decreased 1:2, and serum antibody was 1:320. Five months later, however, myelopathy developed again at the same level. Analysis of his CSF showed 2 WBC (all mononuclear cells), protein of 42 mg/dl, IgG index of 0.25, and negative oligoclonal IgG bands. Brain and thoracic MRI showed no abnormalities. The anti-HSV-1 antibody (IF) in his CSF was 1:8, and serum antibody was 1: 1,280. Serum antibody against HTLV-I was negative. Intravenous methylprednisolone (1 g/day for 3 days) exerted beneficial effects. During the second episode genital herpetic vesicles were observed, and antibody to HSV remained positive in the CSF. He was then administered intravenous acyclovir (750 mg/day for 4 weeks), with improvement in numbness and urinary retention, but the paraparesis persisted. HSV-2 DNA was detected by PCR.

3. Clinical features

Table 2 lists the clinical features of patients with HSM, including our own patients. Klastersky and colleagues (Klastersky et al, 1972) reported the first patient with HSM in 1972, and HSM was only reported as ascending myelitis until the 1980s. The initial symptoms of HSM included lumbar pain, leg pain, and urinary disturbance. Sensory and motor disturbance has been observed to begin in the leg and ascend to the cervicothoracic spinal cord in 1-2 weeks. Like encephalitis or meningitis caused by HSV, disease onset or progression was sometimes accompanied by fever, and in about half of the patients, eczema herpeticum was seen on the lips or genitals. In most patients, the cause of ascending myelitis was HSV-2. During the 1970s and 1980s when these patients were reported, it was difficult to diagnose HSM based on clinical findings. Therefore, pathological diagnosis based on autopsy findings was required for the diagnosis of myelitis and the identification of the causative virus. Many patients with ascending myelitis had such underlying disease as AIDS or immunosuppression due to cancer or diabetes (Koskiniemi et al., 1982; Britton et al., 1985; Tucker et al., 1985; Wiley et al., 1987; Nakagawa et al., 1991; Iwamasa et al., 1991), and HSV-2 myelitis had poor prognosis. Hence, lethal ascending necrotizing myelitis due to HSV-2 in an immunocompromised host was considered the typical clinical feature of HSM, and also HSM was considered an opportunistic infection. In the 1990s, MRI began to be used for diagnostic imaging of the spine, and PCR began to be used for virological diagnosis (Aurelius et al., 1991; Nakajima et al., 2005), which greatly contributed to the diagnosis of HSM. Consequently, clinical features associated with HSM, other than ascending myelitis, were identified. Therefore, patients with transverse myelopathy in the cervicothoracic spinal cord, myelitis without ascending inflammation (non-ascending myelitis), polio-like atrophy that developed as unilateral arm sensory and motor disturbance (Kyllerman, 1993), or recurrence (Shyu, et al., 1993), have been reported. In addition, the frequency of fever and eczema herpeticum has decreased, and the frequency of HSV-1 has increased as a causative virus. Today, it is generally accepted that the frequency of previously reported immunosuppressive underlying diseases in HSM is somewhat low. Moreover, cases of HSM with good prognosis have been reported because of the early diagnosis and the early induction of antiviral agent, acyclovir.

Age/ sex	Neurological symptom Clinical course	Fever	Rash	HSV subtype	Associated condition	Prognosis Sequelae	Author
45/F	Ascending myelitis	+	-	HSV-1	-	Death*	Klastersky 1972
21/F	Ascending myelitis	+	-	HSV**	Pregnancy	Severe	Koskiniemi 1982
M	Subacute ascending myelitis	-	+	HSV-2	AIDS	Death *	Britton 1985
36/M	Ascending myelitis	+	+	HSV-2	AIDS	Death *	Tucker 1985
57/M	Ascending myelitis	+	+	HSV-2	DM	Death *	Wiley 1987
29/F	Ascending myelitis	+	-	HSV-2	-	Severe	Ahmed 1988
64/M	Ascending myelitis	-	-	HSV-2	LK	Death *	Nakagawa 1991
74/F	Ascending myelitis	-	+	HSV-2	ATL	Death *	
64/M	Ascending myelitis	-	-	HSV-2	DM	Death *	Iwamasa 1991
7/M	Non-ascending myelitis	+	-	HSV-1	-	Severe	Kyllerman 1993
72/M	Recurrent ascending myelitis	-	+	HSV-1	-	Severe	Shyu 1993
59/M	Ascending myelitis	+	+	HSV-2	-	Death *	Folpe 1994
76/F	Subacute ascending myelitis	+	-	HSV-2	-	Death	Ellie 1994
51/M	Ascending myelitis	-	-	HSV**	-	Death	Radhakrishnan 1994
42/M	Non-ascending myelitis	-	-	HSV**	-	Recovery	Petereit 1996
44/M	Ascending myelitis	-	+	HSV-2	DM	Severe	Nakajima 1998
39/M	Ascending myelitis	+	-	HSV-2	-	Severe	
69/M	Ascending myelitis	-	-	HSV-2	-	Severe	
50/F	Ascending myelitis	+	-	HSV-2	-	Severe	
68/M	Ascending myelitis	-	-	HSV-2	-	Recovery	
38/M	Subacute ascending myelitis	-	+	HSV-2	-	Severe	
49/F	Recurrent non-ascending myelitis	-	-	HSV-2	-	Recovery	
69/M	Non-ascending myelitis	+	-	HSV-1	-	Severe	
58/M	Subacute non-ascending myelitis	-	-	HSV-1	-	Recovery	
48/M	Ascending myelitis	-	-	HSV-1	-	Recovery	Kuker 1999
6/M	Ascending myelitis	-	-	HSV**	-	Recovery	Galanakis 2001
70/F	Recurrent ascending myelitis	-	+	HSV-2	-	Recovery	Gobbi 2001
60/M	Non-ascending myelitis	-	-	HSV-1	-	Recovery	Azuma 2001
59/M	Encephalo-myelo-radiculitis	+	-	HSV-2	-	Severe	Kusuhara 2002

* Autopsy case, **Unknown HSV subtype, AIDS; Acquired immunodeficiency syndrome, DM; Diabetes mellitus, LK; Lung cancer, ATL; Adult T cell leukemia

Table 2. Clinical features of HSM

4. MRI findings

As MRI findings, spinal lesions of HSM are generally either hypointense or isointense on T1-weighted images and hyperintense on T2-weighted images similar to images obteined in HSV encephalitis (Ellie et al., 1994; Petereit et al, 1996; Nakajima et al., 1998; Kuker, et al., 1999; Galanakis et al., 2001; Gobbi et al., 2001; Azuma et al., 2001) (Fig. 1). Furthermore, spinal lesions occasionally accompany gadolinium enhancement (Fig. 2), and gadolinium enhancement of spinal nerve root and dura mater has been reported (Kuker, et al., 1999). In some cases, spinal lesions were exhibited as hyperintense on both T1 and T2-weighted images, which show hemorrhagic lesions (Nakajima et al., 1998) (Fig. 2). The size of spinal lesions varies, however, lesion in a patient with HSM is single and do not occur in multiple as seen in acute disseminated encephalomyelitis (ADEM) or multiple sclerosis.

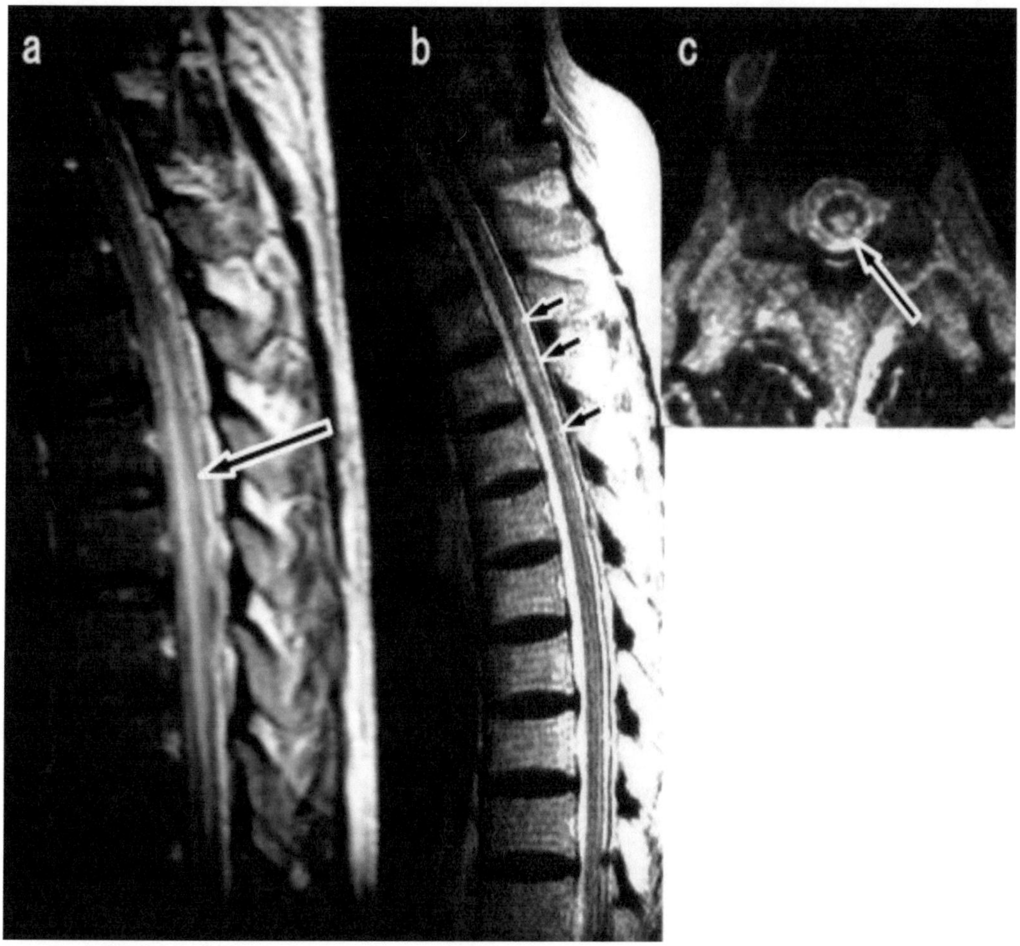

Fig. 1. MRI findings of HSM. Sagittal T2-weighted imageing of HSM (HSV-1) showed cord swellineg and a hyperintense signal in thoracic spinal cord (a). Sagital (b) and axial (c) T2-weighted imageing of HSM (HSV-2) showed hyperintense signal lesion in the posterior portion of thoracic spinal cord.

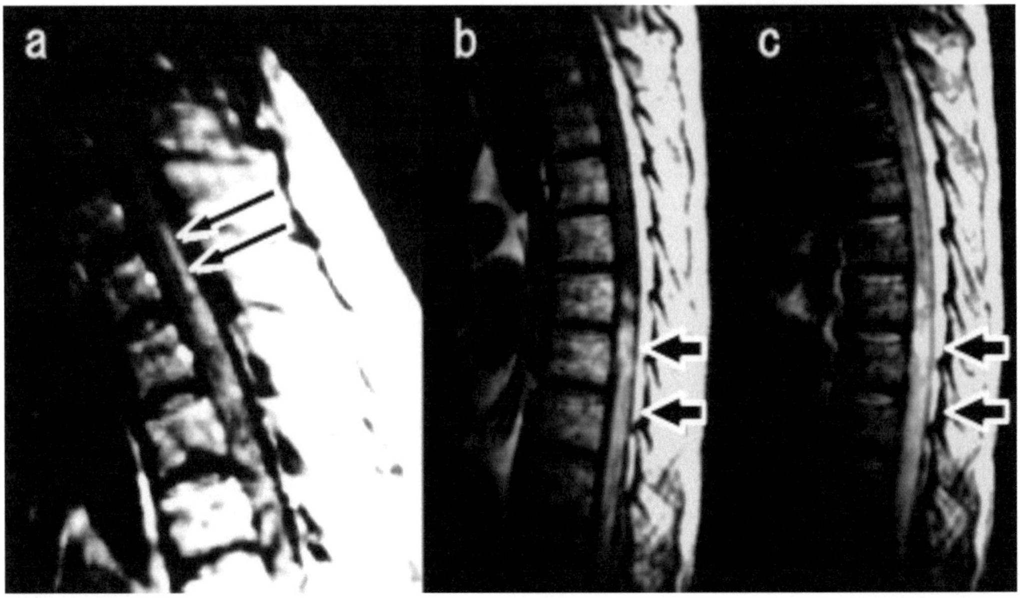

Fig. 2. MRI findings of HSM. Enhanced T1-weighted imageing of HSM (HSV-2) showed an increased signal intensity in the posterior portion of spinal cord at the T2-T4 level (a). T1-weighted imageing (TE600/TR20) (b) and T2-weighted imageing (TE3,000/TR60) (c) of HSM (HSV-2). Both sequences showed a hyperintense signal lesion which was continuous from the T7 level to the lumbosacral spinal cord.

5. Pathogenesis

All 8 reported cases of HSM that autopsy were performed were ascending myelitis (Klastersky et al, 1972; Koskiniemi et al., 1982; Britton et al., 1985; Tucker et al., 1985; Wiley et al., 1987; Nakagawa et al., 1991; Iwamasa et al., 1991; Shyu, et al., 1993). Myelitis was caused by HSV-1 in 1 patient and HSV-2 in 7 patients. Pathological findings showed marked necrosis of both gray and white matters, and such findings as hemorrhage, white blood cell (macrophage) infiltration, perivascular lymphocyte infiltration, and vascular necrosis were confirmed. These inflammatory changes and necrotic lesions were occasionally confirmed in dorsal spinal nerve roots and dorsal root ganglia. Furthermore, in these areas, Cowdry A inclusions, indicating HSV infection, were observed, and electronmicroscopy showed HSV particles. Based on these pathological findings, the onset mechanism for HSM could be deduced as follows: latent HSV-2 infection in the dorsal spinal nerve root of the lumbosacral spinal cord is reactivated by immunosuppression, and the virus enters the spine via the dorsal spinal nerve root. Since 1994, PCR-confirmed myelitis has exhibited various clinical features, such as non-ascending myelitis, recurrent or mild myelitis, and the incidence of HSV-1 has increased. While pathological analysis was not conducted, MRI showed gadolinium enhancement of the spinal nerve root and meninges (Kuker, et al., 1999), thus suggesting inflammation of the dorsal spinal nerve root. Regardless of clinical features and HSV type, myelitis is believed to be induced when HSV enters the spinal cord via the dorsal spinal nerve root or ganglion. It is difficult to ascertain whether HSM is caused by initial infection or reactivation due to latent infection. Most patients with HSM are older than middle age, and in patients in whom serum antibody titer was measured, anti-HSV antibody titer was positive in the early stage, thus suggesting that reactivation of latent HSV in a dorsal spinal nerve root ganglion induces myelitis. Since recurrence for HSV-2 is more frequent than that for HSV-1 in genital herpes, recurrent myelitis may be due to HSV-2. Diagnosis cannot be based solely on serum HSV antibody tier, because there was a case of HSM in whom the progress of serum HSV antibody titer ashowed past infection, while that of CSF titier indicated initial HSV infection (see Case presentation case 1). Recently, one study reported a patient in whom HSV-2 caused genital herpes, while HSV-1 was detected in the CSF from Elsberg syndrome (Yoritaka et al., 2005). This suggests that even in the same host, different HSV types and strains repeat infection and reactivation.

6. Immunological regulation in HSM (animal model)

T-cell-mediated immunities have been shown to be involved in the pathology of HSM. Th1-cell-associated cellular responses (Th1 responses) are known to be essential in the host defence against systemic infections of HSV. Th1 responses are manifested by the increased production of Th1 cytokines (IL-2, IFN-1, etc.) from Th1 cells, while Th2-cell-associated cellular responses (Th2 responses) are manifested by the production of Th2 cytokines (IL-4, L-10, L-13, etc.) released from Th2 cells. Th2 cytokines are known to be inhibitors for the differentiation and expression of Th1 cells. Previously, the pathogenic role of Th2 responses on the severity of HSM was investigated in mice exposed to footpad injection of HSV-2 (Nakajima et al., 2000). Morbidity and mortality of mice with HSM increased when they were treated with a mixture of Th2 (IL-4/IL-10) cytokines (Fig. 3a). The mortality rates of HSM mice were significantly influenced by the IL-4/IL-10 mixture at doses ranging from 1 to 100 pg per mouse. High doses (more than 1000 pg per mouse) of the IL-4/IL-10 mixture did not show significant effects on the mortality of HSM mice. There is an optimum effective dose of the cytokines in these experimental methods (Fig. 3b). Patients with AIDS, malignancy, diabetes mellitus or psychosomatic stress reaction commonly carry dysfunction in T cell functions, and a shift from Th1 responses to Th2 responses has been reported in these patients. Thus, The regulation of Th1/Th2 balance may be a key on the immunological control of HSM.

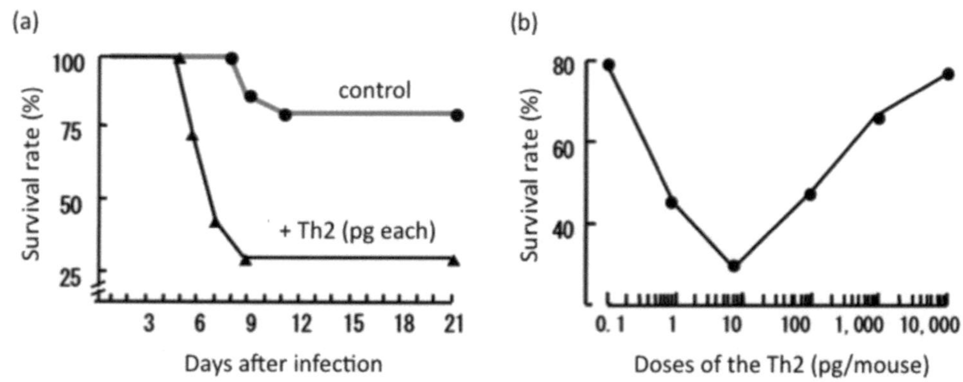

Fig. 3. a: Effect of the IL-4/IL-10 mixture on the morbidity and mortality of HSM mice. b: Effect of various doses of the IL-4/IL-10 mixture.

7. HSV subtyping

Retrospective clinical data was collected on 10 cases of herpes simplex myelitis from 5 institutions in Japan. All cases were diagnosed by using PCR. We assessed differences in clinical presentation, laboratory findings, MRI images, and treatment outcome between HSV-1 and HSV-2 (Table 3).

In most cases, herpes simplex myelitis occurred in immunocompetent persons. In 7 cases, disease onset was marked by sensorimotor disturbances of the lower extremities and urinary disturbances, with the transverse myelopathy ascending to the cervicothoracic

		Number
Age / Sex	51 (29 - 69) / male : female = 8 : 2	
Clinical symptoms		
(Initial Symptoms)	Leg numbness, weakness, urinary disturbance	8
	Unilateral hypesthesia	1
	Unilateral limb sensorimotor disturbances	1
(Maximum)	Transverse myelopathy	10
(Progression)		
	Ascending myelopathy	7
	Non-ascending pattern	3
Associated condition	HIV	1
	Diabetes mellitus	2
Herpes eruption	Genital herpes	3
Therapy	Acyclovir + Steroids	8
	Acyclovir	1
	Steroids	1
Clinical course	Acute	8
		(recurrence 1)
	Subacute	2
		(recurrence 1)
Prognosis	No lethal cases	
	Severe sequelae (paraplegia)	7
	Recovery	3
CSF findings	Cell	11-226 mm3
	Protein	51-276 mg/dl
	Positive oligoclonal band	1
MRI findings	Hyperintense lesions in T2WI	7
	Hyperintense lesions in T1/T2	1
	Gd-enhancement	3
HSV antibodies	IgG elevation	10
	IgM elevation	1
PCR (HSV type)	HSV-1	7
	HSV-2	3

Table 3. Clinical features of 10 patients with HSM

spinal cord level. The other 3 cases demonstrated transverse myelopathy without an ascending pattern. Two cases exhibited recurrent episodes. Nine out of 10 patients had CSF pleocytosis, and MRI demonstrated single lesions that were longitudinal or limited. HSV-2 was detected by PCR at an early stage in all 7 patients with ascending myelitis. HSV-1 DNA was detected in 2 and HSV-2 DNA was detected in 1 of the 3 cases with a non-ascending pattern. All recurrent cases were caused by HSV-2. Anti-herpetic drugs, notably acyclovir, improved mortality. However, because severe sequelae, such as paraplegia, persisted in 7 out of 10 patients, early introduction of acyclovir is necessary. These results demonstrate diverse clinical manifestations of herpes simplex myelitis. The cases of herpes simplex myelitis with an ascending pattern or recurrent course are caused by HSV-2, while those with a non-ascending pattern are mainly caused by HSV-1. Furthermore, a recurrent course is considered to be characteristic of HSV-2 infection (Table 4).

		HSV-1	HSV-2
Case number		n=2	n=8
Clinical symptoms			
Ascending myelopathy	(7 cases)	0	7
Non-ascending pattern	(3 cases)	2	1
Clinical course			
Acute	(8 cases)	1	7
Subacute	(2 cases)	1	1
Recurrence	(2 cases)	0	2
Associated condition			
HIV	(1 case)	1	0
Diabetes mellitus	(2 cases)	0	0
Cases with genital herpes	(3 cases)	0	3
Prognosis			
Severe sequelae	(7 cases)	0	7
Recovery/mild sequelae	(3 cases)	2	1

Table 4. Distinction between HSV-1 and HSV-2

8. PCR methods

PCR represents an important technique for diagnosis and therapeutic planning. PCR is widely utilized by medical institutions and private testing companies. However, because CSF samples collected by lumbar puncture from patients with encephalitis contain very small amounts of HSV DNA, the sensitivity of PCR, nested PCR or real-time PCR must be improved.

8.1 Nested PCR assay

Retrospectively PCR assays were performed as described (Nakajima et al., 1998). The CSF samples were stored at -80°C until PCR. Template DNA was extracted from 300 µl of CSF and HSV DNA was amplified by nested PCR assay. The primer sequences were chosen to flank a conserved region in the HSV-I and HSV-2 DNA polymerase gene. The primers used in the first PCR were as follows: 5'-CAGTACGGCCCCGAGTTCGTGACCGGG-3' and 5'-TACTCGCCGATCACCCCGCG-3'. For the nested PCR, 5'- CATCATCAACTTCGACTGGC-CC-3' and 5'-GGCGTAGTAGGCGGGGATGTCGCG-3' were constructed as the inner primer pair. On the first round of PCR, the profile consisted of DNA denaturation at 94°C for I min, primer annealing at 60°C for 1 min and primer extension at 72°C for I min for 35 cycles. On the second round of PCR, l µl aliquots of the first PCR products were added to 49 pl ofa freshly prepared reaction mixture, followed by 30 cycles of amplihcation at 95°C for 30s, 60°C for 30s, and 72°C for 30s. When HSV-I or HSV-2 DNA was present in the mixture, a 298-bp sequence was amplified by nested PCR. Within this sequence, individual virus strains have unique restriction sites so that amplification product could be typed by digestion with Bgl II and Xho I. As shown in Fig 4, agarose gel electrophoresis showed nested PCR amplified products of HSV-I and HSV-2 strains at a sequence of 298 bp (a). The specific recognition sequence for Xho I is only present in HSV- I DNA, and that for Bgl II is only present in HSV-2 DNA. Xho I yields 209- and 89-bp fragments for HSV-I, whereas Bgl II yields 45- and 253-bp fragments for HSV-2 (b). 1 = HSV-I strain; 2 = HSV-2 strain; 3 = CSF sample from HSM case; 4 = CSF sample from negative control; M = molecular weight makers (Hae III digest of ΦX174).

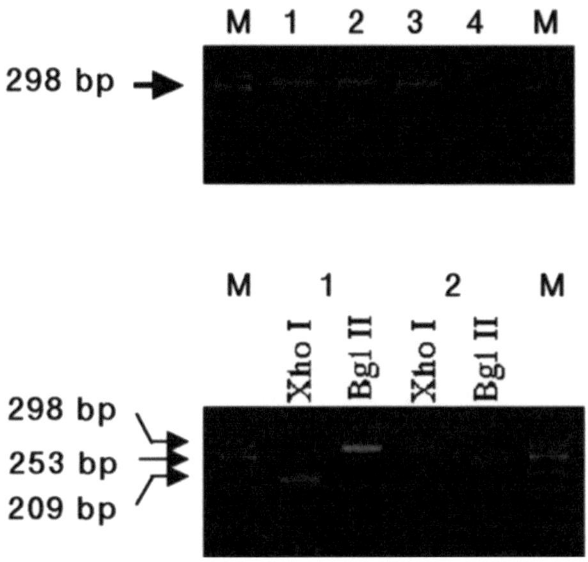

Fig. 4. Defferenciation of HSV-1 and HSV-2 by restriction pattern of PCR pruducts.

8.2 LightCycler PCR

Real-time PCR was performed using a LightCycler (Roche Diagnostics, Mannheim, Germany) and a LightCycler HSV 1/2 Detection Kit (Roche Diagnostics, Mannheim, Germany), which contains the necessary primers, fluorescent-labeled probes, Taq DNA polymerase and reaction buffers for Hybri-probe PCR. Using 20 µl reaction solutions, each containing 2 µl of CSF sample that had been boiled at 100°C. PCR was performed with preprocessing, temperature cycle (amplification) and melting curve analysis. Cycling conditions were as follows: initial denaturation /FastStart Taq DNA polymerase activation at 95°C/10 min, 45 cycles of denaturation at 95°C/10 sec, annealing at 55°C/15 sec and extension at 72°C/15 sec. After amplification was complete, melting curve analysis was performed as follows: starting at 40°C followed by a gradual increase in temperature (transition rate of 0.1°C/sec) to 80°C with continuous fluorescence acquisition. The fragment selected for amplification and detection using the HSV 1/2 Detection Kit includes areas specific to HSV-1 and HSV-2 subtypes and an area common to the two subtypes (the primer region of the DNA polymerase gene is highly conserved for both HSV-1 and HSV-2). Sequence differences between the PCR product and hybridization probes resulted in shifts in the melting temperatures Analysis of the PCR amplification and probe melting curves was accomplished through the use of LightCycler software.

8.3 Sensitivity and selectivity (Comparison with nested PCR)

Using plasmid DNA carrying the HSV DNA polymerase gene that was included in the LightCycler HSV 1/2 Detection Kit as a positive control, serially diluted samples were analyzed. Results showed that fluorescent signals can be detected even at a concentration of 1 copy/tube, and determination was possible up to 10^3 copies/tube (Fig. 5a). Melting analysis was conducted by measuring fluorescent intensity at different melting temperatures after amplifying HSV-1- and HSV-2-positive samples. Fig. 5b shows cumulative fluorescent intensity per unit temperature. Peak melting temperature was 54 °C for HSV-1 and 67 °C for HSV-2, and HSV subtypes could be differentiated based on this difference in melting temperature. By the analysis of CSF samples, detection sensitivity of LightCycler PCR is comparable to that of nested PCR. In addition, subtype differentiation based on melting curve analysis matched that based on restriction band patterns of nested PCR products (Table 5). The process of LightCycler PCR including melting curve analysis took about 50 min to complete.

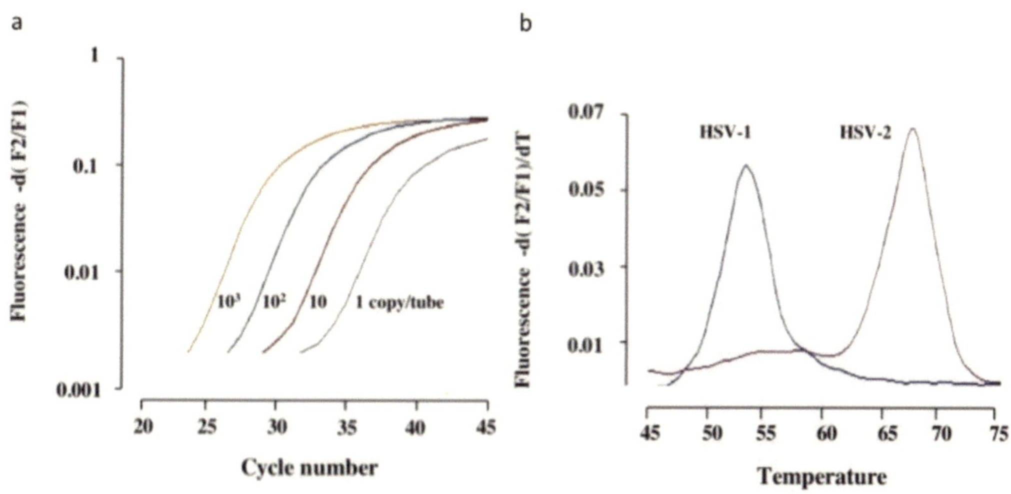

Fig. 5. a: Amplification of HSV DNA by LightCycler PCR. b: Defferenciation of HSV-1 and HSV-2 by melting curve analysis matched.

No.	Diagnosis	Conventional PCR			LightCycler
		Direct	Nested	Subtype*	
1	Encephalitis	-	+	HSV-1	HSV-1
2	Encephalitis	-	+	HSV-1	HSV-1
3	Encephalitis	-	+	HSV-1	HSV-1
4	Encephalitis	-	+	HSV-1	HSV-1
5	Encephalitis	-	+	HSV-1	HSV-1
6	Myelitis	-	+	HSV-2	HSV-2
7	Myelitis	-	+	HSV-2	HSV-2
8	Myelitis	-	+	HSV-1	HSV-1

*Differentiation of HSV types 1 and 2 was made by restriction fragment length of nested PCR productions

Table 5. Comparison of conventional PCR and LightCycler PCR

9. Diagnosis

Table 6 shows the guide for the diagnosis of HSM. In terms of clinical symptoms, ascending myelitis, back pain, and fever can indicate HSV, but it is essential to conduct neurological and virological tests. In the past, eczema herpeticum was identified during disease onset or progression, and as a result, eczema herpeticum is considered a diagnostic clue for HSM. However, according to recent reports, the frequency of eczema herpeticum is not been high, and there has been a report of a patient with Elsberg syndrome in which different HSV types were found in genital rash and cerebrospinal fluid (Yoritaka et al., 2005). Thus, it is considered essential to diagnose HSV infection using a cerebrospinal fluid sample. Table 7 lists diseases that must be differentiated from HSM. If clinical symptoms and MRI findings indicate myelitis and a cerebrospinal fluid test suggests an infection, it is important to conduct a virological test using a cerebrospinal fluid sample in order to rule out HSM. As HSM is rare disease, HSM were previously reported as case presentation, and there is no large-scale epidemiological survey. In Japan, There was a regional questionary survey of the central nervous infection caused by HSV (Kyushu/Okinawa area (the southwestern Japan): 1993-1996). That questionary survey was performed among approximately 100 pediatric

1. Clinical manifestation: neurological symptoms associated with acute or subacute myelitis/myelopathy.
2. Neurodiagnostic tests:
   - MRI shows spinal cord lesions with oedeam or necrosis.
   - CSF analysis demonstrates elevated mononuclear cells and protein.
3. Virologic analysis:
   - PCR of the CSF is the most beneficial diagnostic method.
   - CSF antibody measurements may be useful in retrospective diagnosis
   - Virus cultures are of little value for the diagnosis of HSM

Table 6. Diagnosis of HSM

and/or neurology institutions in Kyushu/Okinawa District between 1993-1996. There were 4 HSM cases among 39 HSV–induced central nerve infections diagnosed by PCR and HSV antibody titers (Table 8). HSM have been increasingly recognized by the diagnostic use of the PCR and the accumulation of the case report. In patients with spinal lesions suggesting the myelitis, virologic examination using CSF specimen should be performed.

- Viral disease
  Varicella-zoster virus, Cytomegalovirus, EB virus, HHV-6, enterovirus (poliomyelitis, Coxsackie, echo), HTLV-1, HIV
- Bacterial disease
  Mycoplasma, Lyme's disease, Syphilis
- Demyelinating disease
  Acute disseminated encephalomyelitis, Neuromyelitis optica, Multiple sclerosis
- Systemic autoimmune disease
  Sjogren's syndrome, Systemic lupus erythematosus, Anti-phospholipid syndrome, Sarcoidosis
- Allergic condition
  Atopic myelitis
- Paraneoplastic syndrome
- Vascular disorder
  Spinal cord infarction, Arteriovenous malformation, Vasculitis
- Spinal tumor
  Malignant lymphoma

Table 7. Differential diagnosis

	Number (n=39)
Temporal lobe/ limbic encephalitis	24
Brainstem encephalitis	1
Diffuse cerebrum	2
Acute disseminated encephalomyelitis	3
Myelitis	4
Meningitis	2
Others	3

Table 8. The clinical form of the central nervous infection caused by HSV: Questionary survey of Kyushu/Okinawa area (the southwestern Japan) (1993-1996)

10. Therapy

HSM was once considered a lethal disease, but in recent years, there have been reports of survival and recovery, primarily due to the use of anti-herpes agents. If HSM is suspected based on clinical findings, diagnostic imaging, and cerebrospinal fluid findings, then acyclovir should be administered. If acyclovir is not effective, even when HSM is confirmed or strongly suggested, concurrent use of vidarabine should be considered. In the past, an antiviral agent and a steroidal agent were concurrently administered in many patients. Of the 9 patients in the above mentioned study, a steroidal agent was administered concurrently: methylprednisolone pulse therapy in 4 patients, betamethasone in 2 patients and predonine in 1 patient (Nakajima et al., 1998). Regarding the use of steroids, while steroids were used after confirming HSM in some patients, they were also used in combination with antiviral agents because of suspected demyelinating disease, such as ADEM or multiple sclerosis; autoimmune/inflammatory diseases, such as, vasculitis; or cryptogenic transverse myelopathy. Due to their anti-edema action, steroids can be used to treat HSM and herpes encephalitis, however, the immunosuppressive effects of steroids may enhance HSV proliferation. In studies using an animal model of herpes encephalitis, steroid administration did not increase the amount of HSV in the brain or exacerbate encephalitis (Thompson et al., 2000; Meyding-Lamade et al., 2003), but because there has not been a controlled clinical study on the concurrent use of steroids for the treatment of herpes encephalitis, no clear therapeutic guidelines for the treatment of herpes encephalitis using steroids have been established. However, one recent study investigated the use of steroids in herpes encephalitis in clinical settings (Kamei et al., 2005). In order to clarify the prognosticators for herpes encephalitis, the study examined age, background factors, clinical symptoms, and treatment, and the results showed that prognosis was more favorable with antiviral and steroid combination therapy than with antiviral monotherapy. Therefore, steroids can improve prognosis by suppressing edema formation, inflammatory cytokine production, and secondary autoimmune mechanisms. As a result, we believe that steroids should be actively combined with antiviral agents for the treatment of HSM.

11. Conclusions

Initially, HSM was reported to be lethal acute ascending myelitis that was likely to occur in immunocompromised hosts; however, with the recent improvements in viral diagnosis, including PCR and diagnostic imaging, it has been shown that the clinical features and onset of HSM greatly vary. With the use of antiviral agents, there have been more reports of survivors, but many patients have experienced severe aftereffects, such as paraplegia and quadriplegia, thus suggesting the importance of early diagnosis and therapy. Immunological mechanisms are involved in the onset and pathogenesis of HSM (Nakajima et al., 2000; Nakajima et al., 2001), and establishing a treatment that suppresses viral proliferation using an antiviral agent and reduces inflammation through immunological control is useful for alleviating organic damage to the central nerve, improving survival, and reducing aftereffects.

12. References

Ahmed I. (1988). Survival after herpes simplex type II myelitis. *Neurology*, Vol. 38, No. 9, (Sep.1988), pp. 1500.

Aurelius, E., Johansson, B., Skoldenberg, B., Staland, A. & Forsgren, M. (1991). Rapid diagnosis of herpes simplex encephalitis by nested polymerase chain reaction assay of cerebrospinal fluid. *Lancet*, Vol. 337, No. 8735, (Jan. 1991), pp. 189-192.

Azuma, K., Yoshimoto, M., Nishimura, Y., Fujimoto, H., Ayabe, M., Shoji, H. & Eizuru, Y. (2001). Herpes simplex virus type 1 myelitis with a favorable outcome. *Intern Med*, Vol. 40, No. 10, (Oct. 2001), pp. 1068-1069.

Britton, CB., Mesa-Tejada, R., Fenoglio CM., Hays, AP., Garvey, GG. & Miller, JR. (1985). A new complication of AIDS: thoracic myelitis caused by herpes simplex virus. *Neurology*, Vol. 35, No. 7, (Jul. 1985), pp.1071-1074.

Eberhardt, O., Kuker, W., Dichgans, J. & Weller, M. (2004). HSV-2 sacral radiculitis (Elsberg syndrome). *Neurology*, Vol. 63, NO. 4, (Aug. 2004), pp. 758-759.

Ellie, E., Rozenberg, F., Dousset, V. & Beylot-Barry, M. (1994). Herpes simplex virus type 2 ascending myeloradiculitis: MRI findings and rapid diagnosis by the polymerase chain method. *J Neurol Neurosurg Psychiatry*, Vol. 57, No. 7, (Jul. 1994), pp. 869-870.

Folpe, A., Lapham, LW. & Smith, HC. (1994). Herpes simplex myelitis as a cause of acute necrotizing myelitis syndrome. *Neurology*, Vol. 44, No. 10, (Oct. 1994), pp. 1955-1957.

Galanakis, E., Bikouvarakis, S., Mamoulakis, D., Karampekios, S. & Sbyrakis, S. (2001). Transverse myelitis associated with herpes simplex virus infection. *J Child Neurol*, Vol. 16, No. 11, (Nov. 2001), pp. 866-867.

Gobbi C., Tosi C., Stadler C., Merenda C. & Bernasconi E. (2001). Recurrent myelitis associated with herpes simplex virus type 2. *Eur Neurol*, Vol. 46, No. 4, (2001), pp. 215-218.

Iwamasa, T., Yoshitake, H., Sakuda, H., Kamada, Y., Miyazato, M., Utsumi, Y. & Nakamura, A. (1991). Acute ascending necrotizing myelitis in Okinawa caused by herpes simplex virus type 2. *Virchows Arch A Pathol Anat Histopathol*, Vol. 418, No. 1, (1991), pp. 71-75.

Kamei, S., Sekizawa, T., Shiota, H., Mizutani, T., Itoyama, Y., Takasu, T., Morishima, T. & Hirayanagi, K. (2005). Evaluation of combination therapy using aciclovir and corticosteroid in adult patients with herpes simplex virus encephalitis. *J Neurol Neurosurg Psychiatry*, Vol. 76, N0. 11, (Nov. 2005), pp. 1544-1549.

Klastersky, J., Cappel, R., Snoeck, JM., Flament, J. & Thiry, L. (1972). Ascending myelitis in association with herpes-simplex virus. *N Engl J Med*, Vol. 287, No. 4, (Jul. 1972), pp. 182-184.

Koskiniemi, ML., Vaheri, A., Manninen, V. & Nikki, P. (1982). Ascending myelitis with high antibody titer to herpes simplex virus in the cerebrospinal fluid. *J Neurol*, Vol. 227, No. 3, (1982), pp. 187-191.

Kuker, W., Schaade, L., Ritter, K. & Nacimiento, W. (1999). MRI follow-up of herpes simplex virus (type 1) radiculomyelitis. *Neurology*, Vol. 52, No. %, (Mar. 1999), pp. 1102-1103.

Kusuhara, T., Nakajima, M., Inoue, H., Takahashi, M. & Yamada, T. (2002). Parainfectious encephalomyeloradiculitis associated with herpes simplex virus 1 DNA in cerebrospinal fluid. *Clin Infect Dis*, Vol. 34, No. 9, (May. 2002), pp. 1199-1205.

Kyllerman, MG., Herner, S., Bergstrom, TB. & Ekholm, SE. (1993). PCR diagnosis of primary herpesvirus type I in poliomyelitis-like paralysis and respiratory tract disease. *Pediatr Neurol*, Vol. 9, No. 3, (May-Jun. 1993), pp. 227-229.

Meyding-Lamade, UK., Oberlinner, C., Rau, PR., Seyfer, S., Heiland, S., Sellner, J., Wildemann, BT. & Lamade, WR. (2003). Experimental herpes simplex virus encephalitis: a combination therapy of acyclovir and glucocorticoids reduces long-term magnetic resonance imaging abnormalities. *J Neurovirol*, Vol. 9, No. 1, (Feb. 2003), pp. 118-125.

Nakagawa, M., Nakamura, A., Kubota, R., Kakazu, T., Kuba, M., Nakasone, K. & Iwamasa, T. (1991). Necrotizing myelopathy associated with malignancy caused by herpes simplex virus type 2: clinical report of two cases and literature review. *Jpn J Med*, Vol. 30, No. 2, (Mar.-Apr. 1991), pp. 182-188.

Nakajima, H., Furutama, D., Kimura, F., Shinoda, K., Ohsawa, N., Nakagawa, T., Shimizu, A. & Shoji, H. (1998). Herpes simplex virus myelitis: clinical manifestations and diagnosis by the polymerase chain reaction method. *Eur Neurol*, Vol. 39, No. 3, (1998), pp. 163-167.

Nakajima, H., Kobayashi, M., Pollard, RB. & Suzuki, F. (2000). A pathogenic role of Th2 responses on the severity of encephalomyelitis induced in mice by herpes simplex virus type 2 infection. *J Neuroimmunol*, Vol. 110, No. 1-2, (Oct. 2000), pp. 106-13.

Nakajima, H., Kobayashi, M., Pollard, RB. & Suzuki, F. (2001). Monocyte chemoattractant protein-1 enhances HSV-induced encephalomyelitiss by stimulating Th2 responses. *J Leukocyte Biol*, Vol. 70, No. 3, (Sep. 2001), pp. 374-380.

Nakajima, H., Hanafusa, T., Nakagawa, T. & Shimizu, A. (2005). Rapid detection and subtyping of herpes simplex virus DNA in CSF by means of LightCycler PCR. *Current Trends in Neurology*, Vol. 1, pp. 134-135.

Petereit, HF., Bamborschke, S. & Lanfermann, H. (1996). Acute transverse myelitis caused by herpes simplex virus. *Eur Neurol*, Vol. 36, No. 1, (1996), pp. 52-53.

Radhakrishnan, VV., Saraswathy, A., Mohan, PK. & Narayanan, SK. (1994). Necrotizing myelopathy--a report of two cases with review of literature. *Indian J Pathol Microbiol*, Vol. 37, No. 4, (Oct. 1994), pp. 439-445.

Shyu, WC., Lin, JC., Chang, BC., Harn, HJ., Lee, CC. & Tsao, WL. (1993). Recurrent ascending myelitis: an unusual presentation of herpes simplex virus type 1 infection. *Ann Neurol*, Vol. 34, No. 4, (Oct. 1993), pp. 625-627.

Thompson, KA., Blessing, WW. & Wesselingh, SL. (2000). Herpes simplex replication and dissemination is not increased by corticosteroid treatment in a rat model of focal Herpes encephalitis. *J Neurovirol*, Vol. 6, No. 1, (Feb. 2000), pp. 25-32.

Tucker, T., Dix, RD., Katzen, C., Davis, RL. & Schmidley, JW. (1985). Cytomegalovirus and herpes simplex virus ascending myelitis in a patient with acquired immune deficiency syndrome. *Ann Neurol*, Vol. 18, No. 1, (Jul. 1985), pp. 74-79.

Tyler, KL. (2004). Herpes simplex virus infections of the central nervous system: encephalitis and meningitis, including Mollaret's. *Herpes*, Vol. 11, Suppl 2, (Jun. 2004), pp. A57-A64.

Wiley, CA., VanPatten, PD., Carpenter, PM., Powell, HC. & Thal, LJ. (1987). Acute ascending necrotizing myelopathy caused by herpes simplex virus type 2. *Neurology*, Vol. 37, No. 11, (Nov. 1987), pp. 1791-1794.

Yoritaka, A., Ohta, K. & Kishida, S. (2005). Herpetic lumbosacral radiculoneuropathy in patients with human immunodeficiency virus infection. *Eur Neurol*, Vol. 53, No. 4, (20005), pp. 179-181.

11

Astrocyte CD38: Links to Neuroinflammation in HAND

Sugato Banerjee and Anuja Ghorpade
Department of Cell Biology and Anatomy, University of North Texas Health Science Center, Fort Worth, TX USA

1. Introduction

Central nervous system (CNS) HIV-1 infection can lead to encephalitis (HIVE), which compromises brain function and presents clinically as HIV-associated dementia [HAD, (Navia et al., 1986; Price et al., 1988; Wiley and Achim, 1994; Brew et al., 1995; Grant, 2008; Letendre et al., 2008; Price and Spudich, 2008)], the most serious form of HIV-associated neurocognitive disorders [HAND, (Grant, 2008; Letendre et al., 2008)]. HAND is associated with various cognitive, behavioral and motor dysfunctions [for details refer (Ances and Ellis, 2007; Grant, 2008)]. Although initiation of combined antiretroviral therapy (cART) has been linked to cognitive improvement and decreased incidence of HAD (Brodt et al., 1997; Sacktor et al., 1999; Foley et al., 2008), the yearly incidence rates for milder forms of HAND are still as high as 10-25% (Woods et al., 2009), and the prevalence of HAD is on the rise due to longer life expectancy of HIV-1-infected individuals (Lindl et al., 2010).

The neuroinflammatory cascade associated with HAND, beginning with the infiltration of HIV-1-infected macrophages and immune activated microglial cells, likely reaches the endpoint of neurodegeneration via glial activation and changes in glial inflammatory responses (Kaul and Lipton, 2006). Reactive astrogliosis, the recruitment to and proliferation of astroglial cells at injury sites, is commonly observed during HIVE (Gonzales and Davis, 1988; Persidsky et al., 1996; Ridet et al., 1997; Wu and Schwartz, 1998; Petito et al., 1999). Astrocytes are the most abundant cell type in the CNS; and yet, their specific roles continue to be unraveled. Thus, characterization of molecules/pathways involving the activated astrocytes during HIVE and HAND, is of high interest.

CD38 expression on peripheral T lymphocytes is a marker for disease progression in HIV-1-infected patients (Savarino et al., 2000; Vigano et al., 2000; Kolber, 2008; Sinclair et al., 2008). CD38 is a 45-kD ectoenzyme involved in the synthesis of potent calcium- (Ca^{2+}) mobilizing agents, cyclic ADP ribose (cADPR) and nicotinic acid adenine dinucleotide phosphate (NAADP+) (Heidemann et al., 2005b; Banerjee et al., 2008). CD38 expression has been detected both in neurons and astrocytes in the cerebral cortex (Mizuguchi et al., 1995; Yamada et al., 1997), while it is primarily expressed by astrocytes in culture (Pawlikowska et al., 1996). Our group has shown that CD38 is one of the most upregulated molecules in IL-1β-activated astroglial cells *in vitro* and is also expressed by astrocytes in HIVE brain tissues

(Kou et al., 2009). However, very little is known about the role of CD38 in HAND. In this review, we will explore the possible mechanistic links between, astrocyte-CD38 upregulation, Ca^{2+} homeostasis and HIV-1 neuropathogenesis.

2. Neuroinflammation during HIVE and astrocytes

HIV-1 enters the brain early, after systemic infection of circulating T cells and macrophages, by crossing the blood brain barrier [BBB (Bell et al., 1998; Bell, 2004)]. Neurons are rarely infected by the virus (Price et al., 1988; Kaul et al., 2001; Ellis et al., 2007), thus most neuronal damage is due to indirect toxicity mediated by activated astrocytes and virus-infected and/or activated mononuclear phagocytes (MP, macrophage/microglia). However, viral proteins like HIV-1 Tat and gp120 released by infected MP may show direct neurotoxicity (Mauermann et al., 2008; Li et al., 2009). Pro-inflammatory cytokines such as tumor necrosis factor (TNF)-α, interleukin (IL)-1β and IL-6, have been implicated in HIV-1 neuropathogenesis (Dickson et al., 1991; Sebire et al., 1993; Gendelman and Tardieu, 1994; Persidsky et al., 1999). Indeed, IL-1β production is one of the first responses observed upon activation of immune cells including MP (Pellegrini et al., 1996). This suggests that immune cell activation during peripheral HIV-1 infection may provide soluble IL-1β that penetrates the BBB (Vitkovic et al., 2000a; Vitkovic et al., 2000b). Brain tissue and cerebrospinal fluid from HIVE patients (Gallo et al., 1991; Tyor et al., 1993; Vitkovic et al., 1995; Boven et al., 1999), as well as brain tissue from simian immunodeficiency virus infected rhesus monkeys (Lane et al., 1996), demonstrated elevated IL-1β levels. Various studies have shown links between IL-1β and astrocyte activation during HIVE (Blumberg et al., 1994; Kaul and Lipton, 2006; Peng et al., 2006). IL-1β is also known to stimulate release of neurotoxic molecules like reactive oxygen species and inducible nitric oxide synthase by astrocytes (Jana et al., 2005; Sharma et al., 2007). Our previous work showed IL-1β-mediated astrocyte Fas ligand expression and subsequent caspase activation in surrounding neurons *in vitro* (Deshpande et al., 2005). We have also shown the effects of IL-1β and HIV-1 gp120, leading to CD38 upregulation in primary astrocyte cultures (Banerjee et al., 2008) and increased CD38 mRNA and protein expression in HIVE brain (Kou et al., 2009). IL-1β-activated astrocytes are known to release cytokines like IL-6 and chemokines like CCL2, CXCL8 and RANTES (Lee and Aarhus, 1993; Zhao and Brinton, 2004; Sharma et al., 2007). Our work showed that CD38 is a partial regulator of chemokine and cytokine signaling by IL-1β-activated astrocytes, thus affecting the inflammatory milieu during HIVE (Kou et al., 2009). IL-1β has also been shown to mediate activation of mitogen activated protein kinases (MAPKs) in primary astrocyte cultures (Parker et al., 2002; Zhao et al., 2004). MAPKs belong to a family of serine threonine kinases [for details refer (Davis, 1995; Chang and Karin, 2001)]. These kinases are involved in inflammation, cell proliferation and differentiation in astrocytes (Rajan and McKay, 1998; Hua et al., 2002; Morita et al., 2003). It is also well established, that the prolonged activation of MAPKs and nuclear factor (NF)-κB may mediate inflammatory conditions during HIVE (Yi et al., 2004; Kaul and Lipton, 2006). Our studies have shown direct involvement of MAPK and NF-κB in the regulation of CD38 expression and signaling in primary astrocytes, thus indicating that CD38 may be a major molecule in astrocyte-mediated inflammatory signaling in HIVE brain (Mamik et al., In Press).

3. Calcium in glial biological functions and HAND

Astrocytes can sense, respond to, and modulate neuronal activity (Cotrina and Nedergaard, 2005; Heidemann et al., 2005a). They provide crucial support for neurons and the other CNS cells through diverse functions, ranging from the production of neurotrophic factors to the elimination of neurotoxins (Ransom et al., 2003). Their ability to respond vigorously to diverse neural insults is commonly referred to as reactive astrogliosis, astrocytosis or astrocyte activation (Eng and Ghirnikar, 1994). Astrogliosis is associated with HAND and also observed in HIV-1 gp120 transgenic mice (Kaul et al., 2001). Since astrocytes are not electrically excitable, they sense changes in the microenvironment through receptors on their plasma membranes. Activation of these transmembrane receptors or ion channels and intracellular endoplasmic reticulum (ER) receptors, as well as mitochondrial Na^+/Ca^{2+} exchangers, increases intracellular calcium concentration ($[Ca^{2+}]_i$) [for details review (Cotrina and Nedergaard, 2005; Reyes and Parpura, 2009)]. Depending on the amplitude, spatial resolution and duration of Ca^{2+} response, genes are up or downregulated (Berridge et al., 2003). Change in free $[Ca^{2+}]_i$ also results in secretion of glutamate and other neuro-active compounds (peptides, eicosanoids, neurotrophins) into the microenvironment. These substances modulate the activity of juxtaposed neurons and other astrocytes (Cotrina and Nedergaard, 2005). In addition, Ca^{2+} waves are also used for long-distance communication between astrocytes via gap junction proteins, which in turn can be modulated by IL-1β (John et al., 1999).

After a physiological task is completed, the cytosolic Ca^{2+} levels return to normal by extrusion of Ca^{2+} either via Na^+/Ca^{2+} exchangers or plasma membrane Ca^{2+}-ATPases (Rojas et al., 2004; Rojas et al., 2007), while Ca^{2+} mobilized from internal stores return to normal via sarco/ER Ca^{2+}-ATPase (Bers, 2002; Wang et al., 2006; Liu et al., 2007). Some recent reports show that mitochondrial Ca^{2+} uniporter may also act as a sink to trap off the excess $[Ca^{2+}]_i$ (Reyes and Parpura, 2008, 2009). Thus, the physiological levels of free $[Ca^{2+}]_i$ are tightly controlled. However, Ca^{2+} overload triggered by excessive influx through plasma membrane voltage and receptor-operated channels, by metabotropic receptors or Ca^{2+} released from intracellular pools, may lead to HIV-1-induced neurotoxicity (Nath and Geiger, 1998; Holden et al., 1999). Mobilization of intracellular Ca^{2+} pools is an important modulator of apoptosis in various cells, including T cells, ventricular myocytes, and cerebellar granule cells (Khan et al., 1996; Jayaraman and Marks, 1997; Lin and Leonard, 1997; Felzen et al., 1998; Herbein et al., 1998). Furthermore, it has been associated with HIV-1 gp120-induced neuronal cell death *in vitro* (Meucci et al., 1998).

4. CD38 function and Ca^{2+} homeostasis

It has been suggested that there is more than one substrate for the enzymatic activity of CD38, including nicotinamide adenine dinucleotide (NAD+) and nicotinamide adenine dinucleotide phosphate (NADP) in astrocytes (Berthelier et al., 1998; Deaglio et al., 2001; Antonelli and Ferrannini, 2004; De Flora et al., 2004; Heidemann et al., 2005a). The CD38-catalyzed cleavage of the nicotinamide-ribose bond eventually leads to the production of cADPR (Berthelier et al., 1998). Despite the fact that CD38 is a very inefficient cyclase because ADPR produced by hydrolysis of cADPR is the major end product (Lee and Aarhus, 1993), it has been demonstrated that this small amount of cADPR is still biologically relevant (Partida-Sanchez et al., 2003).

NADP+, the major alternate substrate to NAD+, leads to the formation of NAADP+ by CD38 primarily in acidic conditions (Heidemann et al., 2005b). While some recent reports have shown that hydrolysis of NAD+ to adenosine may increase $[Ca^{2+}]_i$ in astrocytes (Doengi et al., 2008; Okuda et al., 2010), both cADPR and NAADP+ are potent Ca^{2+} mobilizing metabolites (Lee, 2001; Antonelli and Ferrannini, 2004; De Flora et al., 2004; Heidemann et al., 2005a). These secondary messengers generated by CD38 lead to intracellular Ca^{2+} release by various mechanisms. NAADP+ has been shown to mobilize Ca^{2+} from inositol 1,4,5 trisphosphate (IP3) receptors (IP3R) in astrocytes (Heidemann et al., 2005b), ryanodine (Ry) receptors (RyR) in T cells (Dammermann and Guse, 2005; Steen et al., 2007), or from other uncharacterized intracellular Ca^{2+} stores (Mandi and Bak, 2008). However, cADPR is primarily involved in release of intracellular Ca^{2+} through RyRs in various cell types including myocytes, fibroblasts, smooth muscle cells, T cells, neuronal cells and astrocytes (Bruzzone et al., 2003; Partida-Sanchez et al., 2003; Kunerth et al., 2004; Hashii et al., 2005; Fliegert et al., 2007; Jude et al., 2008). cADPR can also be involved in the extracellular Ca^{2+} influx in T cells and neuroblastoma-derived neuronal cells (Partida-Sanchez et al., 2001; Amina et al., 2010). These evidences suggest that CD38 is a primary regulator of Ca^{2+} signaling in various cell types, including astrocytes.

5. Astrocyte glutamate production vs. glutamate uptake in HAND

Astrocytes are known to regulate glutamate homeostasis in CNS [for details review (Hamilton and Attwell, 2010)]. In the HIV-1-infected brain, multiple factors may impair astrocyte regulation of Ca^{2+} and glutamate levels. Gendelman and co-workers first reported high levels of arachidonic acid and cytokines such as TNF-α and IL-1β, in HIVE brain tissue (Gendelman et al., 1994), which likely lead to reduced glutamate uptake and increased Ca^{+2}-mediated release of glutamate by astrocytes (Parpura et al., 1994; Bezzi et al., 1998). It has also been shown that HIV-1 gp120 may indirectly contribute to impaired astrocyte-glutamate uptake *in vitro* (Schneider-Schaulies et al., 1992; Benos et al., 1994). Thus, in addition to glutamate release, dysreguation of $[Ca^{+2}]_i$ in astrocytes may also contribute to HIV neuropathogenesis through impaired glutamate uptake. Impaired glutamate uptake can lead to further increases in the extracellular glutamate levels. Enhanced glutamate levels in turn activate N-methyl-D-aspartic acid (NMDA) receptors causing increased levels of intracellular Ca^{2+} in neurons as shown both in cultured neurons and acute brain slices (Kaul et al., 2001), and can eventually lead to neuronal apoptosis or necrosis. Excess glutamate may also lead to lipid peroxidation and eventually affect both astrocyte and neuronal viability (Visalli et al., 2007).

Under normal physiological conditions, astrocytes selectively regulate extracellular levels of glutamate to maintain homeostasis in the neuronal microenvironment mainly through glutamate transporters (Rothstein et al., 1996). Previous work on primary human astrocytes has shown downregulation of excitatory amino acid transporter 2 (EAAT2) upon activation of astrocytes with HIV-1 gp120, leading to reduction in glutamate uptake (Wang et al., 2003). Glutamate transporter activity and inhibition of glutamate uptake can also be mediated by MAPKs and NF-κB in astrocytes (Abe and Saito, 2001; Jayakumar et al., 2006). Our laboratory showed that CD38 expression and function in astrocytes, is primarily regulated by NF-κB and MAPKs (Mamik et al., In Press). Thus, it is relevant to propose that CD38 levels may affect astrocyte-mediated glutamate homeostasis during neuroinflammatory conditions.

Both RyR and IP3R blockers can reduce excess glutamate release by astrocytes (Hua et al., 2004; Reyes and Parpura, 2009). This suggests that perhaps both IP3R and RyR may be involved in the increase in $[Ca^{2+}]_i$, an event that plays a major role in glutamate release. We have previously reported CD38-cADPR-mediated increase in $[Ca^{2+}]_i$ in activated astrocytes. Our data suggests that elevated CD38 level leads to production of excess cADPR, which may eventually result in higher Ca^{2+} in activated astrocytes during HIVE (Banerjee et al., 2008). As previously reported by De Flora's group, this rise in $[Ca^{2+}]_i$ by CD38 may lead to increased release of glutamate by astrocytes (Verderio et al., 2001). Studies by Bezzi and co-workers showed that cultured astrocytes may trigger $[Ca^{2+}]_i$-dependent release of

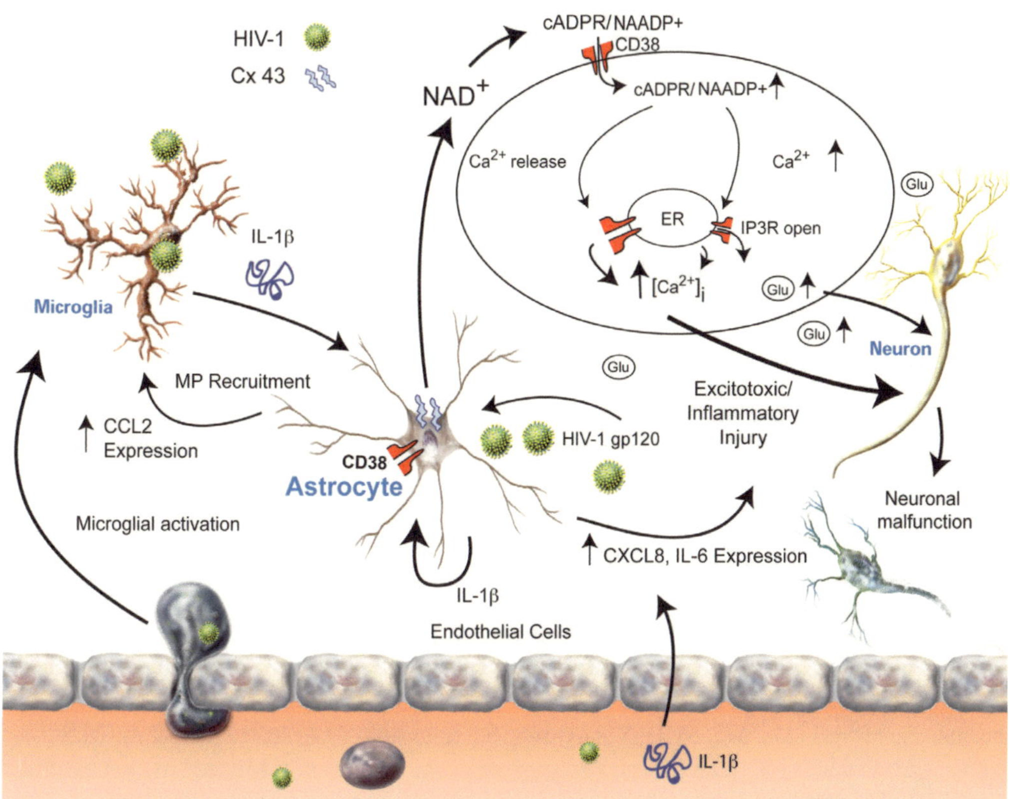

Fig. 1. Schematic representation of CD38-mediated astrocyte-neuron interactions. In HIVE, virus-infected macrophages cross the blood-brain barrier and initiate inflammatory processes in the brain including microglial activation. Activated macrophages and microglia produce IL-1β, which along with viral protein HIV-1 gp120 leads to activation of astrocytes. Inflammatory responses of activated astrocytes may include upregulation of molecules detrimental to neural homeostasis. One of these pathways includes CD38 upregulation, which produces Ca^{2+}-mobilizing metabolites like NAD+. NAD+ upon release through Connexin 43 (Cx 43) hemichannels is hydrolyzed and transported back into the cell as cADPR by membrane bound CD38. cADPR and NAADP+ may regulate release of $[Ca^{2+}]_i$. Astrocyte-mediated release of glutamate and other inflammatory mediators (IL-6 and CXCL8) into the synapse may ultimately lead to excitotoxic neuronal injury.

glutamate, which may lead to NMDA receptor-mediated increased Ca^{+2} levels in neurons (Bezzi et al., 1998). The above evidences suggest that the initial release of glutamate due to increase in $[Ca^{+2}]_i$ by astrocytes, may be influencing the prolonged higher Ca^{2+} levels in neurons during HAND. Taken together, CD38/cADPR-mediated rise of $[Ca^{2+}]_i$ in activated astrocytes (Banerjee et al., 2008) may contribute to increased extracellular glutamate levels, resulting in neuronal excitotoxicity during HAND.

6. Conclusion

6.1 Role of astrocyte-CD38 in HAND: Possible mechanisms

Astrocytes are capable of generating complex changes in $[Ca^{2+}]_i$, allowing them to communicate with each other and with neighboring neuronal cells. The CD38/cADPR system is involved in regulating $[Ca^{2+}]_i$ homeostasis in astrocytes (Banerjee et al., 2008). A paracrine model of interaction has been suggested, involving NAADP+ and cADPR, leading to glutamate-release by astrocytes, affecting neurons (Verderio et al., 2001; De Flora et al., 2004). Our previous data demonstrate that in HIV-1 CNS disease, astrocytes express elevated levels of CD38 (Kou et al., 2009), thus activating these paracrine pathways. The possible connections between HIV-1 infection, neuroinflammation and astrocyte activation, which result in CD38 upregulation and dysregulation of Ca^{2+}/glutamate homeostasis and culminate in neuronal injury (Fig. 1).

7. Acknowledgement

The authors would like to thank Ms. Kathleen Borgmann, Ms. Radhika Suryadevara and Ms. Manmeet Mamik for their suggestions and editing help. We would also like to acknowledge our collaborators Drs. Timothy Walseth, Mathur Kannan and Keshore Bidasee for insightful discussions on CD38 biology.

8. References

Abe, K., and Saito, H. (2001). Possible linkage between glutamate transporter and mitogen-activated protein kinase cascade in cultured rat cortical astrocytes. Journal of neurochemistry 76, 217-223.

Amina, S., Hashii, M., Ma, W.J., Yokoyama, S., Lopatina, O., Liu, H.X., Islam, M.S., and Higashida, H. (2010). Intracellular calcium elevation induced by extracellular application of cyclic-ADP-ribose or oxytocin is temperature-sensitive in rodent NG108-15 neuronal cells with or without exogenous expression of human oxytocin receptors. Journal of neuroendocrinology 22, 460-466.

Ances, B.M., and Ellis, R.J. (2007). Dementia and neurocognitive disorders due to HIV-1 infection. Semin Neurol 27, 86-92.

Antonelli, A., and Ferrannini, E. (2004). CD38 autoimmunity: recent advances and relevance to human diabetes. J Endocrinol Invest 27, 695-707.

Banerjee, S., Walseth, T.F., Borgmann, K., Wu, L., Bidasee, K.R., Kannan, M.S., and Ghorpade, A. (2008). CD38/cyclic ADP-ribose regulates astrocyte calcium signaling: implications for neuroinflammation and HIV-1-associated dementia. J Neuroimmune Pharmacol 3, 154-164.

Bell, J.E. (2004). An update on the neuropathology of HIV in the HAART era. Histopathology 45, 549-559.

Bell, J.E., Brettle, R.P., Chiswick, A., and Simmonds, P. (1998). HIV encephalitis, proviral load and dementia in drug users and homosexuals with AIDS. Effect of neocortical involvement. Brain 121, 2043-2052.

Benos, D.J., Hahn, B.H., Bubien, J.K., Ghosh, S.K., Mashburn, N.A., Chaikin, M.A., Shaw, G.M., and Benveniste, E.N. (1994). Envelope glycoprotein gp120 of human immunodeficiency virus type 1 alters ion transport in astrocytes: implications for AIDS dementia complex. Proc Natl Acad Sci U S A 91, 494-498.

Berridge, M.J., Bootman, M.D., and Roderick, H.L. (2003). Calcium signalling: dynamics, homeostasis and remodelling. Nat Rev Mol Cell Biol 4, 517-529.

Bers, D.M. (2002). Cardiac excitation-contraction coupling. Nature 415, 198-205.

Berthelier, V., Tixier, J.M., Muller-Steffner, H., Schuber, F., and Deterre, P. (1998). Human CD38 is an authentic NAD(P)+ glycohydrolase. Biochem J 330 (Pt 3), 1383-1390.

Bezzi, P., Carmignoto, G., Pasti, L., Vesce, S., Rossi, D., Rizzini, B.L., Pozzan, T., and Volterra, A. (1998). Prostaglandins stimulate calcium-dependent glutamate release in astrocytes. Nature 391, 281-285.

Blumberg, B.M., Gelbard, H.A., and Epstein, L.G. (1994). HIV-1 infection of the developing nervous system: central role of astrocytes in pathogenesis. Virus Res 32, 253-267.

Boven, L.A., Gomes, L., Hery, C., Gray, F., Verhoef, J., Portegies, P., Tardieu, M., and Nottet, H.S. (1999). Increased peroxynitrite activity in AIDS dementia complex: implications for the neuropathogenesis of HIV-1 infection. J Immunol 162, 4319-4327.

Brew, B.J., Rosenblum, M., Cronin, K., and Price, R.W. (1995). AIDS dementia complex and HIV-1 brain infection:clinical-virological correlation. Ann Neurol 38, 563-570.

Brodt, H.R., Kamps, B.S., Gute, P., Knupp, B., Staszewski, S., and Helm, E.B. (1997). Changing incidence of AIDS-defining illnesses in the era of antiretroviral combination therapy. Aids 11, 1731-1738.

Bruzzone, S., Kunerth, S., Zocchi, E., De Flora, A., and Guse, A.H. (2003). Spatio-temporal propagation of Ca2+ signals by cyclic ADP-ribose in 3T3 cells stimulated via purinergic P2Y receptors. The Journal of cell biology 163, 837-845.

Chang, L., and Karin, M. (2001). Mammalian MAP kinase signalling cascades. Nature 410, 37-40.

Cotrina, M.L., and Nedergaard, M. (2005). Intracellular calcium control mechanisms in glia. Neuroglia (BOOK), 229-239.

Dammermann, W., and Guse, A.H. (2005). Functional ryanodine receptor expression is required for NAADP-mediated local Ca2+ signaling in T-lymphocytes. The Journal of biological chemistry 280, 21394-21399.

Davis, R.J. (1995). Transcriptional regulation by MAP kinases. Mol Reprod Dev 42, 459-467.

De Flora, A., Zocchi, E., Guida, L., Franco, L., and Bruzzone, S. (2004). Autocrine and paracrine calcium signaling by the CD38/NAD+/cyclic ADP-ribose system. Ann N Y Acad Sci 1028, 176-191.

Deaglio, S., Mehta, K., and Malavasi, F. (2001). Human CD38: a (r)evolutionary story of enzymes and receptors. Leuk Res 25, 1-12.

Deshpande, M., Zheng, J., Borgmann, K., Persidsky, R., Wu, L., Schellpeper, C., and Ghorpade, A. (2005). Role of activated astrocytes in neuronal damage: potential links to HIV-1-associated dementia. Neurotox Res 7, 183-192.

Dickson, D.W., Mattiace, L.A., Kure, K., Hutchins, K., Lyman, W.D., and Brosnan, C.F. (1991). Microglia in human disease, with an emphasis on acquired immune deficiency syndrome. Lab Invest 64, 135-156.

Doengi, M., Deitmer, J.W., and Lohr, C. (2008). New evidence for purinergic signaling in the olfactory bulb: A2A and P2Y1 receptors mediate intracellular calcium release in astrocytes. The FASEB journal : official publication of the Federation of American Societies for Experimental Biology 22, 2368-2378.

Ellis, R., Langford, D., and Masliah, E. (2007). HIV and antiretroviral therapy in the brain: neuronal injury and repair. Nat Rev Neurosci 8, 33-44.

Eng, L.F., and Ghirnikar, R.S. (1994). GFAP and astrogliosis. Brain pathology 4, 229-237.

Felzen, B., Shilkrut, M., Less, H., Sarapov, I., Maor, G., Coleman, R., Robinson, R.B., Berke, G., and Binah, O. (1998). Fas (CD95/Apo-1)-mediated damage to ventricular myocytes induced by cytotoxic T lymphocytes from perforin-deficient mice: a major role for inositol 1,4,5-trisphosphate. Circ Res 82, 438-450.

Fliegert, R., Gasser, A., and Guse, A.H. (2007). Regulation of calcium signalling by adenine-based second messengers. Biochemical Society transactions 35, 109-114.

Foley, J., Ettenhofer, M., Wright, M., and Hinkin, C.H. (2008). Emerging issues in the neuropsychology of HIV infection. Current HIV/AIDS reports 5, 204-211.

Gallo, P., Laverda, A.M., De Rossi, A., Pagni, S., Del Mistro, A., Cogo, P., Piccinno, M.G., Plebani, A., Tavolato, B., and Chieco-Bianchi, L. (1991). Immunological markers in the cerebrospinal fluid of HIV-1-infected children. Acta Paediatr Scand 80, 659-666.

Gendelman, H., and Tardieu, M. (1994). Macrophages/microglia and the pathophysiology of CNS injuries in AIDS. J of Leukocyte Biology 56, 387-388.

Gendelman, H.E., Genis, P., Jett, M., Zhai, Q.H., and Nottet, H.S. (1994). An experimental model system for HIV-1-induced brain injury. Adv Neuroimmunol 4, 189-193.

Gonzales, M.F., and Davis, R.L. (1988). Neuropathology of acquired immunodeficiency syndrome. Neuropathol Appl Neurobiol 14, 345-363.

Grant, I. (2008). Neurocognitive disturbances in HIV. Int Rev Psychiatry 20, 33-47.

Hamilton, N.B., and Attwell, D. (2010). Do astrocytes really exocytose neurotransmitters? Nature reviews Neuroscience 11, 227-238.

Hashii, M., Shuto, S., Fukuoka, M., Kudoh, T., Matsuda, A., and Higashida, H. (2005). Amplification of depolarization-induced and ryanodine-sensitive cytosolic Ca2+ elevation by synthetic carbocyclic analogs of cyclic ADP-ribose and their antagonistic effects in NG108-15 neuronal cells. J Neurochem 94, 316-323.

Heidemann, A.C., Schipke, C.G., and Kettenmann, H. (2005a). Extracellular application of NAADP+ induces Ca2+ signaling in astrocytes in situ. J Biol Chem.

Heidemann, A.C., Schipke, C.G., and Kettenmann, H. (2005b). Extracellular application of nicotinic acid adenine dinucleotide phosphate induces Ca2+ signaling in astrocytes in situ. J Biol Chem 280, 35630-35640.

Herbein, G., Mahlknecht, U., Batliwalla, F., Gregersen, P., Pappas, T., Butler, J., O'Brien, W.A., and Verdin, E. (1998). Apoptosis of CD8+ T cells is mediated by macrophages through interaction of HIV gp120 with chemokine receptor CXCR4. Nature 395, 189-194.

Holden, C.P., Haughey, N.J., Nath, A., and Geiger, J.D. (1999). Role of Na+/H+ exchangers, excitatory amino acid receptors and voltage-operated Ca2+ channels in human immunodeficiency virus type 1 gp120-mediated increases in intracellular Ca2+ in human neurons and astrocytes. Neuroscience 91, 1369-1378.

Hua, L.L., Zhao, M.L., Cosenza, M., Kim, M.O., Huang, H., Tanowitz, H.B., Brosnan, C.F., and Lee, S.C. (2002). Role of mitogen-activated protein kinases in inducible nitric oxide synthase and TNFalpha expression in human fetal astrocytes. J Neuroimmunol 126, 180-189.

Hua, X., Malarkey, E.B., Sunjara, V., Rosenwald, S.E., Li, W.H., and Parpura, V. (2004). C(a2+)-dependent glutamate release involves two classes of endoplasmic reticulum Ca(2+) stores in astrocytes. J Neurosci Res 76, 86-97.

Jana, M., Anderson, J.A., Saha, R.N., Liu, X., and Pahan, K. (2005). Regulation of inducible nitric oxide synthase in proinflammatory cytokine-stimulated human primary astrocytes. Free Radic Biol Med 38, 655-664.

Jayakumar, A.R., Panickar, K.S., Murthy Ch, R., and Norenberg, M.D. (2006). Oxidative stress and mitogen-activated protein kinase phosphorylation mediate ammonia-induced cell swelling and glutamate uptake inhibition in cultured astrocytes. The Journal of neuroscience : the official journal of the Society for Neuroscience 26, 4774-4784.

Jayaraman, T., and Marks, A.R. (1997). T cells deficient in inositol 1,4,5-trisphosphate receptor are resistant to apoptosis. Mol Cell Biol 17, 3005-3012.

John, G.R., Scemes, E., Suadicani, S.O., Liu, J.S., Charles, P.C., Lee, S.C., Spray, D.C., and Brosnan, C.F. (1999). IL-1beta differentially regulates calcium wave propagation between primary human fetal astrocytes via pathways involving P2 receptors and gap junction channels. Proc Natl Acad Sci U S A 96, 11613-11618.

Jude, J.A., Wylam, M.E., Walseth, T.F., and Kannan, M.S. (2008). Calcium signaling in airway smooth muscle. Proceedings of the American Thoracic Society 5, 15-22.

Kaul, M., Garden, G.A., and Lipton, S.A. (2001). Pathways to neuronal injury and apoptosis in HIV-1-associated dementia. Nature 410, 988-993.

Kaul, M., and Lipton, S.A. (2006). Mechanisms of neuroimmunity and neurodegeneration associated with HIV-1 infection and AIDS. J Neuroimmune Pharmacol 1, 138-151.

Khan, A., Soloski, M., Sharp, A., Schilling, G., Sabatini, D., Li, S., Ross, C., and Snyder, S. (1996). Lymphocyte apoptosis: mediation by increased type 3 inositol 1,4,5-triphosphate receptor. Science 273, 503-507.

Kolber, M.A. (2008). CD38+CD8+ T-cells negatively correlate with CD4 central memory cells in virally suppressed HIV-1-infected individuals. Aids 22, 1937-1941.

Kou, W., Banerjee, S., Eudy, J., Smith, L.M., Persidsky, R., Borgmann, K., Wu, L., Sakhuja, N., Deshpande, M.S., Walseth, T.F., *et al.* (2009). CD38 regulation in activated astrocytes: implications for neuroinflammation and HIV-1 brain infection. J Neurosci Res 87, 2326-2339.

Kunerth, S., Langhorst, M.F., Schwarzmann, N., Gu, X., Huang, L., Yang, Z., Zhang, L., Mills, S.J., Zhang, L.H., Potter, B.V., *et al.* (2004). Amplification and propagation of pacemaker Ca2+ signals by cyclic ADP-ribose and the type 3 ryanodine receptor in T cells. J Cell Sci 117, 2141-2149.

Lane, T.E., Buchmeier, M.J., Watry, D.D., and Fox, H.S. (1996). Expression of inflammatory cytokines and inducible nitric oxide synthase in brains of SIV-infected rhesus monkeys: applications to HIV- induced central nervous system disease. Mol Med 2, 27-37.

Lee, H.C. (2001). Physiological functions of cyclic ADP-ribose and NAADP as calcium messengers. Annu Rev Pharmacol Toxicol 41, 317-345.

Lee, H.C., and Aarhus, R. (1993). Wide distribution of an enzyme that catalyzes the hydrolysis of cyclic ADP-ribose. Biochimica et biophysica acta 1164, 68-74.

Letendre, S., McCutchan, J.A., and Ellis, R.J. (2008). Neurologic Complications of HIV Disease and Their Treatment. Top HIV Med 16, 15-22.

Li, W., Li, G., Steiner, J., and Nath, A. (2009). Role of Tat protein in HIV neuropathogenesis. Neurotoxicity research 16, 205-220.

Lin, J.X., and Leonard, W.J. (1997). Signaling from the IL-2 receptor to the nucleus. Cytokine Growth Factor Rev 8, 313-332.

Lindl, K.A., Marks, D.R., Kolson, D.L., and Jordan-Sciutto, K.L. (2010). HIV-associated neurocognitive disorder: pathogenesis and therapeutic opportunities. Journal of neuroimmune pharmacology : the official journal of the Society on NeuroImmune Pharmacology 5, 294-309.

Liu, X.L., Miyakawa, A., Aperia, A., and Krieger, P. (2007). Na,K-ATPase generates calcium oscillations in hippocampal astrocytes. Neuroreport 18, 597-600.

Mamik, M.K., Banerjee, S., Walseth, T.F., Hirte, R., Tang, L., Borgmann, K., and Ghorpade, A. (In Press). HIV-1 and IL-1β regulate astrocytic CD38 through mitogen-activated protein kinases and nuclear factor-κB signaling mechanisms. J Neuroinflammation.

Mandi, M., and Bak, J. (2008). Nicotinic acid adenine dinucleotide phosphate (NAADP) and Ca2+ mobilization. Journal of receptor and signal transduction research 28, 163-184.

Mauermann, M.L., Angius, D., Spinner, R.J., Letendre, L.J., Amrami, K.K., and Dyck, P.J. (2008). Isolated granulocytic sarcoma presenting as a brachial plexopathy. Journal of the peripheral nervous system : JPNS 13, 153-156.

Meucci, O., Fatatis, A., Simen, A.A., Bushell, T.J., Gray, P.W., and Miller, R.J. (1998). Chemokines regulate hippocampal neuronal signaling and gp120 neurotoxicity. Proc Natl Acad Sci U S A 95, 14500-14505.

Mizuguchi, M., Otsuka, N., Sato, M., Ishii, Y., Kon, S., Yamada, M., Nishina, H., Katada, T., and Ikeda, K. (1995). Neuronal localization of CD38 antigen in the human brain. Brain Res 697, 235-240.

Morita, M., Higuchi, C., Moto, T., Kozuka, N., Susuki, J., Itofusa, R., Yamashita, J., and Kudo, Y. (2003). Dual regulation of calcium oscillation in astrocytes by growth factors and pro-inflammatory cytokines via the mitogen-activated protein kinase cascade. J Neurosci 23, 10944-10952.

Nath, A., and Geiger, J. (1998). Neurobiological aspects of human immunodeficiency virus infection: neurotoxic mechanisms. Prog Neurobiol 54, 19-33.

Navia, B.A., Jordan, B.D., and Price, R.W. (1986). The AIDS dementia complex: I. Clinical features. Annals of Neurology 19, 517-524.

Okuda, H., Higashi, Y., Nishida, K., Fujimoto, S., and Nagasawa, K. (2010). Contribution of P2X7 receptors to adenosine uptake by cultured mouse astrocytes. Glia 58, 1757-1765.

Parker, L.C., Luheshi, G.N., Rothwell, N.J., and Pinteaux, E. (2002). IL-1 beta signalling in glial cells in wildtype and IL-1RI deficient mice. Br J Pharmacol 136, 312-320.

Parpura, V., Basarsky, T.A., Liu, F., Jeftinija, K., Jeftinija, S., and Haydon, P.G. (1994). Glutamate-mediated astrocyte-neuron signalling. Nature 369, 744-747.

Partida-Sanchez, S., Cockayne, D.A., Monard, S., Jacobson, E.L., Oppenheimer, N., Garvy, B., Kusser, K., Goodrich, S., Howard, M., Harmsen, A., *et al.* (2001). Cyclic ADP-ribose production by CD38 regulates intracellular calcium release, extracellular calcium influx and chemotaxis in neutrophils and is required for bacterial clearance in vivo. Nat Med 7, 1209-1216.

Partida-Sanchez, S., Randall, T.D., and Lund, F.E. (2003). Innate immunity is regulated by CD38, an ecto-enzyme with ADP-ribosyl cyclase activity. Microbes Infect 5, 49-58.

Pawlikowska, L., Cottrell, S.E., Harms, M.B., Li, Y., and Rosenberg, P.A. (1996). Extracellular synthesis of cADP-ribose from nicotinamide-adenine dinucleotide by rat cortical astrocytes in culture. J Neurosci 16, 5372-5381.

Pellegrini, P., Berghella, A.M., Di Loreto, S., Del Beato, T., Di Marco, F., Adorno, D., and Casciani, C.U. (1996). Cytokine contribution to the repair processes and homeostasis recovery following anoxic insult: a possible IFN-gamma-regulating role in IL- 1beta neurotoxic action in physiological or damaged CNS. Neuroimmunomodulation 3, 213-218.

Peng, H., Erdmann, N., Whitney, N., Dou, H., Gorantla, S., Gendelman, H.E., Ghorpade, A., and Zheng, J. (2006). HIV-1-infected and/or immune activated macrophages regulate astrocyte SDF-1 production through IL-1beta. Glia 54, 619-629.

Persidsky, Y., Ghorpade, A., Rasmussen, J., Limoges, J., Liu, X.J., Stins, M., Fiala, M., Way, D., Kim, K.S., Witte, M.H., *et al.* (1999). Microglial and astrocyte chemokines regulate monocyte migration through the blood-brain barrier in human immunodeficiency virus-1 encephalitis. Am J Pathol 155, 1599-1611.

Persidsky, Y., Limoges, J., McComb, R., Bock, P., Baldwin, T., Tyor, W., Patil, A., Nottet, H.S., Epstein, L., Gelbard, H., *et al.* (1996). Human immunodeficiency virus encephalitis in SCID mice. Am J Pathol 149, 1027-1053.

Petito, C.K., Kerza-Kwiatecki, A.P., Gendelman, H.E., McCarthy, M., Nath, A., Podack, E.R., Shapshak, P., and Wiley, C.A. (1999). Review: neuronal injury in HIV infection. J Neurovirol 5, 327-341.

Price, R.W., Brew, B., Sidtis, J., Rosenblum, M., Scheck, A.C., and Cleary, P. (1988). The brain in AIDS: central nervous system HIV-1 infection and AIDS dementia complex. Science 239, 586-592.

Price, R.W., and Spudich, S. (2008). Antiretroviral therapy and central nervous system HIV type 1 infection. J Infect Dis 197 Suppl 3, S294-306.

Rajan, P., and McKay, R.D. (1998). Multiple routes to astrocytic differentiation in the CNS. J Neurosci 18, 3620-3629.

Ransom, B., Behar, T., and Nedergaard, M. (2003). New roles for astrocytes (stars at last). Trends Neurosci 26, 520-522.

Reyes, R.C., and Parpura, V. (2008). Mitochondria modulate Ca2+-dependent glutamate release from rat cortical astrocytes. The Journal of neuroscience : the official journal of the Society for Neuroscience 28, 9682-9691.

Reyes, R.C., and Parpura, V. (2009). The trinity of Ca2+ sources for the exocytotic glutamate release from astrocytes. Neurochemistry international 55, 2-8.

Ridet, J.L., Malhotra, S.K., Privat, A., and Gage, F.H. (1997). Reactive astrocytes: cellular and molecular cues to biological function. Trends Neurosci 20, 570-577.

Rojas, H., Colina, C., Ramos, M., Benaim, G., Jaffe, E.H., Caputo, C., and DiPolo, R. (2007). Na+ entry via glutamate transporter activates the reverse Na+/Ca2+ exchange and triggers Ca(i)2+-induced Ca2+ release in rat cerebellar Type-1 astrocytes. Journal of neurochemistry 100, 1188-1202.

Rojas, H., Ramos, M., and Dipolo, R. (2004). A genistein-sensitive Na+/Ca2+ exchange is responsible for the resting [Ca2+]i and most of the Ca2+ plasma membrane fluxes in stimulated rat cerebellar type 1 astrocytes. The Japanese journal of physiology 54, 249-262.

Rothstein, J.D., Dykes-Hoberg, M., Pardo, C.A., Bristol, L.A., Jin, L., Kuncl, R.W., Kanai, Y., Hediger, M.A., Wang, Y., Schielke, J.P., *et al.* (1996). Knockout of glutamate transporters reveals a major role for astroglial transport in excitotoxicity and clearance of glutamate. Neuron 16, 675-686.

Sacktor, N.C., Lyles, R.H., Skolasky, R.L., Anderson, D.E., McArthur, J.C., McFarlane, G., Selnes, O.A., Becker, J.T., Cohen, B., Wesch, J., *et al.* (1999). Combination antiretroviral therapy improves psychomotor speed performance in HIV-seropositive homosexual men. Multicenter AIDS Cohort Study (MACS). Neurology 52, 1640-1647.

Savarino, A., Bottarel, F., Malavasi, F., and Dianzani, U. (2000). Role of CD38 in HIV-1 infection: an epiphenomenon of T-cell activation or an active player in virus/host interactions? Aids 14, 1079-1089.

Schneider-Schaulies, J., Schneider-Schaulies, S., Brinkmann, R., Tas, P., Halbrugge, M., Walter, U., Holmes, H.C., and Ter Meulen, V. (1992). HIV-1 gp120 receptor on CD4-negative brain cells activates a tyrosine kinase. Virology 191, 765-772.

Sebire, G., Emilie, D., Wallon, C., Hery, C., Devergne, O., Delfraissy, J.F., Galanaud, P., and Tardieu, M. (1993). In vitro production of IL-6, IL-1 beta, and tumor necrosis factor-alpha by human embryonic microglial and neural cells. J Immunol 150, 1517-1523.

Sharma, V., Mishra, M., Ghosh, S., Tewari, R., Basu, A., Seth, P., and Sen, E. (2007). Modulation of interleukin-1beta mediated inflammatory response in human astrocytes by flavonoids: implications in neuroprotection. Brain Res Bull 73, 55-63.

Sinclair, E., Ronquillo, R., Lollo, N., Deeks, S.G., Hunt, P., Yiannoutsos, C.T., Spudich, S., and Price, R.W. (2008). Antiretroviral treatment effect on immune activation reduces cerebrospinal fluid HIV-1 infection. Journal of acquired immune deficiency syndromes 47, 544-552.

Steen, M., Kirchberger, T., and Guse, A.H. (2007). NAADP mobilizes calcium from the endoplasmic reticular Ca(2+) store in T-lymphocytes. The Journal of biological chemistry 282, 18864-18871.

Tyor, W.R., Glass, J.D., Baumrind, N., McArthur, J.C., Griffin, J.W., Becker, P.S., and Griffin, D.E. (1993). Cytokine expression of macrophages in HIV-1-associated vacuolar myelopathy [see comments]. Neurology 43, 1002-1009.

Verderio, C., Bruzzone, S., Zocchi, E., Fedele, E., Schenk, U., De Flora, A., and Matteoli, M. (2001). Evidence of a role for cyclic ADP-ribose in calcium signalling and neurotransmitter release in cultured astrocytes. J Neurochem 78, 646-657.

Vigano, A., Saresella, M., Villa, M.L., Ferrante, P., and Clerici, M. (2000). CD38+CD8+ T cells as a marker of poor response to therapy in HIV-infected individuals. Chem Immunol 75, 207-217.

Visalli, V., Muscoli, C., Sacco, I., Sculco, F., Palma, E., Costa, N., Colica, C., Rotiroti, D., and Mollace, V. (2007). N-acetylcysteine prevents HIV gp 120-related damage of human cultured astrocytes: correlation with glutamine synthase dysfunction. BMC Neurosci 8, 106.

Vitkovic, L., Bockaert, J., and Jacque, C. (2000a). "Inflammatory" cytokines: neuromodulators in normal brain? J Neurochem 74, 457-471.

Vitkovic, L., Chatham, J.J., and da Cunha, A. (1995). Distinct expressions of three cytokines by IL-1-stimulated astrocytes in vitro and in AIDS brain. Brain Behav Immun 9, 378-388.

Vitkovic, L., Konsman, J.P., Bockaert, J., Dantzer, R., Homburger, V., and Jacque, C. (2000b). Cytokine signals propagate through the brain. Mol Psychiatry 5, 604-615.

Wang, T.F., Zhou, C., Tang, A.H., Wang, S.Q., and Chai, Z. (2006). Cellular mechanism for spontaneous calcium oscillations in astrocytes. Acta pharmacologica Sinica 27, 861-868.

Wang, Z., Pekarskaya, O., Bencheikh, M., Chao, W., Gelbard, H.A., Ghorpade, A., Rothstein, J.D., and Volsky, D.J. (2003). Reduced expression of glutamate transporter EAAT2 and impaired glutamate transport in human primary astrocytes exposed to HIV-1 or gp120. Virology 312, 60-73.

Wiley, C.A., and Achim, C. (1994). Human immunodeficiency virus encephalitis is the pathological correlate of dementia in acquired immunodeficiency syndrome. Ann Neurol 36, 673-676.

Woods, S.P., Moore, D.J., Weber, E., and Grant, I. (2009). Cognitive neuropsychology of HIV-associated neurocognitive disorders. Neuropsychology review 19, 152-168.

Wu, V.W., and Schwartz, J.P. (1998). Cell culture models for reactive gliosis: new perspectives. J Neurosci Res 51, 675-681.

Yamada, M., Mizuguchi, M., Otsuka, N., Ikeda, K., and Takahashi, H. (1997). Ultrastructural localization of CD38 immunoreactivity in rat brain. Brain Res 756, 52-60.

Yi, Y., Lee, C., Liu, Q.H., Freedman, B.D., and Collman, R.G. (2004). Chemokine receptor utilization and macrophage signaling by human immunodeficiency virus type 1 gp120: Implications for neuropathogenesis. J Neurovirol 10 Suppl 1, 91-96.

Zhao, L., and Brinton, R.D. (2004). Suppression of proinflammatory cytokines interleukin-1beta and tumor necrosis factor-alpha in astrocytes by a V1 vasopressin receptor agonist: a cAMP response element-binding protein-dependent mechanism. The Journal of neuroscience : the official journal of the Society for Neuroscience 24, 2226-2235.

Zhao, M.L., Brosnan, C.F., and Lee, S.C. (2004). 15-deoxy-delta (12,14)-PGJ2 inhibits astrocyte IL-1 signaling: inhibition of NF-kappaB and MAP kinase pathways and suppression of cytokine and chemokine expression. J Neuroimmunol 153, 132-142.

Part 3

Other Agents

12

Encephalitic Angiostrongyliasis

Kittisak Sawanyawisuth
Khon Kaen University
Thailand

1. Introduction

Angiostrongyliasis, caused by *Angiostrongylus cantonensis*, is an emerging infectious disease worldwide (Wang et al., 2008). *A. cantonensis* is a neurotropic nematode. The endemic areas are Southeast Asia, East Asia, and the Pacific Islands. Sporadic outbreaks and report cases are frequently reported globally.

There are three main clinical presentations of angiostrongyliasis including meningitic, encephalitic, and ocular form (Sawanyawisuth & Sawanyawisuth, 2008). Meningitic angiostrongyliasis is the most common form and has a good prognosis. In contrast, encephalitic angiostrongyliasis occurs in a minority of angiostrongyliasis cases but has high mortality rate. Clinicians worldwide should be knowledgeable and have low suspicious level of this condition due to its high mortality.

The chapter will cover the life cycle of *A. cantonensis* and its route of transmission. In addition, risk factors, pathology, clinical manifestations, treatment, prognosis, and prevention of encephalitic angiostrongyliasis will be reviewed.

2. Life cycle and transmission (Figure 1)

The adult worms of *A. cantonensis* or the rat lung worm reside in rat's pulmonary arteries. The young adults migrate to pharynx, pass the esophagus and expose to the environment with the feces. The intermediate hosts are snails where the larvae become the later stages of larvae. Rats ingest the contaminated snails or slugs and the larvae migrate to the brain via gastrointestinal blood vessels. The worms then migrate back to the pulmonary artery and complete its life cycle.

Humans are an accidental host of this parasite and get infected by eating raw snails or other paratenic hosts such as shrimps, frogs, or monitor lizards. Contaminated slugs, vegetables, or juices (Tsai et al., 2004) are other possible sources of the parasites. Similarly to rats, *A. cantonensis* larva migrate to human meninges and brain causing eosinophilic meningitis and encephalitis, respectively. There is a report showed that some larva migrated to human pulmonary artery (Sonakul 1978) and died there.

3. Risk factors

Human angiostrongyliasis caused by *A. cantonensis* has three clinical presentations including eosinophilic meningitis, eosinophilic encephalitis, and ocular angiostrongyliasis. The vast of patients develop meningitic angiostrongyliasis. Gastrointestinal involvement is also possible (Sawanyawisuth et al., 2010). One patient presented with clinical symptoms of gut obstruction and then developed encephalitic angiostrongyliasis afterward.

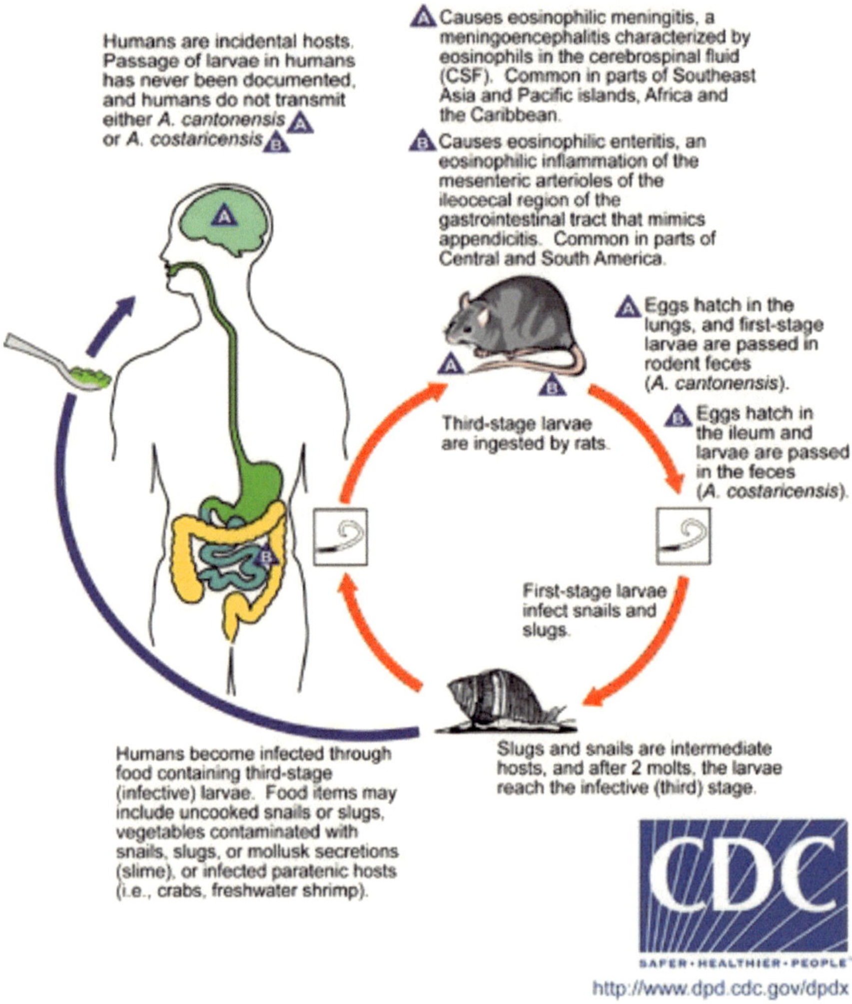

Fig. 1. *Angiostrongylus cantonensis* life cycle
Downloaded from http://www.cdc.gov/parasites/angiostrongylus/biology.html

There is a report comparing clinical presentations between meningitic and encephalitic angiostrongyliasis. The study aimed to find the clinical factors predictive for encephalitic angiostrongyliasis (Sawanyawisuth et al., 2009). The study was done in the Northeastern part of Thailand, the endemic area of angiostrongyliasis. There were 14 encephalitic angiostrongyliasis and 80 meningitic angiostrongyliasis patients in the study. Three significant risk factors for developing encephalitic angiostrongyliasis were older age, prolong headache and having fever with adjusted odds ratio (95% confidence interval) of 1.22 (1.05-1.42), 1.26 (1.03-1.55), and 37.05 (1.59-862.34), respectively.

Unlike bacterial meningitis, fever is not common in meningitic angiostrongyliasis. Fever and neck stiffness are found only 10% and 50% in patients with meningitic angiostrongyliasis. In constrast to meningitic angiostrongyliasis, having fever and neck stiffness are more common in encephalitic angiostrongyliasis (71% and 86%, respectively).

Even though coma is a presenting symptom for encephalitic angiostrongyliasis, patients with encephalitic angiostrongyliasis always have preceding headache before an abrupt onset of coma. The median duration of headache in encephalitic angiostrongyliasis was significantly longer than those with meningitic angiostrongyliasis (18.5 vs 7 days). Finally, every a year of age increases a risk of being encephalitic angiostrongyliasis for 22% comparing to those who have meningitic angiostrongyliasis.

In summary, people who get infected with *A. cantonensis* may develop encephalitic angiostrongyliasis if one is elderly or has fever or long duration of preceding headache.

4. Pathology

A previous study showed that *A. cantonensis* larva might take about two or three days to reach human brain from gastrointestinal tract. The patient developed encephalitic angiostrongyliasis approximately two to three days after having localized peritonitis (Sawanyawisuth et al., 2010).

There are at least eleven proved cases of encephalitic angiostrogyliasis (Ko et al., 1987; Nye et al., 1970; Sonakul 1978). All cases had at least one *A. cantonensis* larva in the brain. The numbers of worm in autopsy cases vary and range from one to numerous larvae. Worms may be alive or dead and worm sizes are between 50-120 micron. Locations of worms were random. Of those, worms were also detected in cerebrospinal fluid examination in two cases. Seven cases were Thai and four cases were reported from Hong Kong.

Gross pathology showed diffused brain swelling, leptomeningitis, mild ventricular dilatation, and several small focal hemorrhage. On microscopic examination, there are four major findings including worm tracks, hemorrhagic spot, cell infiltration with granuloma, and parts of worms. The worm track size are between 0.1-1 mm in length and approximately 1 mm in diameter. Hemorrhagic spot may be found but not all cases, mostly are small in size. The cell infiltrations may be plasma cells, lymphocytes, and eosinophils. The granuloma is also presented. Charcot-Leyden crystals, an evidence of eosinophils, may be found. Parts of worm may also be shown in particular section. Vascular changes such as vessel wall edema, perivascular infiltration with lymphocytes and eosinophils. The granuloma and vascular changes are identical to a case of gastrointestinal involvement of *A. cantonensis* (Sawanyawisuth et al., 2010).

5. Clinical manifestations

The clinical manifestations of encephalitic angiostrongyliasis are similar to viral encephalitis (Sawanyawisuth et al., 2009). The main symptoms are acute fever with abrupt onset of alteration of consciousness to coma stage without significant motor weakness. Unlike viral encephalitis, seizures are rare.

Clinical clues for encephalitic angiostrongyliasis are history of exposure to *A. cantonensis* larva, cerebrospinal fluid eosinophils, and history of preceding headache prior to coma (Chotmongkol & Sawanyawisuth, 2002; Sawanyawisuth et al., 2009). The first two factors are very crucial. History of eating raw freshwater snails, slugs, frogs, shrimps, monitor lizards, contaminated vegetables, contaminated juice or even playing with snails (Wan & Weng, 2004) within the range of 90 days is the major risk factor for angiostrongyliasis.

Cerebrospinal fluid eosinophils more than 10% of the total white blood cells is also suggesttive for encephalitic angiostrongyliasis. Even though there are several causes of cerebrospinal fluid eosinophils, history of exposure to *A. cantonensis* may support the diagnosis of encephalitic angiostrongyliasis.

In some patients, history of preceding headache before developing coma may be obtained from patients' relatives. This finding support the mechanism of developing encephalitic angiostrongyliasis that encephalitic angiostrongyliasis may be the progression of meningitic angiostrongyliasis. The median duration of headache is about 18 days (range 1-30 days).

The alteration of consciousness after the headache may take approximately two days to coma stage (range 1-4 days). Fever may develop before or together with the occurrence of alteration of consciousness. The duration of fever may range between 1-21 days.

The other histories or physical findings in encephalitic angiostrongyliasis are history of paresthesia (8%), vomiting (8%), sixth cranial nerve palsy (14%), seventh cranial nerve palsy (7%), papilledema (21%), and neck stiffness (86%) as shown in Table 1 (Sawanyawisuth et al., 2009). Most affected patients are male in either encephalitic or meningitic angiostrongyliasis (approximately 80%) due to habit of eating raw foods. Rare manifestations include radiculomyelitis (Graber et al., 1997; Kliks et al., 1982), localized peritonitis (Sawanyawisuth et al., 2009), or ocular blindness (Sawanyawisuth et al., 2007).

Variables	N (%) or median (range)
Baseline characteristics	
Males	11 (79)
Age (years)	51 (26-78)
Summer season admitted	7 (50)
Incubation (days)	12 (1-30)
Duration of preceding headache (days)	18.5 (1-30)
Duration to coma stage (days)	2.3 (1-4)
Paresthesia	1/13 (8)
Vomiting	1/13 (8)
Physical signs	
Fever	10 (71)
Sixth cranial nerve palsy	2 (14)
Seventh cranial nerve palsy	1 (7)
Papilledema	3 (21)
Stiff neck	12 (86)

Table 1. Clinical manifestations of encephalitic angiostrogyliasis (Adapted from Sawanyawisuth et al., 2009).

The laboratory tests in encephalitic angiostrongyliasis are not diagnostic with the exception of the predominant of cerebrospinal fluid eosinophils. The median peripheral white blood cell counts is 10,850 cells/mm^3 (range 5,350-20,800) with percent of eosinophils of 8% (range 0-33) as shown in table 2. The cerebrospinal fluid findings are comparable with meningitic angiostrongyliasis. The median opening pressure of cerebrospinal fluid was 225 mmH$_2$O. The median of cerebrospinal fluid white blood cell was 623 cells/mm^3 but may be high as 1,500 cells/mm^3. The percentage of cerebrospinal fluid eosinophils may range from 16-70%. The cerebrospinal fluid protein and glucose range are 61-254 mg/dL and 17-240 mg/dL, respectively. The cerebrospinal fluid glucose/plasma glucose ratio can be low as 19% (Sawanyawisuth et al., 2009).

Variables	Median (range)
Blood tests	
White blood cell (cells/mm^3)	10,850 (5,350-20,800)
Percent eosinophils	8 (0-33)
Cerebrospinal fluid findings	
Opening pressure (mmH2O)	225 (140-580)
White blood cell (cells/mm^3)	623 (57-1,500)
Percent eosinophils	44 (16-70)
Protein (mg/dL)	133 (61-254)
Glucose (mg/dL)	41 (17-240)
Cerebrospinal fluid glucose/plasma glucose ratio (%)	35 (19-53)

Table 2. Laboratory findings in encephalitic angiostrogyliasis (Adapted from Sawanyawisuth et al., 2009).

The measurement of serum and cerebrospinal fluid immunoglobulin may be an additional diagnostic tool for encephalitic angiostrongyliasis. The intrathecal level of immunoglobulin particularly immunoglobulin E by using quotient diagram (Reibergram) comparing between cerebrospinal fluid and serum has been reported to be diagnostic (Dorta-Contreras & Reiber, 1998; Padilla-Docal et al., 2008).

The neuroimaging studies in encephalitic angiostrongyliasis are not specific (Jin et al., 2005; Jin et al., 2008; Kanpittaya et al., 2000; Tsai et al., 2003). The computed tomography of the brain always shows diffuse brain swelling, small area of attenuation with surrounding hypodense area, or meningeal enhancement. The magnetic resonance imagings may give some information but still not diagnostic. The lesions might be scattered or diffuse high-, or iso-, or low-signal on T1 weighted and high-signal on T2 weighted imagings. After the gadolinium injection, the lesions usually become nodular or stick-shaped enhancement. The involved area may be random in the brain such as basal ganglia, mudulla oblongata, globus pallidus, or cerebral peduncles. High signal on periventricular area, linear small hemorrhagic tract, or linear enhancement in the leptomeninges may be found. The MRI intensity in T1-weighted imaging may correlate with severity of headache, cerebrospinal fluid pleocytosis, and cerebrospinal fluid and blood eosinophilia (Tsai et al., 2003). Finally, communicating hydrocephalus may be the late complication of encephalitic angiostrongyliasis (Graber et al., 1997; Sawanyawisuth et al., 2006). Electroencephalogram in encephalitic angiostrongyliasis may reveal abnormal slow dysrhythmia or slow alpha rhythm (Ko et al., 1987; Wang et al., 2002).

Serological tests for *A. cantonensis* have been developed and are very useful in situations of equivocal diagnosis between angiostrongyliasis and other parasites; mostly gnathostomiasis and cysticercosis. There are various serological techniques for angiostrongyliasis such as Enzyme-Linked ImmunoSorbent Assay (ELISA), polymerase chain reaction (PCR), immunoblotting, or antigen detection (Chye et al., 2004; Eamsobhana et al., 2006; Eamsobhana & Yong, 2009; Eamsobhana et al., 2009, Intapan et al., 2003; Maleewong et al., 2001). The sensitivity, specificity, and cross-reaction are varied on each technique. Another concern about serologic test is its availability in health-care facilities. Most serological tests have very high specificity for human angiostrongyliasis. The two most common diagnostic bands are 29- and 31-kDa antigenic polypeptide of *A. cantonensis* (Eamsobhana et al., 2006; Eamsobhana & Yong, 2009; Intapan et al., 2003).

6. Diagnosis

The definite diagnosis of encephalitic angiostrogyliasis is the detection of *A. cantonensis* larva in the cerebrospinal fluid or in any part of the brain by the pathological examination. However, the chance of the identification of *A. cantonensis* larva in the cerebrospinal fluid is extremely rare (Punyagupta et al., 1970). Therefore, the diagnosis of encephalitic angiostrogyliasis can be made by clinical criteria.

For patients who presenting with clinical of acute encephalitis or acute fever with alteration of consciousness, *A. cantonensis* may be the causative agent if meet the following clinical criteria: cerebrospinal fluid white blood cell count of more than 10 cells/mm^3, cerebrospinal fluid eosinophils accounts for at least 10%, negative results of cerebrospinal fluid Gram, acid-fast, and India ink staining, cryptococcal antigen, and cultures, plus history of expose to *A. cantonensis* larva.

Some features may decrease the likelihood of encephalitic angiostrogyliasis including history of eating raw fish, history of migratory swelling, clinical diagnosis of subarachnoid hemorrhage or myeloencephalitis, positive serologic test for gnathostomiasis or cysticercosis, brain computed tomography or magnetic resonance imaging suggestive of gnathostomiasis, symptomatic or serology-positive HIV infection, and active or previous history of tuberculosis or malignancy (Sawanyawisuth et al., 2009).

Serodiagnosis may be helpful tool for equivocal case between angiostrogyliasis and other neuroparasitoses such as gnathostomiasis, cysticercosis, or paragonimiasis.

7. Differential diagnosis

There are several causes of cerebrospinal fluid eosinophils such as neurognathostomiasis, cysticercosis, paragonimiasis, toxocariasis, tuberculosis, or malignancy. However, clinical manifestations of each condition are quite obviously different.

Neurognathostomiasis is almost always presenting with radicular pain, bloody CSF, and pertinent neurological deficit such as hemiparesis or paraparesis (Ramirez-Avila et al., 2009 ; Schmutzhard et al., 1988). Seizures may be the predominant symptom of neurocysticercosis. Eosinophilic cerebrospinal fluid due to Paragonimus infection is rare, usually accompanied with pleuro-pulmonary lesions, and less likely to cause alteration of consciousness (Solomon et al., 2006). Eating raw freshwater crab is a risk factor for paragonimiasis. Exposure to dog and raccoon feces may be risk factor for neurotoxocariasis and *Baylisascaris procyonis* infection, respectively. The last two diseases are predominant in children (Solomon et al., 2006). Active tuberculosis and malignancy may also cause eosinophilic cerebrospinal fluid but fluid, but they are rarely reported to have cerebrospinal fluid eosinophils.

8. Treatments

Even though meningitic angiostrongyliasis will be successfully treated with corticosteroid (Chotmongkol et al., 2000), there is no effective treatment for encephalitic angiostrogyliasis. The combination between corticosteroid and anthelminthic agents may be beneficial.

Albendazole may be the preferred combination regimen due to its high absorbable throgh gastrointestinal tract and high concentration in cerebrospinal fluid. A report from China showed that the regimen of dexamethasone (20 mg, qid), gamma-globulin (0.5 g/kg), 20% mannitol, and Chinese herbs (Xing Nao Wan) was an effective treatment regimen for a patient with encephalitic angiostrogyliasis. The patient recovered from coma stage quickly and had only mild memory loss at discharge (Li et al., 2008).

9. Prognosis

Generally, the prognosis of encephalitic angiostrogyliasis is poor (Ko et al., 1987; Martínez-Delgado et al, 2000; Pascual et al., 1981; Chotmongkol & Sawanyawisuth, 2002). The mortality rate is approximately 80% and the rest are likely to be bed-ridden stage. The causes of death are hospital acquired infections or severe brain edema and herniation.

10. Prevention

The effective prevention is to avoid contaminated foods particularly raw freshwater snails, slugs, frogs, shrimps, contaminated vegetables and juice including playing or contact with snails.

11. Conclusion

Encephalitic angiostrongyliasis, a rare manifestation of human angiostrongyliasis, can be diagnosed by clinical criteria. Clinical clue for this condition are history of exposure to *A. cantonensis* larva, evidence of eosinophils in cerebrospinal fluid more than 10% without other possible causes of eosinophils in cerebrospinal fluid. Serological tests may be used as a confirmatory test. Currently, there is no effective treatment. Corticosteroid, anthelminthics, or gamma-globulin may be optional treatments. Due to the high mortality rate, prevention is the most important strategy.

12. References

Chotmongkol, V.; Sawanyawisuth, K. & Thavornpitak, Y. (2000). Corticosteroid treatment of eosinophilic meningitis. *Clinical Infectious Diseases*, Vol.31, No.3, pp.660-662, ISSN 1058-4838.

Chotmongkol, V. & Sawanyawisuth, K. (2002). Clinical manifestations and outcome of patients with severe eosinophilic meningoencephalitis presumably caused by Angiostrongylus cantonensis. *Southeast Asian Journal of Tropical Medicine and Public Health*, Vol.33, No.2, pp.231-234, ISSN 0125-1562.

Chye, S.M.; Lin, S.R.; Chen, Y.L.; Chung, L.Y. & Yen, C.M. (2004). Immuno-PCR for detection of antigen to *Angiostrongylus cantonensis* circulating fifth-stage worms. *Clinical Chemistry*, Vol.50, No.1, pp.51-57, ISSN 1530-8561.

Dorta-Contreras, A.J. & Reiber, H. (1998). Intrathecal synthesis of immunoglobulins in eosinophilic meningoencephalitis due to Angiostrongylus cantonensis. *Clinical and Diagnostic Laboratory Immunology*, Vol.5, No.4, pp.452-455, ISSN 1556-6811.

Eamsobhana, P.; Yoolek, A. & Kreethapon, N. (2003). Blinded multi-laboratory evaluation of an in-house dot-blot ELISA kit for diagnosis of human parastrongyliasis. *Southeast*

Asian Journal of Tropical Medicine and Public Health, Vol.34, No.1, pp.1-6, ISSN 0125-1562.

Eamsobhana, P., &Yong, H.S. (2009). Multi-immunodot for rapid differential diagnosis of eosinophilic meningitis due to parasitic infections. *International Journal of Infectious Diseases,* Vol.13, No.4, pp.425-431, ISSN 1201-9712.

Eamsobhana, P. Ongrotchanakun, J., Yoolek, A., Punthuprapasa, P., Monkong, N., & Dekumyoy, P. (2006). Immunological diagnosis of human angiostrongyliasis due to *Angiostrongylus cantonensis* (Nematoda: Angiostrongylidae). *Journal of Helminthology,* Vol.80, No.3, pp.249-254, ISSN 0022-149X.

Graber, D.; Jaffar, M.C.; Attali, T.; Poisson, J.; Renouil, M.; Alessandri, J.L. & Combes, J.C. (1997). [Angiostrongylosis in infants in Reunion and Mayotte. Apropos of 3 cases of eosinophilic meningitis including 1 fatal radiculo-myeloencephalitis with hydrocephalus]. *Bulletin of the Exotic Pathology Society,* Vol.90, No.5, pp.331-333, ISSN 0037-9085.

Intapan, P.M.; Maleewong, W.; Sawanyawisuth, K. & Chotmongkol, V. (2003). Evaluation of human IgG subclass antibodies in the serodiagnosis of angiostrongyliasis. *Parasitology Research,* Vol.89, No.6, pp.425-429, ISSN 0932-0113.

Jin, E.; Ma, D.; Liang, Y.; Ji, A. & Gan, S. (2005). MRI findings of eosinophilic myelomeningoencephalitis due to Angiostrongylus cantonensis. *Clinical Radiology,* Vol.60, No.2, pp.242-250, ISSN 0009-9252.

Jin, E.H.; Ma, Q.; Ma, D.Q.; He, W.; Ji, A.P. & Yin, C.H. (2008). Magnetic resonance imaging of eosinophilic meningoencephalitis caused by Angiostrongylus cantonensis following eating freshwater snails. *Chinese Medical Journal (English),*Vol.121, No.1, pp.67-72, ISSN 21511918 2151 1918.

Kanpittaya, J.; Jitpimolmard, S.; Tiamkao, S. & Mairiang, E. (2000). MR findings of eosinophilic meningoencephalitis attributed to Angiostrongylus cantonensis. *AJNR American Journal of Neuroradiology,* Vol.21, No.6, pp.1090-1094, ISSN 0195-6108.

Kliks, M.M.; Kroenke, K. & Hardman, J.M. (1982). Eosinophilic radiculomyeloencephalitis: an angiostrongyliasis outbreak in American Samoa related to ingestion of Achatina fulica snails. *American Journal of Tropical Medicine and Hygiene,* Vol.31, No.6, pp.1114-1122, ISSN 0002-9637.

Ko, R.C.; Chan, S.W.; Chan, K.W.; Lam, K.; Farrington, M.; Wong, H.W. & Yuen, P. (1987). Four documented cases of eosinophilic meningoencephalitis due to Angiostrongylus cantonensis in Hong Kong. *Transactions of the Royal Society of Tropical Medicine and Hygiene,* Vol.81, No.5, pp.807-810, ISSN 0035-9203.

Li, H.; Xu, F.; Gu, J.B. & Chen, X.G. (2008). A severe eosinophilic meningoencephalitis caused by infection of Angiostrongylus cantonensis. *American Journal of Tropical Medicine and Hygiene,* Vol.79, No.4, pp.568-570, ISSN 0002-9637.

Maleewong, W.; Sombatsawat, P.; Intapan, P.M.; Wongkham, C. & Chotmongkol V. (2001). Immunoblot evaluation of the specificity of the 29-kDa antigen from young adult female worms *Angiostrongylus cantonensis* for immunodiagnosis of human angiostrongyliasis. *Asian Pacific Journal of Allergy and Immunology,* Vol.19, No.4, pp.267-273, ISSN 0125-877X.

Martínez-Delgado, J.F.; González-Cortiñas, M.; Tápanes-Cruz, T.R. & Ruiz-Méndez, A. (2000). Eosinophilic meningoencephalitis in Villa Clara (Cuba). A study of 17 patients. *Revista de Neurología,* Vol.*31,*No.5, pp.417-421, ISSN 0210-0010.

Nye, S.W.; Tangchai, P.; Sundarakiti, S. & Punyagupta, S. (1970). Lesions of the brain in eosinophilic meningitis. *Archives of Pathology*, Vol.89, No.1, pp.9-19, ISSN 0004-1955.

Padilla-Docal, B.; Dorta-Contreras, A.J.; Bu-Coifiu-Fanego, R.; Hernández, H.F.; Barroso, J.C. & Sanchez-Martinez, C. (2008). Intrathecal synthesis of IgE in children with eosinophilic meningoencephalitis caused by Angiostrongylus cantonensis. *Cerebrospinal Fluid Research*, Vol.25, No.5, pp.18, ISSN 17438454.

Pascual, J.E.; Bouli, R.P. & Aguiar, H. (1981). Eosinophilic meningoencephalitis in Cuba, caused by Angiostrongylus cantonensis. *American Journal of Tropical Medicine and Hygiene*, Vol.30, No.5, pp.960-962, ISSN 0002-9637.

Punyagupta, S.; Bunnag, T.; Juttijudata, P. & Rosen, L. (1970). Eosinophilic meningitis in Thailand. Epidemiologic studies of 484 typical cases and the etiologic role of Angiostrongylus cantonensis. *American Journal of Tropical Medicine and Hygiene*, Vol.19, No.6, pp.950-958, ISSN 0002-9637.

Ramirez-Avila, L. ; Slome, S.; Schuster, F.L.; Gavali, S.; Schantz, P.M.; Sejvar, J. & Glaser, C.A. (2009). Eosinophilic meningitis due to Angiostrongylus and Gnathostoma species. *Clinical Infectious Diseases*, Vol.48, No.3, pp.322-327, ISSN 1058-4838.

Sawanyawisuth, K.; Thammaroj, J.; Limpawattana, P.; Intapan, P.M.; Tiamkao, S. & Jitpimolmard, S. (2006). Communicating hydrocephalus as a complication of eosinophilic meningoencephalitis. *Journal of the Medical Association of Thailand*, Vol.89, No.7, pp.1024-1028, ISSN 0025-7036.

Sawanyawisuth, K.; Kitthaweesin, K.; Limpawattana, P.; Intapan, P.M.; Tiamkao, S.; Jitpimolmard, S. & Chotmongkol, V. (2007). Intraocular angiostrongyliasis: clinical findings, treatments and outcomes. *Transactions of the Royal Society of Tropical Medicine and Hygiene*, Vol.101, No.5, pp.497-501, ISSN 0035-9203.

Sawanyawisuth, K. & Sawanyawisuth, K. (2008). Treatment of angiostrongyliasis. *Transactions of the Royal Society of Tropical Medicine and Hygiene*, Vol.102, No.10, pp.990-996, ISSN 0035-9203.

Sawanyawisuth, K.; Takahashi, K.; Hoshuyama, T.; Sawanyawisuth, K.; Senthong, V.; Limpawattana, P.; Intapan, P.M.; Wilson, D.; Tiamkao, S.; Jitpimolmard, S. & Chotmongkol, V. (2009). Clinical factors predictive of encephalitis caused by Angiostrongylus cantonensis. *American Journal of Tropical Medicine and Hygiene*, Vol.81, No.4, pp.698-701, ISSN 0002-9637.

Sawanyawisuth, K.; Pugkhem, A.; Mitchai, J.; Intapan, P.M.; Anunnatsiri, S.; Limpawattana, P. & Chotmongkol, V. (2010). Abdominal angiostrongyliasis caused by Angiostrongylus cantonensis: a possible cause of eosinophilic infiltration in human digestive tract. *Pathology Research and Practice*, Vol.206, No.2, pp.102-104, ISSN 0344-0338.

Schmutzhard, E.; Boongird, P. & Vejjajiva, A. (1988). Eosinophilic meningitis and radiculomyelitis in Thailand, caused by CNS invasion of Gnathostoma spinigerum and Angiostrongylus cantonensis. *Journal of Neurology, Neurosurgery and Psychiatry*, Vol.51, No.1, pp.80-87, ISSN 0022-3050.

Solomon, T.; Danesi M.; Bia, F.J. & Plekc, T.P. (2006) Neurologic disease, In: *Tropical infectious diseases: Principles, Pathogens & Practice*, Guerrant, R.L.; Walker, D.H. & Weller, P.F., (Ed.), 1601-1608, Churchill Livingstone, ISBN 978-0-7020-3935-5, Philadelphia, USA.

Sonakul, D. (1978). Pathological findings in four cases of human angiostrongyliasis. *Southeast Asian Journal of Tropical Medicine and Public Health*, Vol.9, No.2, pp.220-227, ISSN 0125-1562.

Tsai, H.C.; Liu, Y.C.; Kunin, C.M.; Lai, P.H.; Lee, S.S.; Chen, Y.S.; Wann, S.R.; Lin, W.R.; Huang, C.K.; Ger, L.P.; Lin, H.H. & Yen, M.Y. (2003). Eosinophilic meningitis caused by Angiostrongylus cantonensis associated with eating raw snails: correlation of brain magnetic resonance imaging scans with clinical findings. *American Journal of Tropical Medicine and Hygiene*, Vol.68, No.3, pp.281-285, ISSN 0002-9637.

Tsai, H.C.; Lee, S.S.; Huang, C.K.; Yen, C.M.; Chen, E.R. & Liu, Y.C. (2004). Outbreak of eosinophilic meningitis associated with drinking raw vegetable juice in southern Taiwan. *American Journal of Tropical Medicine and Hygiene*, Vol.71, No.2, pp.222-226, ISSN 0002-9637.

Wan, K.S. & Weng, W.C. (2004). Eosinophilic meningitis in a child raising snails as pets. *Acta Tropica*, Vol.90, No.1, pp.51-53, ISSN 0001-706X.

Wang, Q.P.; Lai, D.H.; Zhu, X.Q.; Chen, X.G. & Lun, Z.R. (2008). Human angiostrongyliasis. *Lancet Infectious Diseases*, Vol.8, No.10, pp.621-630, ISSN 1473-3099.

Wang, X.; Huang, H.; Dong, Q.; Lin, Y.; Wang, Z.; Li, F.; Nawa, Y. & Yoshimura, K. (2002). A clinical study of eosinophilic meningoencephalitis caused by angiostrongyliasis. *Chinese Medical Journal (English)*, Vol.115, No.9, pp.1312-1315, ISSN 21511918 2151 1918.

13

Clinical and Therapeutic Aspects of *Cryptococcal Meningitis* in West Africa

A.A. Oumar[1,2], A.S. Hammond[2], B. Diarra[2],
A.I. Maiga[2], G.K. Taboue[1], S. Dao[1,2,3] and A. Tounkara[1,2]
[1]*Faculty of Medicine, Pharmacy and Odontostomatology, University of Bamako*
[2]*HIV/TB Research and Training Center, University of Bamako*
[3]*Infectious Diseases Service, Hospital Point G, Bamako*
Mali

1. Introduction

Cryptococcus meningitis is the most severe form of cryptococcal infections that infects the brain parenchyma and sub-arachnoid space. It often progresses to fatal disease states when it goes untreated. The clinical presentation and disease course of cryptococcal infection is partially marked by changes that occur as a result of certain medical conditions including, use of glucocorticoids or other immunosuppressive drugs, diabetes, as well as the immune status of the host (Chuck, 1989; Dismukes, 1988). Mostly, the disease affects people with a compromised immune system and is found in people with advanced HIV infection and AIDS, with the major burden in South-East Asia and Africa (Mwaba, 2001; Maher, 1994; Moosa, 1997).

The infection itself is caused by inhalation of a yeast-like round fungus with a polysaccharide capsule, known as *Cryptococcal neoformans,* and disseminates from the lungs. This fungus is the only pathogenic species of the genus *Cryptococcus*. Based on the capsule components four serotypes of *C. neoformans* (A, B, C and D) have been isolated, and the species is divided into two forms. Each serotype has different epidemiologic and pathogenic profile and their presence suggests an environmentally unfriendly atmosphere for people with a defective T cell function. Consequently, the common forms of *C. neoformans* that affect humans in Europe and parts of US is *C. neoformans* var *neoformans,* whereas in tropical areas such as the Far East, Africa and Australia, *C. neoformans* var *gattii* is the common form of cryptococcal infection (Gari-Toussaint,1996). *C. neoformans* var *gattii* is also thought to be ecologically resident on Eucalyptus trees (Ellis, 1990). An outbreak of Cryptococcosis in healthy humans and animals in Vancouver Island, Canada, and the subsequent isolation of *C. neoformans* var *gattii* in Washington and Oregon in the US, have now led to the understanding that this species is not restricted to tropical and sub-tropical climates alone (Datta, 2009). Rather it has a wider geographic distribution and can also thrive in temperate climates, as well as on species of trees other than Eucalyptus (Datta, 2009).

Estimates indicate that worldwide, the burden of human cryptococcal infections ranges between 2 to 30 % and most infected patients have HIV/AIDS (Bicanic, 2006; French, 2002). An observation in the US in 1990 showed an increase to 5000 cases of *cryptococcal meningitis* infection in AIDS patients, compared to 300 cases in 1980 where half of these cases were apparently without signs of immune suppression. In most nations, the effective adoption of antiretroviral therapy (ART) has led to a dramatic decrease in *C. neoformans* infection (Mirza, 2003). In the US for instance, only 7 % of 2087 AIDS patients were found to have cryptococcoses whereas, in France the incidence dropped to 100 cases per year due to the introduction of triple antiretroviral therapy (Steven, 1989). In most parts of Africa however, the HIV epidemic led to the emergence and resurgence of many opportunistic infections including *cryptococcal meningitis*, mycobacteria, and cytomegalovirus. Lack of full access to ART in West Africa, resulted in *cryptococcal meningitis* becoming the second opportunistic infection to cause fatal disease, after mycobacteria in late stage HIV-infected patients (Okongo, 1998; Mwaba, 2001). For instance, between 1993 and 2006, *C. neoformans* accounted for 0.7 % of meningitis cases in Dakar, Senegal and 2.5 % at Point G Teaching Hospital in Mali (Soumare, 2005c; Coulibaly,2005). By comparison, in 2006, 33 cases out of 3655 (0.9 %) hospitalized patients were found to be infected with *cyptococcal meningitis* in Cameroon (Mbuagbaw, 2006).

In West Africa, diagnosis and treatment of c*ryptococcal meningitis* is particularly faced with many difficulties including problems associated with efficiency of the healthcare system in these countries, poverty rate and educational status of those infected In the text that follows we summarize our understanding of the current challenges faced in the clinical diagnosis and treatment of this disease in this region, and make suggestions for future consideration.

2. Epidemiology

Although considerable efforts have been made to estimate the number of cases of *cyptococcal meningitis* and the percentage of those infected by *Cryptococcal neoformans*, there is still gaps in the knowledge of true estimates worldwide (Harrison, 2009). Current reports show that globally there are approximately 957, 900 cases of *cyptococcal meningitis* occurring every year, with majority of these infections found in areas of high HIV prevalence (Park, 2009). Of this figure, lack of adequate resources and funding, lack of early diagnosis, access to treatment and an ineffective distribution of ART results in the deaths of between 125,000 and 1,124,900 cases shortly (3 months) after the infection (Park, 2009). In Uganda *cyptococcal meningitis* disease was found to cause 17 % of deaths among HIV-1-infected adults. In South Africa, between 13-44% of all deaths among 3 HIV-seropositive cohorts were reported to be associated with *Cryptococcus neoformans* infection (Bicanic, 2006). Globally, the incidence rates among people with HIV/AIDS are estimated to have risen to 12 % per year (Park, 2009). Although HIV and other immune compromised individuals are implicated in this disease, reports indicate that there are a few cases of *cyptococcal meningitis* unrelated to HIV infection (Mirza, 2003).

With the introduction of antiretroviral therapy (ART) rates in parts of the US decreased substantially from 23.6 per 1000 persons in 1993 to 1.6 per 1000 persons in the year 2000 (Mirza, 2003) despite ongoing debates about the best timing to start ART. Though the optimal timing to initiate ART is not clear, it is known that current ART regimens and adherence to treatment are capable of suppressing viremia and thereby create an environment that enhances the functions of the immune system of patients undergoing treatment (Bisson, 2008; Zolopa, 2009; Makadzange, 2010). Consequently, the effective provision of ART has caused significant reductions in morbidity and mortality associated with severe immune suppression and has led to a reduction in the incidence of *cyptococcal meningitis* in HIV/AIDS patients. Such reduction is observed more in countries where there is early access to HIV care and prophylaxis for *cyptococcal meningitis* as well as early diagnosis during initial stages of the infection.

Current trends indicate that, most cases of *cyptococcal meningitis* found in Africa are among HIV-infected people with <100 cells/µl CD4 T cell count. Based on reported figures it is known that *cyptococcal meningitis* causes between 10-20 % deaths in Africa (French, 2002; Okongo, 1998; Park, 2009). Recently, a study in Malawi found *cyptococcal meningitis* to be the most common cause of meningitis disease with 40 % of cases from HIV-infected people. In West Africa, the disease is thought to be the most common opportunistic infection after mycobacteria. Data from West Africa are scanty due probably to a number of logistic problems and inefficiency with the health systems of the countries in this region, and as a result only a few of the cases in this region are reported here. Based on 2009 estimates 6 countries can be ranked from first to sixth in terms of total numbers of *cyptococcal meningitis* cases in West Africa. At the top of this hierarchy is Senegal, followed by Burkina Faso, Cote d'Ivoire, Mali, Niger and Ghana, with approximately 0.7-2.5 % patients with AIDS having cryptococcal infection.

Countries	**Years of Study**	**Prevalence (%)**	**Study Place**
Senegal (Soumare,2005)	2005	3.9 - 32.5	Infectious Diseases department of the Teaching Hospital of Fan
Burkina Faso (Ki-Zerbo,1996;Millogo,2004)	1996 to 2004	1.16 - 20.5	Internal medicine department of the Teaching Hospital of Ouagadougou
Cote D'Ivoire (Ouedraogo,2007)	2007	4.3 - 16.5	Internal medicine and Infectious Diseases departments of the Teaching Hospital of Coccody
Mali (Oumar,2008)	2008	8.3	Infectious Diseases of the Teaching Hospital of Point-g, Bamako
Niger (Seybou,2008)	2008	6.3	National Hospital of Niamey
Ghana (Frimpong,1998)	1998	0	Microbiology Laboratory of Kumasi

Note: Hierarchical list showing prevalence of *Cryptococcal meningitis* in West Africa obtained from different studies in this region.

Table 1. Prevalence of *Cryptococal meningitis* in West Africa

3. Clinical & diagnostic profiles of *Cryptococcal meningitis*

3.1 Clinical features

Cryptococcal meningitis is an insidious disease. Following infection, cryptococcus spread to other organs particularly the central nervous system (CNS) which is the main site in either immune competent or immune suppressed individuals. Most patients present with no symptoms and only report fever and mild headaches as a result of intracranial pressure. Reports from Burkina Faso showed that between 1996 and 1998, the major symptoms in patients with cryptococcal infection were headache and fever with 3 out of 7 patients having no neck stiffness (Millogo, 2004). However, patients who reported with the same disease in 2004 showed signs of neck stiffness, and headache. For patients with HIV/AIDS, the meningitis may spread rapidly to many organs. Records from Cote d'Ivoire showed that a number of hospitalized patients on admission presented with nonspecific severe symptoms that were associated with progression of *cryptococcal meningitis* disease including weight loss (44-62 %), chronic diarrhea (22-44.2 %), fever (50-85 %), chronic coughs (14 %), coma, convulsions and neck stiffness (24.4-85%) (Eholie, 2000). In Mali, 15 of 17 (88.2 %) cases with *cryptococcal meningitis* had signs of some abnormality while the remaining 2 had isolated fever. Overall, 14 of these patients had HIV-1 infection and their median CD4 T cell counts were <200 cells/µl (range 1-237 cells/µl). The CD4 T cell counts for the remaining 3 immune competent individuals were between 347 and 899 cells/µl (Minta, 2008). In Senegal, common symptoms reported were headache (86.7 %), fever (73.3 %), vomiting (66.7 %) and general weight loss (75.6 %). Most patients also presented with neurological signs including altered consciousness, seizures, motor deficits (paraplegia, flaccid hemi paresis and paraparesis), cranial nerve problems and coma at different stages of the disease. In 27 patients meningeal syndrome characterized by neck stiffness was followed by the presence of positive Kernig and/ or Bradzinski sign (Soumare, 2005a). There were no records for CD4 T cell counts of the patients studied here (Soumare, 2005b; 2005c). Data from Niger showed that all 8 HIV-1-infected patients with cryptococcosis had both fever and headache, 3 of 8 (37.5 %) had coma, and 1 (12.5 %) had seizures. The average CD4 T cell count for these patients was 41 cells/µl.

3.2 Diagnostic features

Diagnosis of the disease is easy and requires no sophisticated methods or equipment. Specimens for laboratory diagnosis are collected based on the symptoms presented by the patient. Although most body fluids, including cerebro-spinal fluid (CSF), sputum, bronchoalveolar lavage (BAL), bronchial washings, biopsy tissues, prostatic fluid and blood, can be used for performing the test, the most common specimen used in many areas around the world is CSF. In West Africa, diagnosis is commonly performed by microscopic examination of CSF for yeast cells.

3.2.1 Direct microscopy

The conventional method for laboratory diagnosis involves direct examination of CSF deposits by use of Indian ink/Nigrosin wet mount coloration to detect yeast cells. Direct microscopy of samples from HIV-infected individuals often yields positive results in 90% of cases (Desmet, 1989). It is more useful to perform blood culture for disseminated cases. To confirm diagnosis, CSF is cultured on Sabouraud agar plates for > 36 h. This allows cultures to grow and the method can be utilized for evaluating disease burden by diluting aliquots of CSF and enumerating the number of colony-forming units for the fungal load in the specimen (Eholie, 2000; Ki-Zerbo, 1996; Millogo, 2004; Soumare, 2005c). With a little modification, the method can also be used for assessing efficacy of anticryptococcal regimens (Bicanic, 2009).

3.2.2 Serology

Some reports have indicated that, due to changes in the epidemiology of the infection, detection of small capsules of the antigen make recognition difficult with India ink staining (Bottone, 1986). A second method for diagnosing *C. meningitis* infection is therefore by use of latex agglutination test to detect cryptococcal polysaccharide capsular antigens of *C. neoformans*. This test can be performed on CSF and serum and there are commercially available kits (example Crypto-LA [International Biological Labs. Inc., Cranbury, N.J.], MYCO-Immune [American MicroScan, Mahwah, N.J.], and IMMY [Immuno-Mycologics, Inc., norman, Okla], or CALAS [Meridian Diagnostics Inc., Cincinnati, Ohio]) with high sensitivity and specificity for carrying out this test. In most AIDS or other severely immune compromised patients, it is not useful to perform antibody detection tests.

Country	Different Studies	Diagnostic Methods		
		Culture of CSF	Serology	Direct Microscopy
Burkina Faso	Ki-Zerbo, 1996	+	-	+
	Millogo, 2004	+	-	+
Cote d'Ivoire	Eholie, 1997	-	+	+
	Eholie, 2000	+	+	+
	Eholie, 2004	+	+	+
	Ouedraogo, 2007	+	-	+
Mali	Oumar, 2008	-	-	+
	Minta, 2008	+	-	+
Senegal	Soumare, 2005a	+	+	+
	Soumare, 2005b	+	+	+
	Soumare, 2005c	+	+	+
Niger	Seybou, 2008	-	+	-
Ghana	Frimpong, 1998	+	-	+

Note: (+) is Used and (-) not Used

Table 2. Different Methods Used for Cryptococcus Diagnosis in West Africa

4. Therapeutic aspects

Much progress has been made in the management of *Cryptococcal meningitis* in the developed world. For immune compromised patients with *Cryptococcal meningitis* three phases of therapy (induction for 2 weeks, consolidation for 8 weeks and maintenance for prolonged period) for receiving antifungal treatment have been suggested based on results from a clinical trial (van der Horst, 1997). Also, based on guidelines endorsed by the Infectious Diseases Society of America a higher dose of amphotericin B followed by fluconazole can be used to treat AIDS patients with cryptococcal meningitis. Of importance is that, although oral fluconazole is known to provide some initial relief from cryptococcal meningitis, it takes a longer duration to cleanse the cerebrospinal fluid of its fungal pathogens (Brouwer, 2004; Larsen, 1990; van der Horst, 1997).

It is now known that use of fluconazole alone, for treatment of the disease in AIDS patients is not enough, and that other approaches such as the use of amphotericin B combined with flucytosine, as well as increased immunological responses due to the use of antiretroviral drugs, are also required (Larsen, 1990). Thus, for immune suppressed patients with *cryptococcal meningitis,* treatment regimens include < 1.0 mg/kg/day amphotericin B deoxycholate (AmB) given intravenously plus 100 mg/kg/day flucytosine for 2 weeks followed by 400 mg oral Fluconazole for 8 weeks. In most countries in Africa however, due to a number of reasons including, cost, lengthy regulatory approval to import antifungal drugs, difficulty of administration and blood monitoring of amphotericin B-based therapy to avoid toxicity, fluconazole is used as primary therapy for the treatment of the disease (Bicanic 2009; Bicanic, 2005). Fluconazole causes fewer, less severe side effects, including skin rashes and liver enzyme abnormalities. Even with the use of fluconazole alone, problems with access to expert medical care and the management of complications of AIDS still exist in this region (Mwaba, 2001; Wertheimer, 2004). In most countries of West Africa fluconazole monotherapy was used.

Some reports have suggested that initial monotherapy with fluconazole led to relapse of HIV-associated cryptococcal meningitis. To prevent relapses, most doctors recommend that people who have had cryptococcal meningitis take fluconazole daily. Other drugs used include intravenous amphotericin B taken weekly or biweekly (Jackson, 2010).

Amphotericin B has many side effects, including kidney damage, high fever, low blood pressure, decreased numbers of red or white blood cells, nausea, vomiting, and chills. A newer formulation of the drug, in which the active compound is encased in a fatty substance, has been under study for a while and may have fewer side effects (Sharkey, 1996). However, more research is needed to assess the safety and effectiveness of this new form of amphotericin B. Flucytosin also may cause serious side effects, including decreased numbers of red or white blood cells, liver damage, nausea, diarrhoea, seizures, abdominal discomfort, or rash. In Mali treatment with amphotericin B and fluconazole injection is known to have had such side effects in 13 out of 17 patients (Oumar, 2008). Before the administration of amphotericin B, patients were injected with chlorpromazine (one hour before) and acetylsalicylic acid (30 min earlier). Then the infusions of amphotericin B were followed by an infusion of between 1.5-2 liters of 0.9% saline. This procedure was to reduce adverse effects associated with the use of amphotericin B (Oumar, 2008). In immune competent people, treatment is done using injectable amphotericin B alone, or followed by infusion of fluconazole treatment for some cases. In other cases, patients received amphotericin B in association with injectable ceftriaxon (Minta, 2008).

In Senegal fluconazole alone was the most commonly used antifungal in at least 93% of cases. It was used together with amphotericin B in one case (Soumare, 2005c). Here, the treatment strategy was the administration of fluconazole at 400 to 800 mg/day by intravenous infusion for 8 weeks, followed by a maintenance dose of 200 mg daily for a month. The maintenance treatment was however, continued until the CD4 count rose above 200 cells/µl for a period of 6 months (Soumare, 2005a). In Niger 3 out of 4 patients diagnosed in 2007 received monotherapy consisting of 400mg/day fluconazole (Seybou, 2008). The average duration of treatment was 25.2 days (range, 2-72 days). Although no HIV patients died during emergency periods, 165 cases (53%) were hospitalized and 147 patients were allowed to return home after the emergency care (47%) (Tanon, 2006). In a patient aged 66 years, cognitive functions declined partly from the 10th day. The delirium in a second patient aged 49 years, declined by the 10th day, and complete neurological recovery was observed at 3 months (Kouame, 2007). Overall, hospital stay period lasted for 25 days and between 1-50 days for those associated with cryptococcal meningitis. The severity of the prognosis was related to the combination of two or more opportunistic infections (Ouedraogo, 2007). In Burkina Faso, fluconazole was initially effective in two patients with a dose of 400mg/day, which was started on the eve of the death of a patient (Millogo, 2004).
The paucity of prospective data on the management of cryptococcal meningitis in patients without AIDS is the most challenging aspect of formulating treatment guidelines, but the principles of induction, consolidation, and maintenance were still applied. For patients with a predisposition to renal dysfunction a combination antifungal therapy with a lipid formulation of amphotericin B plus flucytosine was generally indicated.

5. Early diagnosis, Importance and challenges of ART initiation in the management of cryptococcal meningitis

During HIV infection, because the CD4+ T cells are the primary target of the virus, progressive loss of these cells leads to increasing immunodeficiency and risk of opportunistic diseases, progression to AIDS and ultimately death (O'Brien, 1996) The resurgence of HIV in resource poor settings in Africa and the complications associated with management of AIDS has led to a number of deaths attributable to cryptococcal meningitis. The good news is that reduction in CD4 cells can be reversed with effective antiretroviral therapy early in the course of infection and slow down its spread (Bisson, 2008). Despite this, it is important to note that often some proportion of patients who start therapy when their CD4 T cell counts are below 100 cells/µl are unable to gain restoration of their cells with ART and therefore pose additional challenges in treatment (Kelley, 2009). In addition to an increase in CD4 cell count, early initiation of therapy also increases general immune function, is cost-effective and facilitates the reduction in a number of clinical events, including lowering of incidence or risk of opportunistic infections. And although a number of guidelines are available for early initiation of ART in patients with AIDS-defining illnesses, the implementation of these guidelines in itself is a further challenge for resource-limited regions such as West Africa. Here, treatment poses additional financial burden because, under such guidelines ART will have to be provided for a large number of patients. Another concern is that, the use of ART comes with some complex challenges. Most notably is the possibility of developing immune reconstitution inflammatory syndrome (IRIS), a condition that occurs following rapid restoration of immune function after ART

Countries	Different Studies	Antifungal and adjuvant therapy						
		AmB	FCZ	KTZ	AmB ; ASA	FCZ; ASA	AmB ; FCZ	AmB ;FCZ ; SS CPMZ
Burkina Faso	Ki-Zerbo, 1996	-	+	+	-	-	-	-
	Millogo,2004	-	+	-	-	-	-	-
Cote D'Ivoire	Eholie,1997	+	-	-	-	-	-	-
	Eholie,2004	+	-	-	-	-	-	-
	Ouattara, 2007	-	-	-	-	+	-	-
	Ouedraogo, 2007	+	-	-	-	-	-	-
Mali	Oumar,2008	-	-	-	-	-	-	+
	Minta,2008	+	-	-	-	-	+	-
Senegal	Soumare, 2005a	-	+	-	-	-	+	-
	Soumare, 2005b	-	+	-	-	-	-	-
	N'diaye,2008	+	+	-	-	-	-	-
Niger	Seybou, 2008	-	+	-	-	-	-	-
Ghana	Frimpong , 1998	No Treatment as they didn't recovered the fungus						

(+) is Used and (-) not Used
AmB : Amphotericin B ; FCZ : Fluconazol ; KTZ: Ketoconazole; CPMZ: Chlorpromazin; ASA: acetyl salicylic acid; SS: Saline solution

Table 3. Treatment Regimens used for Cryptococcus in West Africa administration. In South Africa, cryptococcal reconstitution disease was associated with 6 of 22 deaths in a HIV-infected cohort within 3 months of starting ART (Bicanic, 2009; Lawn, 2005). Recent data also suggests potential drug interactions between nevirapine-based ART and high levels of fluconazole and the handling of any toxicities associated with this interaction may pose additional management difficulties in the West African context (Manosuthi, 2007).

6. The lethality of cryptococcal meningitis in West Africa

Cryptococcal meningitis is a disease that has a high chance of causing death. In West Africa, reported deaths associated with this disease are between 42 and 80% (Sow, 1998; Millogo, 2004, Eholie, 2000, Bissagnene, 1994, Ki-Zerbo, 1996, Soumare, 2005a, Kadjo, 2007, Oumar, 2008). The disease progresses to fatal states quickly. In 80% of cases, patients died before day 15 after hospitalization (Millogo, 2004, Seybou 2008). Such high mortality is correlated with an increased number of Cryptococcal pathogens similar to that seen with *Mycobacterium tuberculosis* (Eholié, 2000, Ouedraogo, 2007). One study noted that a lowered CSF glucose provides poor prognosis for *Cryptococcal meningitis* in West Africa (Ki-Zerbo, 1996). Pronounced immune deficiency and hematological abnormalities such as hyponatremia are also factors of poor prognosis (Eholié, 1997; Ki-Zerbo, 1996). Others noted that the lethality of the disease is significantly higher in patients with a CD4 T cell count below 20 cells/µl (Ki-Zerbo, 1996; Soumare, 2005a). Recent studies in the region indicate that the lethality of *Cryptococcal meningitis* is significantly associated with delay in diagnosis and initiation of appropriate treatment as well as non-compliance to drug therapy due to financial reasons (Eholié, 2000; Kadjo, 2007; Millogo, 2004; Ouattara, 2007; Oumar, 2008; Soumare, 2005b). The high lethality may also be due to inadequate treatment regimens used in the region (Oumar, 2008, Soumare, 2005a, Kadjo, 2007). The high fatality rate found in most countries of West Africa could be due to the fact that people consult with end-stage disease.

7. Conclusion

Impaired immunity associated with HIV infection has led to many complications. Effective introduction of anti-retroviral therapy has played a significant role in the reductions of Cryptococcosis in HIV/AIDS patients in most developed nations. The resurgence of HIV in developing countries has however, exposed many inadequacies in the management and control of cryptococcal meningitis in West Africa and elsewhere. Inadequate resources and an ineffective distribution of ART in this region could lead those with HIV to be more at risk of infection with Cryptococcus species. For those already having Cryptococcus disease, lack of early diagnosis offers an environment to progress to more fatal disease states.

Given that laboratory diagnosis of *Cryptococcal meningitis* is easy to perform and does not require extensive equipment, it is vital that the resources and capacity to perform this test is made available in centers of HIV care. An increasing number of studies have shown that relapses to initial treatment to cryptococcal disease is a possibility and can lead to further complications, including immune reconstitution inflammatory syndrome. Despite this knowledge, little is known of surveillance studies related to drug susceptibility to resistant cases of *Cryptococcal meningitis* in West Africa. More education at community and other grass root levels must be stepped up to increase awareness of the importance of early screening for Cryptococcus disease. In most resource-poor settings studied in West Africa, the standard of care for HIV/AIDS patients with acute cryptococcal meningitis are dependent on availability of resources and access to anti-fungal drugs. Logically, as a first step, and if available it is necessary to sterilize the CSF of patients with amphotericin B, since this regimen is known to minimize resistance to fluconazole (Bicanic, 2006). As an alternative approach, it will be beneficial in this setting to give higher doses of fluconazole bearing in mind that better clinical and microbiological responses to fluconazole have been observed in some studies (Berry, 1992; Hossain, 2002). In addition, there is an urgent need for policy makers to step up capabilities for managing complications associated with HIV patients progressing to AIDS. Finally, given the impact of effective antiretroviral therapy in reducing HIV-associated morbidity and mortality it will be more supportive if in West Africa, governments and care-givers find easier alternative ways to reach patients with these drugs (ART) taking into consideration travel times to the health care centers which often deters patients from seeking care. Clearly, more work is needed in this region for the management of cryptococcal meningitis and includes a focus on effective diagnosis, therapeutic use of available medications and monitoring to avoid toxicity levels.

8. Acknowledgment

We thank Dr Yeya Sarro Sadio, Professor Ibrahim Maiga and Professor Amadou Diallo for valuable assistance during this work. We are grateful to the University of Bamako for their support of this work. Funding for this chapter was obtained from DCR/NIAID/NIH.

9. References

Berry, A.J., Rinaldi M.G., & Graybill J.R. 1992. Use of high-dose fluconazole as salvage therapy for cryptococcal meningitis in patients with AIDS. *Antimicrob Agents Chemother* 36:690-692.

Bicanic T, Brouwer AE, Meintjes G, Rebe K, Limmathurotsakul D, Chierakul W, Teparrakkul P, Loyse A, White NJ, Wood R, Jaffar S & Harrison T. 2009. Relationship of cerebrospinal fluid pressure, fungal burden and outcome in patients with cryptococcal meningitis undergoing serial lumbar punctures. *AIDS*. Mar 27;23(6):701-6.

Bicanic, T., Harrison T., Niepieklo A., Dyakopu N., & Meintjes G. 2006. Symptomatic relapse of HIV-associated cryptococcal meningitis after initial fluconazole monotherapy: the role of fluconazole resistance and immune reconstitution. *Clin Infect Dis* 43:1069-1073.

Bicanic T, Wood R, Bekker LG, Darder M, Meintjes G & Harrison TS. 2005. Antiretroviral roll-out, antifungal roll-back: access to treatment for cryptococcal meningitis. *Lancet Infect Dis* 5:530-1

Bissagnene E, Ouhon J, Kra O, & Kadio A. 1994. Aspects actuels de la cryptococcose neuroméningée à Abidjan. Med Mal Infect; 24 (Spécial): 580-5

Bisson GP, Lukes J, Thakur R, Mtoni I & MacGregor RR. 2008. Cryptococcus and lymphocytic meningitis in Botswana. *S Afr Med J.* Sep;98(9):724-5.

Bottone, E.J., & Wormser G.P. 1986. Poorly encapsulated Cryptococcus neoformans from patients with AIDS. II. Correlation of capsule size observed directly in cerebrospinal fluid with that after animal passage. *AIDS Res* 2:219-225.

Brouwer, A.E., Rajanuwong A., Chierakul W., Griffin G.E., Larsen R.A., White N.J., & Harrison T.S. 2004. Combination antifungal therapies for HIV-associated cryptococcal meningitis: a randomised trial. *Lancet* 363:1764-1767.

Chuck, S.L., & Sande M.A. 1989. Infections with Cryptococcus neoformans in the acquired immunodeficiency syndrome. *N Engl J Med* 321:794-799.

Coulibaly I. 2005. Cryptococcose neuroméningée à l'Hôpital du Point G, Bamako, Mali [Thesis] Medicine University of Bamako

Datta, K., Bartlett K.H., Baer R., Byrnes E., Galanis E., Heitman J., Hoang L., Leslie M.J., MacDougall L., Magil S.S.l, Morshed M.G., & Marr K.A. 2009. Spread of Cryptococcus gattii into Pacific Northwest region of the United States. *Emerg Infect Dis* 15:1185-1191.

Datta, K., Bartlett K.H., & Marr K.A. 2009. Cryptococcus gattii: Emergence in Western North America: Exploitation of a Novel Ecological Niche. *Interdiscip Perspect Infect Dis* 2009:176532.

Desmet, P., Kayembe K.D., & De Vroey C. 1989. The value of cryptococcal serum antigen screening among HIV-positive/AIDS patients in Kinshasa, Zaire. *AIDS* 3:77-78.

Dismukes, W.E. 1988. Cryptococcal meningitis in patients with AIDS. *J Infect Dis* 157:624-628.

Eholie, S.P., Adou-Brynh D., Domoua K., Kakou A., Ehui E., Gouamene A., Bonnard D., Aoussi E., Bissagnene E., & Kadio A. 2000. [Adult non-viral lymphocytic meningitis in Abidjan (Cote d'Ivoire)]. *Bull Soc Pathol Exot* 93:50-54.

Eholie SP, N'gbocho L, Bissagnene E, Coulibaly M, Ehui E, Kra O, Assoumou A, Aoussi E, & Kadio A. 1997. Mycoses profondes au cours du SIDA à Abidjan (Côte d'Ivoire). *Bull Soc Pathol Exot* 90: 307 – 11.

Ellis, D.H., & Pfeiffer T.J. 1990. Natural habitat of Cryptococcus neoformans var. gattii. *J Clin Microbiol* 28:1642-1644.

French, N., Gray K., Watera C., Nakiyingi J., Lugada E., Moore M., Lalloo D., Whitworth J.A., & Gilks C.F. 2002. Cryptococcal infection in a cohort of HIV-1-infected Ugandan adults. *Aids* 16:1031-1038.

Frimpong, E.H., & Lartey R.A. 1998. Study of the aetiologic agents of meningitis in Kumasi, Ghana, with special reference to Cryptococcal neoformans. *East Afr Med J* 75:516-519.

Gari-Toussaint M & Mondain-Mitton V. 1996. Cryptococcose. *Encycl Méd Chir*, Maladies infectieuses.

Harrison, T.S. 2009. The burden of HIV-associated cryptococcal disease. *Aids* 23:531-532.

Hossain, M.A., Mukherjee P.K., Reyes G., Long L., & Ghannoum M.A. 2002. Effects of fluconazole singly and in combination with 5-fluorocytosine or amphotericin B in the treatment of cryptococcal meningoencephalitis in an intracranial murine model. *J Chemother* 14:351-360.

Jackson A & Hosseinipur MC. 2010. Management of Cryptococcal Meningitis in Sub-Saharan African. *Curr HIV/AIDS Rep*,7:134-142.

Kadjo K, Ouattara B, Kra O, Yao H, Diby K, Toure M, Toutou T,& Nlamkey EK. 2007. La cryptococcose neuroméningée dans les services de Médecine interne et de maladies infectieuses du CHU de Treichville (Côte d'Ivoire). *Méd Afr Noire* 54 : 65-8.

Kelley CF, Kitchen CM, Hunt PW, Rodriguez B, Hecht FM, Kitahata M, Crane HM, Willig J, Mugavero M, Saag M, Martin JN& Deeks SG. 2009. Incomplete peripheral CD4+ cell count restoration in HIV-infected patients receiving long-term antiretroviral treatment. *Clin Infect Dis,* 48, 6:787-94

Ki-Zerbo G., Sawadogo A , Millogo A, Andonaba JB,Yameogo A, Ouedraogo I, Tamini M,& Durand G. 1996. La cryptococcose neuromeningee au cours du SIDA : étude préliminaire à l'hôpital de Bobo-Dioulasso (Burkina Faso). *Méd Afr Noire* 43: 13-8.

Kouame-Assouan, A.E., Cowppli-Bony P., Aka-Anghui Diarra E., Assi B., Doumbia M., Diallo L., Adjien K.C., Akani E., Sonan T., Diagana M., Boa Y.E., & Kouassi B. 2007. [Two cases of cryptococcal meningitis revealed by an ischemic stroke]. *Bull Soc Pathol Exot* 100:15-16.

Larsen, R.A., Leal M.A., & Chan L.S. 1990. Fluconazole compared with amphotericin B plus flucytosine for cryptococcal meningitis in AIDS. A randomized trial. *Ann Intern Med* 113:183-187.

Lawn, S.D., Bekker L.G., Myer L., Orrell C., & Wood R. 2005. Cryptococcocal immune reconstitution disease: a major cause of early mortality in a South African antiretroviral programme. *Aids* 19:2050-2052.

Maher, D., & Mwandumba H. 1994. Cryptococcal meningitis in Lilongwe and Blantyre, Malawi. *J Infect* 28:59-64.

Makadzange AT, Ndhlovu CE, Takarinda K, Reid M, Kurangwa M, Gona P & Hakim JG. 2010. Early versus delayed initiation of antiretroviral therapy for concurrent HIV infection and cryptococcal meningitis in sub-saharan Africa. *Clin Infect Dis.* Jun 1;50(11):1532-8.

Manosuthi, W., Athichathanabadi C., Uttayamakul S., Phoorisri T., & Sungkanuparph S. 2007. Plasma nevirapine levels, adverse events and efficacy of antiretroviral therapy among HIV-infected patients concurrently receiving nevirapine-based antiretroviral therapy and fluconazole. *BMC Infect Dis* 7:14.

Mbuagbaw J, Biholong,& Njamnshi A K. 2006. La cryptococcose neuroméningée et l'infection au VIH dans le service de médecine du centre hospitalier et universitaire de Yaoundé, Cameroun. *Afr J Neurol Sc* ; 25: 13-9.

Millogo, A., Ki-Zerbo G.A., Andonaba J.B., Lankoande D., Sawadogo A., Yameogo I., & Sawadogo A.B. 2004. [Cryptococcal meningitis in HIV-infected patients at Bobo-Dioulasso hospital (Burkina Faso)]. *Bull Soc Pathol Exot* 97:119-121.

Minta, D.K., Dembele M., Diarra A.S., Sidibe A.T., Konate A., Diarra M., Coulibaly I., Maiga II, Traore A.K., Maiga M.Y., Doumbo O.K., Traore H.A., Pichard E., & Chabasse D. 2008. [Neuromeningeal cryptococcosis in non-HIV patients to CHU ward of Point G in Bamako (Mali): 3 case report]. *Bull Soc Pathol Exot* 101:308-310.

Mirza, S.A., Phelan M., Rimland D., Graviss E., Hamill R., Brandt M.E., Gardner T., Sattah M., de Leon G.P., Baughman W., & Hajjeh R.A. 2003. The changing epidemiology of cryptococcosis: an update from population-based active surveillance in 2 large metropolitan areas, 1992-2000. *Clin Infect Dis* 36:789-794.

Moosa, M.Y., & Coovadia Y.M. 1997. Cryptococcal meningitis in Durban, South Africa: a comparison of clinical features, laboratory findings, and outcome for human immunodeficiency virus (HIV)-positive and HIV-negative patients. *Clin Infect Dis* 24:131-134.

Mwaba, P., Mwansa J., Chintu C., Pobee J., Scarborough M., Portsmouth S., & Zumla A. 2001. Clinical presentation, natural history, and cumulative death rates of 230 adults with primary cryptococcal meningitis in Zambian AIDS patients treated under local conditions. *Postgrad Med J* 77:769-773.

O'Brien WA, Hartigan PM, Martin D, Esinhart J, Hill A, Benoit S, Rubin M, Simberkoff MS & Hamilton JD.1996. Changes in plasma HIV-1 RNA and CD4+ lymphocyte counts and the risk of progression to AIDS. Veterans Affairs Cooperative Study Group on AIDS. *N Engl J Med,334*,7:426-31.

Okongo, M., Morgan D., Mayanja B., Ross A., & Whitworth J. 1998. Causes of death in a rural, population-based human immunodeficiency virus type 1 (HIV-1) natural history cohort in Uganda. *Int J Epidemiol* 27:698-702.

Ouattara B, Eholie S, Adou-Bryn K. D,Kra O,Tia H, Kouadio-Yapo CG, Edo V, & Ouhon J. 2007. Etude rétrospective des méningites bactériennes et à cryptocoques chez des sujets adultes infectés par le VIH à Abidjan (Côte d'Ivoire). *J Mycol Méd* 17: 82-6.

Ouedraogo S. M, Ouedraogo M, Dagnan N. S, & Adom A. H. 2007. Infections opportunistes au cours du Sida au CHU de Treichville. *Mali Med* 22(1): 26-8.

Oumar, A.A., Dao S., Ba M., Poudiougou B., & Diallo A. 2008. [Epidemiological, clinical and prognostic aspects of cryptococcal meningitis in hospital area of Bamako, Mali]. *Rev Med Brux* 29:149-152.

Park, B.J., Wannemuehler K.A., Marston B.J., Govender, N. Pappas P.G., & Chiller T.M. 2009. Estimation of the current global burden of cryptococcal meningitis among persons living with HIV/AIDS. *Aids* 23:525-530.

Sharkey PK, Graybill JR, Johnson ES, Hausrath SG, Pollard RB, Kolokathis A, Mildvan D, Fan-Havard P, Eng RH, Patterson TF, Pottage JC Jr, Simberkoff MS, Wolf J, Meyer RD, Gupta R, Lee LW & Gordon DS.1996. Amphotericin B lipid complex compared with amphotericin B in the treatment of cryptococcal meningitis in patients with AIDS. *Clin Infect Dis*. Feb;22(2):315-21

Seybou O, De Truchis P, Adamou A, Nouhou Y, Tiousso B, Madougou B, Adehossi E, Bougnoux ME, Mouala C,Rouveix E, & Ide M. 2008. Epidémiologie de la cryptococcose au Niger: étude prospective chez des patients infectés par le VIH à Niamey. *ICASA*. Abstract N° 670/ SOB09

Soumare, M., M. Seydi, C.T. Ndour, Y. Dieng, A.M. Diouf, & B.M. Diop. 2005. [Update on neuromeningeal cryptococcosis in Dakar]. *Med Trop (Mars)* 65:559-562.

Soumare, M., Seydi M., Ndour C.T., Dieng Y., Ngom-Faye N.F., Fall N., & Diop B.M. 2005. [Clear-fluid meningitis in HIV-infected patients in Dakar]. *Bull Soc Pathol Exot* 98:104-107.

Soumare, M., Seydi M., Ndour C.T., Fall N., Dieng Y., Sow A.I., & Diop B.M. 2005. [Epidemiological, clinical, etiological features of neuromeningeal diseases at the Fann Hospital Infectious Diseases Clinic, Dakar (Senegal)]. *Med Mal Infect* 35:383-389.

Sow P S, Diop B M, Dieng Y, Dia N M, Seydi M, Dieng T, Badiane S, & Coll-Seck AM. 1998. Cryptococcose neuroméningée au cours de l'infection à VIH à Dakar. *Med Mal Infect* 28:511-5.

Steven L, Chuck D, Merle A & Sande MD. 1989. Infectious with *Cryptococcus neoformans* in the acquired immunodeficiency syndrome. *N Engl J Med* ; 321:794-9.

Tanon, A., S. Eholie, Y. Binan, E. Ehui, E. Zana, C. Maurice, E. Bissagnene, E. Aoussi, A. Kakou, & A. Kadio. 2006. [Medical emergencies related to HIV/AIDS in tropical zones: a prospective study in Cote d'Ivoire (1999-2000)]. *Med Trop (Mars)* 66:162-166.

van der Horst, C.M., Saag M.S., Cloud, G.A. Hamill R.J., Graybill J.R., Sobel J.D., Johnson P.C., Tuazon C.U., Kerkering T., Moskovitz B.L., Powderly W.G., & Dismukes W.E. 1997. Treatment of cryptococcal meningitis associated with the acquired immunodeficiency syndrome. National Institute of Allergy and Infectious Diseases Mycoses Study Group and AIDS Clinical Trials Group. *N Engl J Med* 337:15-21.

Wertheimer, A.I., Santella T.M., & Lauver H.J. 2004. Successful public/private donation programs: a review of the Diflucan Partnership Program in South Africa. *J Int Assoc Physicians AIDS Care (Chic)* 3:74-79, 84-75.

Zolopa A, Andersen J, Powderly W, Sanchez A, Sanne I, Suckow C, Hogg E & Komarow L.2009. Early antiretroviral therapy reduces AIDS progression/death in individuals with acute opportunistic infections: a multicenter randomized strategy trial. *PLoS One*.4(5):e5575. Epub 2009 May 18.

14

Clostridium Septicum Encephalitis: A Case Report

Bernadette Calabek, Georg Hinterholzer, Gabriele Neuwirth-Senautka, Harald Kirschner, Barbara Horvath-Mechtler and Wolfgang Grisold
Kaiser Franz Josef-Spital, SMZSüd, Department of Neurology, Ludwig Boltzmann-Institute of Neurooncology, Vienna Austria

1. Introduction

Clostridium septicum is one of the agents causing gas gangrene, and was notorious in injuries in battlefield. Infections of the CNS are very rare. Here, we present a 69year-old patient who died from a cerebral clostridium septicum infection.
Clostridium septicum is an anaerobic, spore-forming, gram-positive bacillus. Its virulence depends on toxin building. Spontaneous clostridium septicum infections are rare and are associated with a high mortality (Khan AA et al., 2006, Marangou et al., 1992). Associations with this bacterium and colorectal malignancies have been reported (Khan et al., 2006, Kolbeinsson et al., 1991, Mirza et al., 2009). C. septicum causes disease in mammals and birds, and it was recognized historically as one of the causes of gas gangrene arising from battlefield injuries (Smith, 1984). In the 1960s and 1970s, it became apparent that those patients with hematologic malignancies were susceptible for this kind of infection (Alexander et al., 2010). The number of cases attributable to other malignancies, particularly colonic neoplasms, has increased.

2. Case presentation

A 69-year-old man suffering from myelodysplastic syndrome developed chills, fever and altered state of consciousness within a few hours. The patient was admitted at the intensive care unit in a comatose state with hypotension and tachycardia, intubation was necessary. The neurological examination did not show focal signs. The patient´s past medical history revealed in addition to the myelodysplastic syndrome diabetes mellitus and chronic renal insufficiency. Laboratory data showed leukocytosis and high-elevated CRP. The CT-scan of the brain showed two atypical intracerebral hemorrhages located right parietally and left occipitally, and two gas-filled lesions right frontal and left occipital. There were no traumatic injuries or cranial fractures. The patient received antibiotic therapy with metronidazol, ceftriaxon, fosfomycin and ampicillin. A cerebral abscess or bleeding metastasis had been considered as differential diagnosis.
The next day the cranial MRI showed enormous gas-filled inclusions on both parietal sides, right frontal and of the periventricular white matter on each side. Both anterior horns of the lateral ventricles showed levels of a fluid gas border. Gas lesions were also found in the

venous sinus. The size of all lesions showed progression compared to the previous scan. Twelve hours after admission the blood culture revealed clostridium septicum. The echocardiography was normal. Ultrasound of the upper abdomen revealed a cholecystolithiasis and the kidneys were unremarkable.

Developing a septic shock the patient died of multiple organ failure three days after admission.

The autopsy showed a hyperemic brain. The brainstem and cerebellum were unremarkable. In the frontal sections there was a diffluent area near the left central sulcus, the anterior horns of the lateral ventricles were filled with blood. There was a remarkable crepitation by palpation of the unfixed brain tissue, particularly in the left parietal and occipital region. We

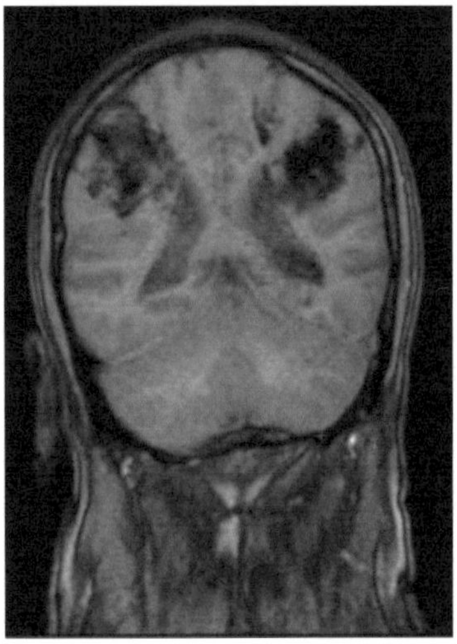

Fig. 1. Levels of fluid-gas in both anterior horns of the lateral ventricles.

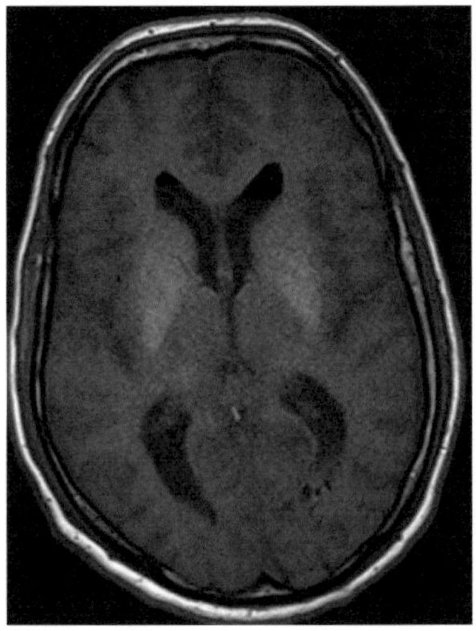

Fig. 2. Gas-filled lesions on both parietal sides.

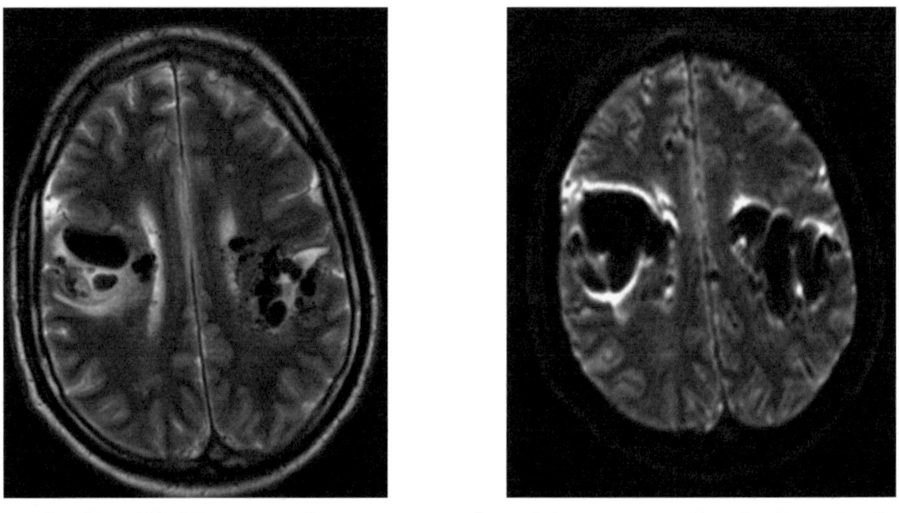

Fig. 3 and 4. Gas-filled lesions in the periventricular white matter and on both parietal sides

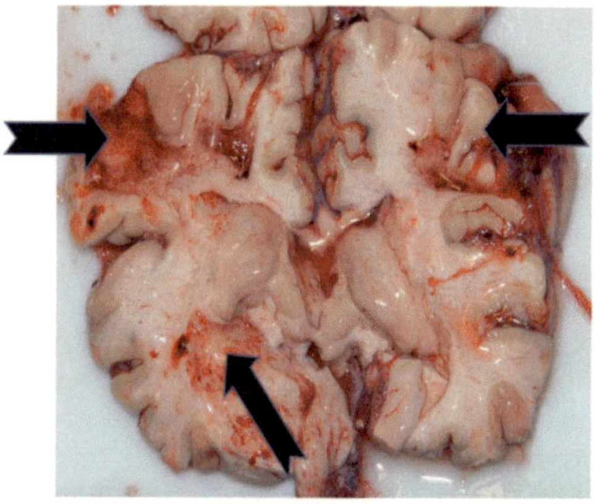

Fig. 5. Hemorrhagic areas on both parietal sides and left temporal

assume this crepitation was caused by escaping of gas bubbles due to the infection. The dissection of the brain revealed hemorrhagic lesions on both parietal sides, left temporal and left occipital. The left parietal lesions also showed suppurative components. These lesions corresponded with the lesions described in the cranial MRI. The swabs we obtained from the parietal lesions verified a clostridium septicum infection. Considering the clinical course and results of the MRI multiple cerebral abscesses must have been assumed.

The autopsy of the body revealed a rectal ulcerated adenoma with low-grade dysplasia associated with an extensive colitis. This colitis is considered a possible source of infection. Interestingly, no further organs had been affected by clostridium septicum.

3. Conclusion

Due to these atypical gas lesions we primarily assumed a traumatic event, which could not be verified. The intracerebral hemorrhages and gas lesions increased within 2 days, an infection with a gas-forming organism was likely. The results of the swabs and blood cultures confirmed the suspicion and revealed clostridium septicum.

Pneumocephalus is commonly seen after head and facial trauma, tumors of the skull base, after neurosurgery or otorhinolaryngology, and rarely spontaneously.

Clostridium septicum is an anaerobic, gas-forming, gram-positive organism, which is found ubiquitous in the soil but is usually not present in the human intestinal flora (Moore et al., 1974). Its virulence is based on protein toxicity. Clostridium septicum is forming alpha-toxin, a lethal and necrotizing pore-forming cytolysin (Kennedy et al., 2005).

Clostridium septicum is a highly virulent but poorly characterized pathogen that is being increasingly recognized as a major contributor to serious clostridial infections. It is the primary aetiological agent of spontaneous gas gangrene or atraumatic myonecrosis. Often malignancy is identified as a result of an investigation following the diagnosis of a clostridium septicum. It is suggested that under such conditions the bacterium is allowed to entry the bloodstream and to establish an infection at a distant site in the body (Kennedy et al., 2005). The condition is rapidly fulminating and often fatal, with reported mortality rates of approximately 60%. A possible explanation for this association is that the anaerobic glycolysis of the tumor may provide a hypoxic and acidic environment that favors proliferation of clostridium septicum (Alpern and Dowell, 1969).

A review of clostridial bacteremia examined blood cultures of 24 hospitalized patients. The review demonstrated that the source of clostridium species was a gastrointestinal site in 24 patients (52.2%). The most frequently identified clostridium species was Clostridium perfringens (in 10 [21.7%] of patients), followed by Clostridium septicum (in 9 [19.6%]). Thirty-one patients (67.4%) were aged > 65 years, 13 patients (28.3%) had diabetes mellitus, and underlying malignancy was present in 22 patients (47.8%) (Rechner et al., 2001).

Although nontraumatic infections in normal hosts do occur, they would appear to be quite rare, based upon our review of the available literature.

In this case the rectal ulcerated adenoma and extensive abscesses of the rectal wall are considered being the source of infection. It would appear likely that our patient's infection arose from his compromised gastrointestinal tract. The rapid progression of disease associated with these atypical gas lesions possibly depends on the immunosuppression by the myelodysplastic syndrome.

In summary, the coincidence of the immunosuppressed situation and the rectal ulcerated adenoma as source of infection just can be suspected. In the long run we do not know the exact coherences between the infection and its real cause in this case.

Key points:

- Clostridium septicum is a gram-positive, spore-forming organism, which is not usually present in the normal intestinal flora of humans. Infection with this organism is most commonly associated with spontaneous gas gangrene.
- Clostridium septicum infections are often associated with a colorectal malignancy or hematologic disease.
- Clinicians should search for an underlying colonic cancer in cases of clostridium septicum infection.

4. References

Alexander B. Granok, Patrick A. Mahon, Genesio W. Biesek, Clostridium septicum Empyema in an Immunocompetent Woman, Case Report Med. 2010;2010:231738.

Alpern RJ, Dowell VR. Clostridium septicum infections and malignancy. Journal of the American Medical Association. 1969; 209(3):385–388.

Kennedy CL, Krejany EO, Young LF, O'Connor JR, Awad MM, Boyd RL, Emmins JJ, Lyras D, Rood JI The alpha-toxin of Clostridium septicum is essential for virulence. Mol Microbiol. 2005 Sep;57(5):1357-66.

Khan AA, Davenport K. A reminder of the association between Clostridium septicum and colonic adenocarcinoma. Int Semin Surg. Oncol. 2006 Apr 28;3:12.

Kolbeinsson ME, Holder WD Jr., Aziz S. Recognition, management, and prevention of Clostridium septicum abscess in immunosuppressed patients, Arch. Surg. 1991 May; 126(5):642-5

Marangou AG, Joske RA, Kaard AO, Thomas W. Cerebral abscess due to Clostridium septicum. J R Soc Med. 1992 Oct;85(10):641.

Mirza NN, McCloud JM, Cheetham MJ. Clostridium septicum sepsis and colorectal cancer, a reminder. World J Surg Oncol. 2009; 6. Oktober 2009; 7:73.

Moore WE, Holdeman LV. Human fecal flora: the normal flora of 20 Japanese-Hawaiians. Appl Microbiol 1974;27:961-79.

Rechner PM, Agger WA, Mruz K., Cogbill TH, Clinical features of clostridial bacteremia: a review from a rural area. Clin Infect Dis. 2001 Aug 1;33(3):349-53.

Smith DL. The Pathogenic Anaerobic Bacteria, Clostridium septicum; pp. 245–255.

15

Superantigen-Mediated Encephalitis

A. Emmer[1], K. Gerlach[1], M. S. Staege[2] and M. E. Kornhuber[1]
[1]Martin-Luther-University, Halle (Saale), Department of Neurology
[2]Martin-Luther-University, Halle (Saale), Department of Paediatrics
Germany

1. Introduction

Encephalitis may result from the interaction between a pathogen and the host brain, such as in bacterial, viral or fungal infection of the CNS. There are, however, different states of aseptic encephalitis, which may be induced e.g. by way of (i) self-directed immune attacks as in experimental autoimmune encephalomyelitis or (ii) by certain substances like the copper chelating agent cuprizone (Torkildsen et al., 2008).

In fact, in encephalitis, infectious and non-infectious processes do not mutually exclude each other. Many pathogens such as bacteria or viruses encode for immune stimulating peptides, better known as superantigens for their enormous potency to stimulate immune cells (Kappler et al., 1989; Fleischer, 1991). T-cell superantigens have been developed twice during the evolution, namely independently by bacteria and by viruses. Not all bacteria or viruses do, however, possess a superantigen. - Superantigens act in a T-cell receptor V(beta) dependent manner (Figure 1). Thereby, up to 10% or even 20% of the T-cell repertoire may become activated, sometimes resulting in a fulminant inflammatory response. The latter depends also on the specific repertoire of the host's antigen-detection apparatus, e.g., the human-leucocyte-antigen (HLA) molecules.

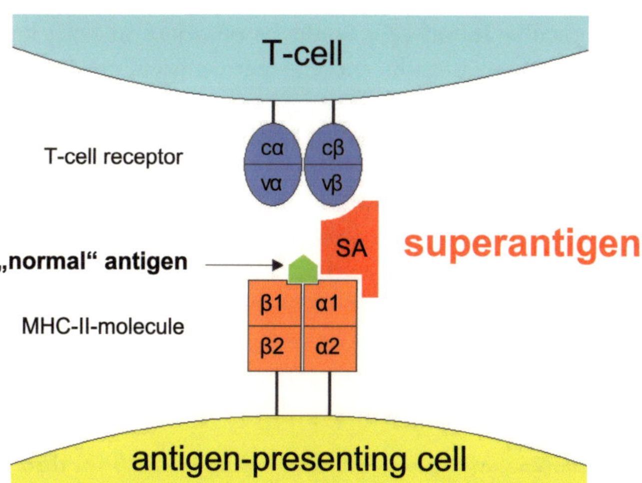

Fig. 1. Antigen and superantigen recognition via the MHC/T-cell receptor complex.

Taken together, superantigens are expected to take part in the inflammatory events induced by their pathogenic source. In florid bacterial or viral encephalitis, the detrimental effects that may be attributed to the pathogen or to its superantigen may be hardly discerned, while both may contribute to the final outcome. However, in case of slowly progressing encephalitides of e.g. viral origin, the superantigenic stimulus might be responsible for the initial and leading symptoms while the consequences of viral degeneration could be compensated for for a considerable time period and may become symptomatic later during the disease course. This is what has been suggested to happen in multiple sclerosis (MS) (Kornhuber et al., 2002, Kornhuber 2006, Emmer et al., 2008, 2010). In this respect, it may be of significance that the initial events of MS plaque generation seem to develop in the absence of tissue inflammation (Filippi et al., 1998; Barnett and Prineas, 2004). Although the etiology for slow progression in MS remains to be established, it has been speculated on a possible role e.g. for human endogenous retroviruses such as MSRV (Garson et al., 1998; Perron and Lang, 2010; Antony et al., 2010).
Our knowledge about the cerebral actions of T-cell superantigens, e.g. Staphylococcal enterotoxin A (SEA), relies on but a few experiments and, thus, is far from being comprehensive. Nevertheless, the results outlined below may be useful for future studies to further characterize the role of superantigens per se or in the context of bacterial or viral encephalitis, respectively.

2. Effects of intracerebral T-cell superantigen

Intracerebrally expressed superantigen induces a perivascular and periventricular inflammation (Kornhuber et al., 2002; Emmer et al., 2010). Fourty-microliter aliquots of superantigen or saline were slowly injected intracerebrally through a small burr hole in isoflurane-anesthetized male 300-g Lewis rats, 2.5 mm lateral from the midline at the bregma at a depth of 3.5 mm. Horizontal hematoxylin/eosin stained sections of the rat brains were investigated after fixing the brains with 4% buffered paraformaldehyde. Sections were obtained at the corpus callosum and at the level of the lateral ventricles. Cuffings of perivascular round cells were identified scattered around the injection canal. In the first 3 days, perivascular round cells could be observed in both hemispheres with a preponderance in the corpus callosum and the periventricular white matter. Thereafter perivascular round cells were confined to the injected hemisphere up to 12 days after SEA injection. Maximum response in the injected hemisphere was identified up to 8 days after injection (Fig. 1).
We wondered why the response to superantigen was relatively variable and usually low. It is well known that relapses in MS are often precipitated by some nonspecific immune stress such as infection. Furthermore, it is known that only activated immune cells are capable to invade the CNS (Wekerle et al., 1986). For these reasons we tried to imitate the stress by loading the blood with activated immune cells.

3. Activated splenocytes amplify superantigen encephalitis

Activated syngeneic splenocytes were injected in volumes of 0.5 ml through the penis vein of 300 g male Lewis rats on the third day after intracerebral injection of the superantigen SEA (see above). Activation of splenocytes was achieved in the following way under sterile conditions: A syngeneic spleen was cut and the content passed through a sieve into isotonic NaCl-solution. Cells were washed three times and the pellet finally resuspended in RPMI-medium with 5 % heat-inactivated fetal calf serum and with a final concentration of 2 μg/ml concanavalin A (ConA). Cells were harvested and washed after 3 days in culture when they were maximally stimulated. They were kept in NaCl on crushed ice for injection purposes. Usually 10^7 cells were injected i.v. under brief general isoflurane anesthesia. The time course of the tissue reaction to 1 mg/ml SEA was investigated (Kornhuber et al., 2002). In general, perivascular round cell infiltrates were more numerous and more reproducible than without adding activated splenocytes. In the first up to 3 days after splenocyte injection, reactive vessels could be identified in both cerebral hemispheres with a preponderance on the injected side. Thereafter, inflamed blood vessels were confined to the injected hemisphere. The response was short-lived and could last for further 3 up to 12 days. Thereafter, no reactive vessels could be identified. On day 5 after i.v.-injection, on average 18.5±11.4 vessels with round cell cuffs were observed. When compared with the corresponding numbers obtained without i.v.-injection of activated splenocytes, the difference was statistically significant ($p < 0.05$; two-sided U-test). When the amount of activated splenocytes was kept constant at 10^7 per animal, the number of reactive blood vessels increased linearly with the concentration of SEA. When the injected SEA was kept constant at a concentration of 1 mg/ml, the number of reactive blood vessels increased linearly with the number of intravenously injected activated splenocytes.

4. Immunohistochemical characterization of round cell cuffing

Immunohistochemical investigations of the SEA-encephalitis were performed using shock-frozen brains fixed at -80 °C. Six μm kryocut sections were made at -14 °C. Neighboring tissue sections that showed both, the cerebral ventricles and the stitch canal were taken for further evaluation. The avidin–streptavidin–biotin (ABC)-method was used throughout for immunohistochemical staining purposes. All used antibodies were ordered by BD Biosciences Pharmingen. After preincubation with goat serum for 20 min, incubation with the primary antibody (1:50, 1 h) was followed by incubation with the secondary antibody (1:50, 30 min). After 30 min in the pre-diluted streptavidin–horseradish–peroxidase (HRP) all tissue sections were finally incubated with diaminobenzidine (DAB) solution until the desired colour intensity was obtained. Sections were dehydrated three times on increasing grades of alcohol and covered with Roti-Histokit. Spleen tissue slices served as the positive controls. All used primary antibodies were highly specific for their target antigen. Negative controls included substitution of primary antibodies by antibodies of the same isotype with specificities against non-host antigens.

12 h after i.v. injection of ConA-activated spleen cells (i.e. 3 days after intracerebral injection of SEA), relatively high numbers of immunoreactive CD3+, CD4+ and CD8+ T-cells were present in a perivascular distribution and also scattered in the parenchyma around the stitch canal of the injected hemisphere (Fig. 3). The perivascular cuffs consisted of several layers of round cells. The amount of immunoreactive cells within the perivascular infiltrates, i.e. CD3+, CD4+ and CD8+ T-cells decreased gradually thereafter (Figs. 3 and 4) and amounted merely to usually 1 complete layer of immunopositive cells 3 days after i.v. injection of splenocytes and some loosely grouped perivascular cells after 5 days. Thus, the

inflammatory response was less large than in the previous experiments (see above). Among the different T-lymphocyte subsets, CD8+ T-cells were generally the most numerous ones (Figs. 3 and 4). The number of CD3+ T-cells within slices of the injected right hemisphere made up only about one quarter of the sum of the T-cells found to express CD8 or CD4 (Figs. 3 and 4). The relative numbers of reactive blood vessels remained more or less constant within the investigated time period (not shown). In the non-injected left hemisphere, the inflammatory activity was generally less prominent (Fig. 4). In fact, notable numbers of CD4+ and CD8+ T-cells within perivascular cuffs were identified only 3 days after i.v. injection of ConA-activated spleen cells (Fig. 4). In the brains of control animals, T-cells expressing CD4, CD8 or CD3 were not detected except for isolated immunopositive cells in the area of the stitch canal 0.5 days after the i.v. injection of ConA-activated splenocytes (not shown). Five days after the i.v. injection, no stained T-cells were found in the investigated brain slices of both control animals.

The cerebral inflammatory reaction was short-lived, presumably due to the rapid disappearance of the injected superantigen, e.g. by non-specific binding to cell surfaces. Differences in the duration of the inflammation in the order of several days may be due to different preparations of the superantigen, which may impact the immunostimulatory potency of the SEA reagent.

The cerebral inflammation induced by SEA was most prominent within the injected hemisphere and consisted initially mainly of CD8+ T-cells, which made up about 65% of the perivascular round cell population (Fig. 4). As no similar inflammatory response could be identified in the brains of the control animals that had received saline intracerebrally, the results do not appear to be due to the stitch trauma. Furthermore, only relatively small numbers of T-cells were found within the non-injected left hemisphere 0.5 days after i.v. injection of the ConA-activated splenocytes. As the number of the perivascular round cells detected in the left hemisphere peaked after 3 days following the i.v. injection of the ConA-activated splenocytes (Fig. 4), migration from the injected right hemisphere via the corpus callosum is the presumable reason for their occurrence contralateral to the injection site as has been suspected previously (Kornhuber et al., 2002). How does the superantigen expressed in the brain tissue lead to local recruitment and activation of T-cells? Presumably, the unprocessed superantigen was presented by MHC molecules on the surface of perivascular cells, microglial cells or dendritic cells, which are known to express MHC-class II constitutively within the CNS (Sedgwick et al., 1993; Stoll, 2002). By way of contrast, MHC-class I is not present on cell surfaces in the cerebral parenchyma unless its expression is specifically induced (Sedgwick et al., 1993; Redwine et al., 2001). When the injected ConA-activated cells appear in the circulation in high numbers after i.v. injection, namely 3 days after the intracerebral SEA-injection, free superantigen seems unlikely to be present in the cerebral extracellular fluid. Therefore, direct binding of SEA to the T-cell receptor (TCR) of ConA-activated splenocytes that come to traverse the blood–brain barrier does not seem to play a major role for T-cell activation in the present case (Fleischer, 1991; Herrmann et al., 1990; Yagi et al., 1990). However, only relatively small numbers of T-cells migrate through the cerebral blood vessels as part of a surveillance process, unless specific stimuli force them to stay on the abluminal side (Wekerle et al., 1986). The persistence of T-cells within the parenchyma after intracerebral injection of SEA may be taken as evidence that a specific stimulus forced them to stay within the CNS, therefore. After local expression of SEA, the majority of the T-cells detected within the intracerebral perivascular infiltrates was CD8+, while a minority was CD4+ (Figs. 1 and 2). Although superantigens presented via MHC II are well known to stimulate CD4+ T-cells, it has been demonstrated that SEA may activate CD8+ T-cells in a TCR-dependent manner (Müller-Alouf et al., 2001; Stinissen et al., 1995). Results obtained by gene expression analysis for the SEA encephalitis are in line with a CD8+ T-cell driven immune response (see below; Emmer et al., 2008). At a first glance it seemed to be curious that the numbers of T-cells expressing CD8 or CD4 detected within the right hemisphere in sum outnumbered the CD3+ ones at each investigated time point. The immunostaining for CD3 like that for CD4 and CD8 was of sufficient quality to allow a clear distinction between positive and negative cells (Fig. 3). Therefore, it does not seem likely that the mismatch between the results for CD3 and CD8 was artificial in nature. Actually, a diminished expression of CD3 but not of CD4 or CD8 has been reported previously for T-cells that had been challenged by superantigen (Damle et al., 1993; Niedergang et al., 1995; Makida et al., 1996; Von Essen et al., 2004). Therefore, the finding of a lower expression of CD3 in comparison to CD8 on T-lymphocytes like in the present investigation can be taken as evidence for the presence of a previous superantigenic stimulus.

Taken together, it has been demonstrated that the round cells that take part in perivascular cuffing of the encephalitis induced by the superantigen SEA are primarily composed of T-cells, especially of CD8+ T-cells. This result may be of importance with respect to the pathogenesis of inflammatory diseases of the central nervous system. The fact that upon the superantigenic stimulus T-cells become CD3-negative in significant numbers, leaving the expression of e.g. CD8 unaltered, may be used to demonstrate the involvement of a superantigenic stimulus in different states of encephalitis.

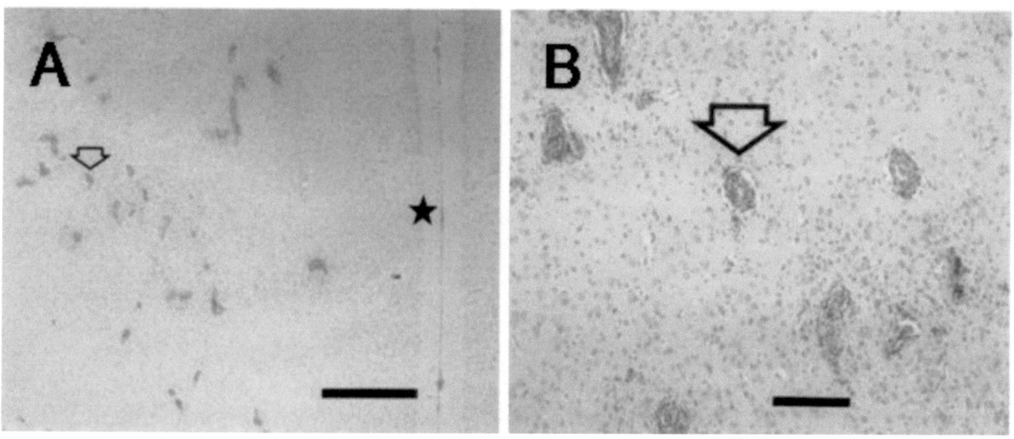

Fig. 2. The figure illustrates the effect of intracerebral superantigen. Frontal sections of the rat brain at the level of the corpus callosum, hematoxylin and eosin stain. The interhemispheric cleft has been marked by a star. (A) Five days after intracerebral SEA-injection and 8 days after i.v. injection ConA-activated splenocytes. (B) Part A at a higher magnification.

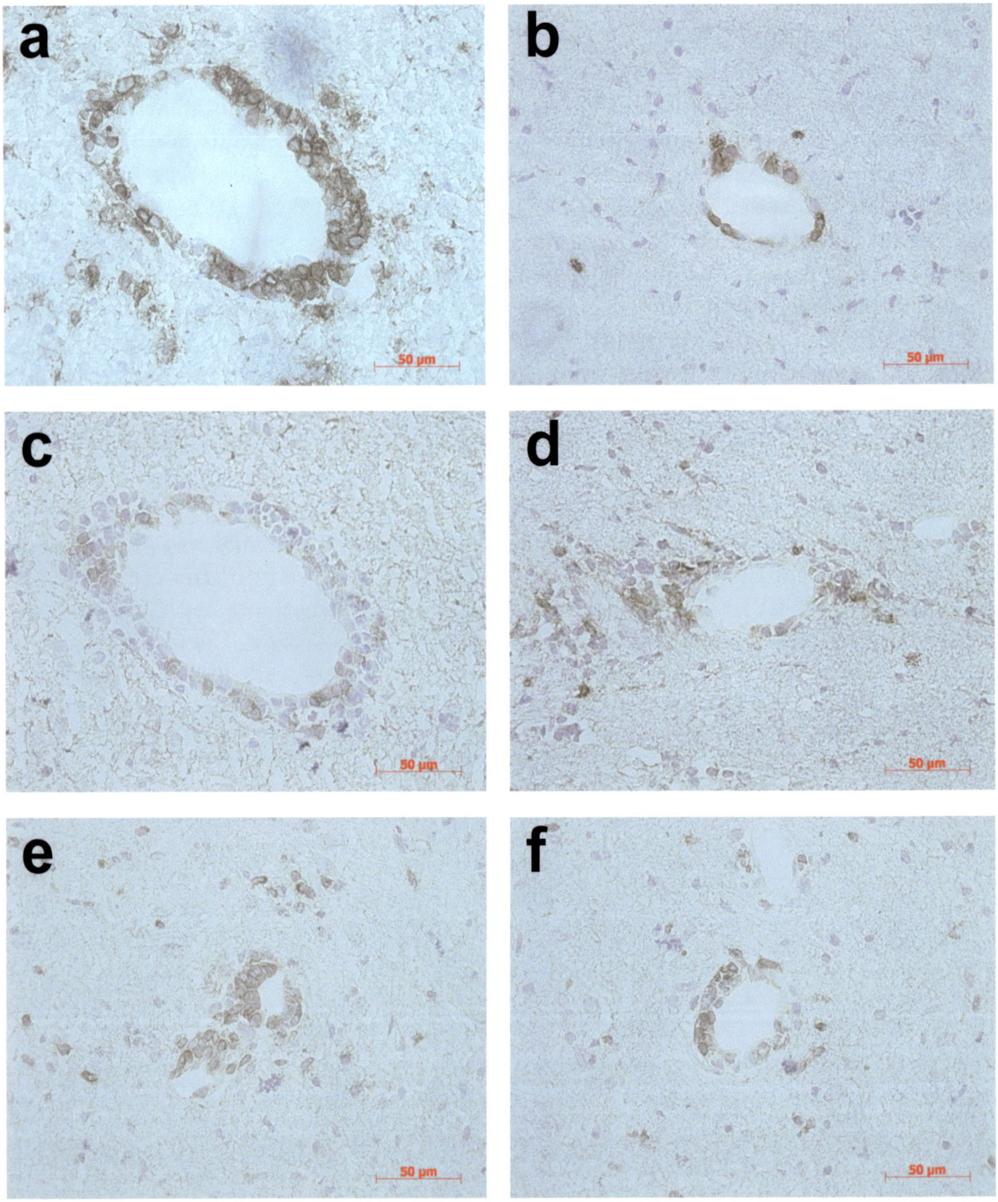

Fig. 3. Representative immunohistochemical stains of rat brain slices of the right hemisphere (streptavidin-biotin-method) after intracerebral injection with Staphylococcal enterotoxin A (SEA). Slices obtained 0.5 and 3 days after i.v. injection of ConA-activated splenocytes show expression of the antigens CD8 (a, day 0.5; b, day 3), CD4 (c, day 0.5; d, day 3), and CD3 (e, day 0.5; f, day 3). Note the special preponderance of CD8+ T-cells (a) in comparison with CD4+ T-cells (c). With time, the perivascular round cell count decreased as exemplified by the T-cells expressing CD8, CD4 or CD3, 3 days after i.v. injection of ConA activated splenocytes (b, d, f) compared with those detected after 0.5 days (a, c, e) (Emmer et al., 2010).

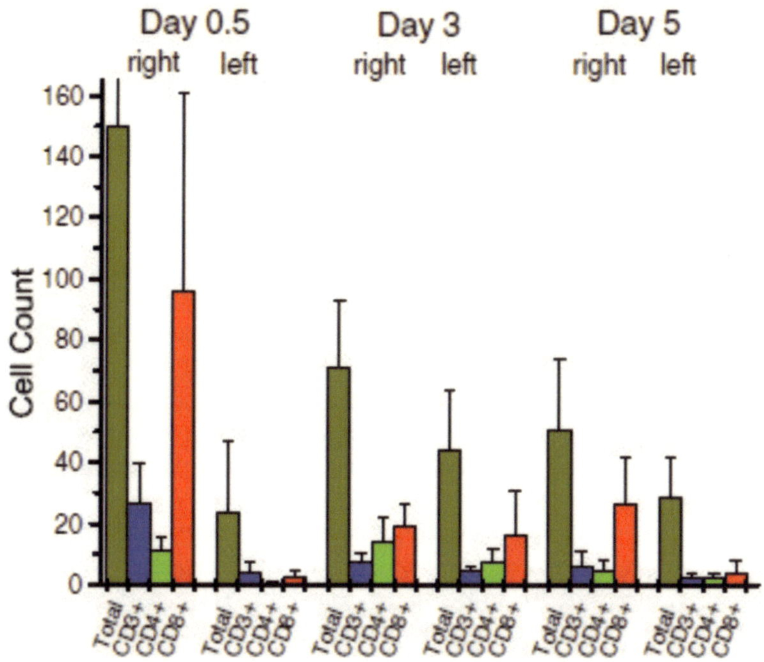

Fig. 4. Summary of the perivascular round cell counts (columns) are given together with the standard deviation (bars) for the entirety of the cells per tissue slice and hemisphere (olive green) and for the cells positively stained with CD3 (blue), CD4 (green) and CD8 (red), after injection of the superantigen Staphylococcal enterotoxin A (SEA) into the right hemisphere followed by intravenous loading of ConA-activated splenocytes 3 days later. The bar of the first left-sided column has been cut. Its value amounts to 58 cells. The 3 investigated time points, i.e. 0.5 days, 3 days and 5 days, refer to the interval between intravenous splenocyte injection and sacrification of the animals (Emmer et al., 2010).

5. Gene expression profile of superantigen encephalitis

Of 5 male 300 g Lewis rats, two animals received 50 µl of 1 mg/ ml SEA and two animals were injected with saline into the right brain hemisphere during deep anaesthesia. Injections were placed 2.5 mm lateral to the midline and 2 mm behind the bregma. One rat was sham operated. Three days after this procedure, 1.5*10^7 ConA-activated splenocytes (see above), were injected into the penis vein of each animal. Eight days after the initial surgical procedure, brains were taken from all Lewis rats. A coronar disk (2 mm) including the injection channel was prepared and divided into an injected half and a non-injected half. The samples were snap frozen in isopropanol and stored at -80 °C. Microarray analysis was performed as described previously (Staege et al., 2004). Data analyses were performed by using Statistical Analysis of Microarrays (SAM) (Tusher et al., 2001). Results from the 4 rat brain hemispheres of the two 'SEA' animals were compared with the 4 hemispheres of the 2 'saline' animals. Furthermore, the differential gene expression after saline injection versus sham operation was calculated. Due to the small sample size, a relatively conservative approach was followed with $\Delta = 0.75$, a false discovery rate of 0.099 and a minimum change factor of three. To be acceptable, the signal intensities had to be above 30. Validation of microarray data was done by real-time PCR. To validate the results of the microarray analysis, the transcriptional regulation of nine genes [CCL5 (RANTES), TIMP-1, osteopontin, CD74, RT1-Da, complement component 3, tenascin C, CD8 and CCL2 (MCP-1)] that showed significant differential expression in rat brains with SEA encephalitis was measured also using real-time PCR. Total RNA was extracted from brain tissue using Trizol (Invitrogen, Karlsruhe, Germany) or the RNeasy kit (Qiagen, Hilden, Germany). Quantitative RT-PCR (qRT-PCR) was performed by using the QuantiTect SYBR Green RT-PCR Kit (Qiagen) using the following conditions: 94 °C, 45 s; 62 °C, 45 s; 72 °C, 60 s. Each reaction was subjected to melting temperature analysis to confirm presence of the expected products. Specific gene amplification was normalized to GAPDH. Target genes and GAPDH were amplified with 40 cycles using a ROTOR GENE RG-3000 (Corbett Research, Sydney, Australia) and ROTOR GENE 6 software. The threshold cycle (CT) value was defined as the fraction cycle number and set at 10 times the standard deviation above the mean baseline fluorescence calculated from cycles 3 to 15. The fold changes in the target genes normalized to actin 22 (as house keeping gene) and relative expression of controls (1 uninjected rat brain) was calculated by using standard ΔΔCT method.

Of the 8800 investigated genes, 106 were at least 3-fold increased with SEA over saline, while 29 genes were decreased at least 3-fold. The respective microarray data of differentially overexpressed *genes* are summarized in Table 1. Genes with increased expression were grouped in the following order: antigen presentation, lymphocytes, chemokines / chemokine receptors, microglial reaction / macrophages, phagocytosis / opsonization, extracellular matrix / cell adhesion, anti-inflammatory reaction and miscellaneous/ compound to inflammation. Some of the genes with decreased expression (not shown) presumably belong to cerebral cell elements such as neurons or astrocytes, e.g. genes encoding for neurotransmitter receptors or ion channels. In fact, the expression for the genes encoding for CCL5 (RANTES), TIMP-1, osteopontin, CD74, RT1-Da, complement component 3, tenascin C, CD8 and CCL2 (MCP-1) in relation to the house keeping gene for actin 22 as measured by real-time PCR showed a high level of conformity in comparison with the results obtained by using microarrays. Differential gene expression after saline injection versus sham operation revealed at least 3-fold overexpression of six genes and underexpression of 40 genes (not shown). The relatively mild differences observed in the gene expression between both conditions may reflect the consequences of the injection trauma and are considered of minor relevance for the SEA encephalitis.

When data were first analysed, it became obvious that after intracerebral SEA injection versus saline injection, expression of several genes was markedly increased in the injected hemisphere and also displayed considerable overexpression in the non-injected contralateral hemisphere as well. This finding might correspond to the bilateral perivascular inflammatory reaction observed by using histology in the first days of SEA encephalitis (see above). Due to this finding, it was decided to analyse both hemispheres together. This approach certainly reduces absolute values of differential gene expression and at the same time it might reduce detection of false-positive data, e.g. resulting from the small number of samples. The results are in conformity with the light microscopy findings of a perivascular inflammation.

Among the genes with elevated expression, there was a considerable number of genes encoding for MHC class II molecules, which are constitutively expressed on microglial cells in the brain. In a state of encephalitis, they may be detected on astrocytes as well.

Superantigen is presented in the context of MHC class II. However, 8 days after intracerebral injection of the superantigen, it might be doubted whether the elevated expression of genes for MHC class II molecules is still a direct consequence of the superantigenic stimulus. Antigen-presenting cells present in the inflammatory area may comprise microglial elements, monocytes and astrocytes [elevated expression of genes for: Serping1, CD53 antigen, CCAAT/ enhancer binding protein (C / EBP) delta, glial fibrillary acidic protein (GFAP) and calcium binding protein S100A4]. T lymphocytes seem to play a major role among the hematogenous cellular infiltrates of the SEA encephalitis. While the genes for CD3 and CD8 were found to be significantly elevated, this was not the case with the gene for CD4. This fits to immunohistochemical results showing that the perivascular round cell cuffs are dominated by CD8+ T lymphocytes on days 3.5, 6 and 8 after intracerebral SEA injection (see above). This finding was unexpected as usually CD4+ T cells are activated by T-cell superantigen presented in the context of MHC class II molecules (Fields et al., 1996). By way of contrast, CD8+ T cells are predominantly stimulated in the context of MHC class I molecules (Jelonek et al., 1998). As the latter ones are not constitutively presented in the brain, it seems unlikely that these molecules play a major role in the induction of the SEA encephalitis. Rather SEA may have been presented in the context of MHC class II. Previously, a similar stimulation of CD8+ T cells via superantigen bound to MHC class II as found in the present investigation has been reported (Fraser, 1989). Of interest, there exists a parallel to MS, where CD8+ T cells have been reported to predominate among perivascular inflammatory infiltrates (Liu et al., 2007; Jilek et al., 2007). Further proteins involved in antigen presentation or in signalling cascades were significantly overexpressed with SEA comprise sialoprotein CD43, cathepsin C, and CD 72. Similar to other states of cerebral inflammation such as in MS or EAE, there was a profound increase in the expression of the genes for the following proteins involved in chemotaxis after SEA injection: RANTES (CCL5), osteopontin, MCP-1 (CCL2) and CXCL10. Furthermore, the gene for the receptor of MCP-1 (CCR2) showed a significantly increased expression. In contrast to the elevated chemokine levels, cytokines, such as interleukin-2, tumour necrosis factor alpha or interferon gamma, did not reveal significantly increased differential expression levels. As these cytokines belong to the group of substances which are released early in the course of an inflammation, it is quite plausible that the genes for these cytokines are not expressed any more differentially 8 days after injection of SEA. Intracerebral injection of SEA was followed by an enhanced expression of genes encoding different complement factors such as C3, C4a, C1q, B, D (adipsin) and serping 1. These factors may be released from microglial cells (Raivich and Banati, 2004) or from macrophages. Complement factors were suggested to play a role in opsonization and phagocytosis. Complement factors 1q, 3 and 4a showed a high expression in microarray studies in EAE and MS (Tajouri et al., 2003; Lock et al., 2002). Actually, increased expression was detected for genes that are also related to phagocytosis. These were Fc-gamma receptor, Vav1, galectin 3 (Wilkinson et al., 2006; Rotshenker, 2003). These genes were previously shown to display increased expression in EAE (Lock et al., 2002; Reichert and Rotshenker, 1999; Carmody et al., 2006). A number of genes with increased expression levels after SEA injection were related to the extracellular matrix. These were lysyl oxidase, tenascin C, alpha-1- collagen type III, syndecan 1, alpha-1-collagen, alpha-1- procollagen type I, vimentin, matrix-gla-protein, periostin, oxidized LDL-receptor-1 and alpha-tubulin. The gene for tenascin C was measured with elevated expression in EAE and in MS (Lock et al., 2002, Carmody et al., 2006), while a similar increase for the gene of alpha-tubulin was present in MS (Carmody et al., 2006). Not all of the above summarized genes that showed enhanced expression after intracerebral superantigen injection did so in EAE or MS. Furthermore, the gene for integrin alpha M was detected with elevated expression in the present study. Integrin alpha M mediates cellular adhesion to the extracellular matrix (Friedl and Brocker, 2000). It is also upregulated in EAE and in MS (Lock et al., 2002, Carmody et al., 2006). Whether the enhanced gene expression of components of the extracellular matrix reflects alterations in the context of the encephalitis or reflects reparative activity remains to be established. Increased expression of the following genes may be regarded as part of an anti-inflammatory tissue reaction: alpha-2-macroglobulin, metallothionein, heat shock protein 27 (HSP27), haeme oxygenase-1, C/ EBP-related transcription factor beta, coeruloplasmin and pleckstrin. The gene products take part in the inactivation of proteolytic enzymes (alpha-macroglobulin), in the reduction in oxidative stress (methallothionein, haeme oxygenase 1, coeruloplasmin) or in the apoptosis induction (HSP27). Several of these genes have been observed with increased expression in EAE or in MS (Table 3), such as metallothionein (Tajouri et al., 2003; Lock et al., 2002; Penkowa and Hidalgo, 2003; Espejo et al., 2005; Espejo and Martinez-Caceres, 2005), haeme oxygenase 1 (Levine and Chakrabarty, 2004; Tan et al., 2004) and HSP27 (Tajouri et al., 2003). Furthermore, there was a significant increase for the genes of the metalloproteinase 9 (MMP9) and its inhibitor, the tissue inhibitor of metalloproteinase 1 (TIMP-1). Both genes were reported to be upregulated in EAE and in plaque tissue from patients with MS (Steinman, 1999; Pagenstecher et al., 1998). While MMP9 is e.g. required for the migration of lymphocytes through the basilar membrane and thus for invading the CNS, the much more pronounced upregulation of TIMP-1 may be regarded as an anti-inflammatory response. Other genes with increased expression levels in the SEA encephalitis are genes encoded for different cytochromes (P450 type 1b1, b558 and b245), granulin, lipocalin and STAT1. The role of the proteins during the course of the SEA encephalitis is not entirely clear. At least the elevated gene expression for STAT1 was noted previously in EAE (Jee et al., 2001) and in MS (Frisullo et al., 2006). Furthermore, the gene for granulin was observed with elevated expression in MS (Tajouri et al., 2003).

Genes with decreased expression: The number of genes with significantly and at least threefold decreased expression was small (n = 29), in comparison with the number of genes showing an increased expression (n = 106). Among the former genes, there was a number of genes related to cerebral cellular functions such as neurotransmitter receptors, ion channel proteins, ion pumps or growth factor receptors: retinoid-X-receptor gamma, cholinergic receptor (nicotinic, alpha polypetide 2, neuronal), potassium voltage-gated channel, subfamily H member 8 (ATPase), proton pump (H+ transporting, V1 subunit G, isoform 3 and H+/K+ ATPase), calbindin and oncomodulin. Expression of these genes was not observed to be decreased in EAE or MS. Nevertheless, in EAE and MS, genes with decreased expression levels were observed to encode proteins with similar functions. These included myosin VIIA, phosphatidylinositol 4- kinase (Tajouri et al., 2003), TGF beta 3, cadherin-7 (Lindberg et al., 2004), somatostatin and kinesin (Lock et al., 2002). Taken together, the gene expression data in the present study support previously reported light microscopy findings of the encephalitis developing after superantigen injection into the rat brain (Kornhuber et al., 2003). The peculiar gene expression pattern found 8 days after superantigen injection is compatible with a CD8+ T lymphocyte driven process leading to different cerebral inflammatory and anti-inflammatory reactions. As superantigens were implicated in the pathogenesis of human autoimmune diseases, such as MS, the comparison of the presented data with those gathered with EAE or MS may be of general interest. Actually, there is considerable conformity between the gene expression profile of the SEA encephalitis and EAE or MS (Table 2). This accordance between the three different states of inflammation may be due to the fact that a T-cell-driven pathogenesis is common to all of them.

Accession no.	Description	SEA	NaCl	Ratio
Antigen presentation				
X13044	MHC-II (CD74 antigen)	3542	130	27.2
X14254	MHC-II (invariant chain)	1209	45	26.9
X07551	MHC-II B-alpha gene	1384	113	12.2
X56596	MHC-II B-1 beta chain	1014	168	6.0
X53054	MHC-II (protein complex)	1322	219	6.0
M64795	MHC-I (CRT 1-u)	620	106	5.8
U31599	MHC-II (DM beta)	433	82	5.3
M36151	MHC-II A-beta gene (RT1 class II locus Bb)	794	154	5.2
K02815	MHC-II (locus Ba)	1982	387	5.1
M15562	MHC-II	1180	231	5.1
X57523	TGF-beta (activated)	310	83	3.7
AI171966	MHC-II (DM beta)	1619	440	3.7
X67504	MHC-I (locus Aw2)	205	61	3.3
U31599	MHC-II	215	69	3.1
Lymphocytes				
X03015	CD8 antigen (alpha chain)	282	35	8.1
S79711	CD3 gamma-chain	68	14	4.9
X14319	T-cell receptor (beta chain)	282	61	4.6
M10072	CD45 antigen	130	32	4.1
U24441	Matrix metallopeptidase 9	198	49	4.0
D90404	Cathepsin C	476	148	3.2
AI045440	Sialophorin	75	24	3.1
Chemokine/chemokine receptor				
M14656	Secreted phosphoprotein 1 (osteopontin)	1694	94	18
AI009658	CCL5 (RANTES)	1345	88	15.3
AA892854	CXCL13	442	63	7
X17053	CCL2 (MCP-1)	226	38	5.9
AA945737	CXCR4	60	11	5.5

Accession no.	Description	SEA	NaCl	Ratio
U17035	CXCL10	175	40	4.4
X52498	TGF beta1	414	132	3.1
Microglial reaction/macrophages				
U18729	Cytochrome b558 alpha subunit	985	169	5.8
U09540	Cytochrome P450 type 1b1	223	40	5.6
AF028784	GFAP (alternatively spliced form)	4474	1030	4.3
AI176856	Cytochrome P450 (Cyp1b1)	289	70	4.1
AA800318	Serping1	1085	285	3.8
M57276	CD53 antigen	537	158	3.4
M65149	CCAAT/enhancer binding protein (C/EBP)	257	77	3.3
M24067	Serpin E1	180	59	3.1
U10894	Allograft inflammatory factor 1	669	219	3.1
Phagocytosis/opsonization				
J02962	IgE-binding protein (Galectin 3)	1220	87	14.0
M29866	Complement component 3	1358	122	11.1
X52477	Pre-pro-complement component 3	935	103	9.1
X71127	Complement C1q beta chain	3632	649	5.6
M92059	Adipsin	138	25	5.5
X73371	Fc gamma-receptor	209	41	5.1
AA892775	Lysozyme	4526	919	4.9
AA891576	Complement component 1q	98	20	4.9
AA893280	Adipose differentiation related protein	563	135	4.2
AI639117	Complement factor B	268	65	4.1
AI639117	Complement factor B	268	65	4.1
M32062	Fc-gamma-receptor 3	433	117	3.7
M32062	Fc gamma-receptor II beta	597	173	3.5
U42719	Complement component 4a	1453	416	3.5
D10757	Proteosome (macropain) subunit, beta type 9	277	80	3.5
U39476	Vav 1 oncogene	106	31	3.4
D88666	Fatty acid-binding protein (adipocyte)	131	40	3.3
Extracellular matrix/cell adhesion				
S66184	Lysyl-oxidase; fibroblast	140	16	8.8
U15550	Tenascin-C	61	10	6.1
S61865	Syndecan 1	105	20	5.3
X70369	Collagen type III alpha 1	862	165	5.2
U59801	Integrin alpha M	84	18	4.7

Accession no.	Description	SEA	NaCl	Ratio
U75405UTR#1	Alpha-1 collagen mRNA	2804	624	4.5
M27207	Procollagen, type 1, alpha 1	2070	568	3.6
X62952	Vimentin	2652	763	3.5
AI012030	Matrix Gla protein	1932	561	3.4
AA894092	Periostin, osteoblast specific factor (predicted)	47	14	3.4
AI231472	Procollagen, type 1, alpha 1	999	308	3.2
AI071531	Oxidized low density lipoprotein receptor 1	63	20	3.2
AA892333	Tubulin, alpha 6	1662	553	3.0
Antiinflammatory reaction				
AI169327	Tissue inhibitor of metalloproteinase 1	940	20	47.0
M22670	Alpha-2-macroglobulin	219	9	24.3
AI045030	CCAAT/enhancer binding protein delta	118	22	5.4
AA998683	Heat shock 27-kDa protein 1	1386	273	5.1
AA817854	Ceruloplasmin	183	39	4.7
AI169327	TIMP-1	1671	362	4.6
S77528	NF-IL6 (C/EBP-related transcription factor beta)	74	16	4.6
L33869	Ceruloplasmin	391	92	4.3
AI176456	Metallothionein	11045	2980	3.7
M86389	Heat shock 27-kDa protein 1	1563	444	3.5
AA799323	Pleckstrin	99	29	3.4
M65149	CCAAT/enhancer binding protein delta	257	77	3.3
J02722	Haeme oxygenase (decycling) 1	194	58	3.3
M23566	Alpha-2-macroglobulin	3153	989	3.2
AA900582	Alpha-2-macroglobulin	1000	330	3.0
Miscellaneous/compound to inflammation				
L07114	Apolipoprotein B complex	378	23	16.4
AA946503	Lipocalin 2	629	45	14.0
M80367	Guanylate nucleotide binding protein	132	25	5.3
X06916	Protein p9Ka, (S100 calcium binding Prot. A4)	774	153	5.1
AA892553	STAT-1	261	54	4.8
D26393	Hexokinase II	143	33	4.3
X62322	Granulin	4118	1048	3.9
AA946044	Yamaguchi sarcoma viral (v-yes-1) oncogene	79	21	3.8
D21215	Coagulation factor 10	44	12	3.7
AA894029	Cytochrome b-245 beta polypeptide)	116	31	3.7

Accession no.	Description	SEA	NaCl	Ratio
L13192	Forkhead box D1	114	32	3.6
M18349	Protein tyrosine phosphatase, receptor type, C	80	22	3.6
J02869	Cytochrome P450 (Cyp2d9)	153	43	3.6
S66024	CAMP responsive element modulator	68	19	3.6
K03039	Leukocyte common antigen	35	10	3.5
X61381	Interferon-induced trans-membrane protein 3	2347	671	3.5
AI233219	Endothelial cell-specific molecule 1	38	11	3.5
M33648	Coenzyme A synthase 2	192	56	3.4
M19257	Retinol binding protein 1, cellular	653	199	3.3
D30649	Ectonucleotide pyrophosphatase 3	56	17	3.3
E00903	Natriuretic peptide precursor type A	362	112	3.2
J05495	Macrophage galactose lectin 1	88	28	3.1
S67722	Prostaglandin-endoperoxide synthase 2	595	192	3.1
U77038	Protein tyrosine phosphatase type 6	68	22	3.1

Table 1. Absolute and relative signal intensities measured with Affymetrix Rat Genome U34A are given for individual genes that exhibited significantly and at least 3-fold increased differential expression after intracerebral (i.c.) SEA injection compared with saline injection.

Description	MS	EAE	SEA encephalitis
MHC-II	↑ [Lock et al., 2002]	↑ [Carmody et al., 2006]	↑
MHC-I	↑ [Tajouri et al., 2003]		↑
Matrixmetallopeptidase 9	↑ [Steinman, 1999]		↑
CD8 antigen alpha chain	↑ [Liu et al., 2007]		↑
T-cell receptor beta chain	↑ [Lock et al., 2002]	↑ [Carmody et al., 2006]	↑
CD3 gamma-chain	↑ [Liu et al., 2007]		↑
CD 45 antigen	↑ [Liu et al., 2007]		↑
Leukocyte common antigen	↑ [Liu et al., 2007]		↑
Cathepsin C (dipeptidyl peptidase I)		↑ [Carmody et al., 2006]	↑
Sialophorin (CD43)		↑ [Ford et al., 2003]	↑
Secreted phosphoprotein 1 (osteopontin)	↑ [Lock et al., 2002] ↓ [Lindberg et al., 2004]	↑ [Kim et al., 2004]	↑
Chemokine (C-C-motiv ligand) 5, RANTES	↑ [Boven et al., 2000]	↑ [Dos Santos et al., 2005]	↑
Early response JE gene (chemokine C-C motiv ligand 2 (MCP-1)	↑ [Tanuma et al., 2006]	↑ [Hofmann et al., 2002]	↑
Chemokine (C-X-C motif) ligand 10 (CXCL10)	↑ [Tajouri et al., 2003]	↑ [Tajouri et al., 2003]	↑
Transforming growth factor,	↓ [Lindberg et al., 2004]	↑ [Carmody et al., 2006]	↑

beta 1 (TGF beta1)	↑ [Lock et al., 2002]		
CD53 antigen		↑ [Carmody et al., 2006]	↑
IgE-binding protein (Galectin 3)		↑ [Reichert, 1999]	↑
Vav 1 oncogene		↑ [Carmody et al., 2006]	↑
Fc gamma-receptor	↑ [Lock et al., 2002]		↑
Lysozym	↑ [Lock et al., 2002]		↑
Complement C1q	↑ [Tajouri et al., 2003]		↑
Complement component 3	↑ [Lock et al., 2002]		↑
Complement component 4a		↑ [Tajouri et al., 2003]	↑
Fatty acid-binding protein (adipocyte)		↑ [Carmody et al., 2006]	↑
Integrin alpha M	↑ [Lock et al., 2002]	↑ [Carmody et al., 2006]	↑
Tenascin-C	↑ [Lock et al., 2002]	↓ [Carmody et al., 2006]	↑
Collagen type III alpha 1	↓ [Tajouri et al., 2003]	↓ [Tajouri et al., 2003]	↑
Tubulin, alpha 6	↑ [Tajouri et al., 2003]	↓	↑
Haeme oxygenase 1		↑ [Tan et al., 2004]	↑
TIMP-1		↑ [Steinman, 1999]	↑
Alpha 2 macroglobulin		↑ [Hunter et al., 1991]	↑
Heat shock 27-kDa protein 1		↑ [Tajouri et al., 2003]	↑
NF-IL6(C / EBP-related transcription factor beta);	↑ [Lock et al., 2002]		↑
Metallothionein	↑ [Tajouri et al., 2003]	↑ [Espejo et al., 2005]	↑
GFAP (alternatively spliced form)		↑ [Tani et al., 1996]	↑
Granulin	↑ [Tajouri et al., 2003]		↑
STAT-1	↑ [Frisullo et al., 2006]	↑ [Carmody et al., 2006]	↑
Coagulation factor 10		↑ [Carmody et al., 2006]	↑
Hexokinase II		↑ [Carmody et al., 2006]	↑
Protein tyrosine phosphatase, receptor type, C		↑ [Carmody et al., 2006]	↑
Guanylate nucleotide binding protein		↑ [Carmody et al., 2006]	↑

Table 2. Comparison of the differential expression of individual genes for which data were available for the SEA encephalitis (present investigation) and from EAE and MS.

6. B-Cell superantigens and oligoclonal bands

When the role of superantigens is considered with respect to encephalitis, B-cell superantigens have to be taken into consideration in addition T-cell superantigens. A prominent representative for B-cell superantigens is gp120, which forms part of the envelope of the human immune-deficiency virus (HIV) (Neshat et al., 2000; Patke and Shaerer, 2000; Zouali, 2007). Like T-cell superantigens, B-cell superantigens stimulate their target cells in a clonal manner (Müller and Köhler, 1997; Goodyear and Silverman, 2005). As more than 1 B-cell clone is expected to be stimulated by a B-cell superantigen, it may be speculated whether this type of stimulus would result in the presence of oligoclonal IgG bands on isoelectric focussing. Indeed, oligoclonal IgG bands have been identified in various encephalitic diseases in the cerebrospinal fluid (CSF), including e.g. different forms of viral or bacterial encephalitis. Usually, all the antibodies forming oligoclonal bands in these diseases are directed against proteins of the encephalitogenic pathogen. However, there are states of encephalitis like in MS, where the presence of oligoclonal bands cannot be attributed to a certain pathogen. In fact, the antigen specificities present in MS oligoclonal bands comprise almost any antigen that has been tested. Therefore, these oligoclonal antibodies in MS have been termed as "nonsense antibodies" (Mattson et al., 1980). Among this nonsense-spectrum of antigen specificities, frequently an intrathecal antibody sythesis against measles, rubella, varizella zoster virus, herpes simplex virus, Epstein-Barr virus, and Chlamydia pneumoniae have been found (Reiber et al., 1998; Skorstad et al., 2009; Franciotta et al., 2010; Fainardi et al., 2009). It may be interesting to mention here, that antibodies specific for myelin proteins form only a small part of the oligoclonal IgG antibodies in MS (Owens et al., 2009). If nonsense antibodies like in MS would be due to a B-cell superantigenic stimulus, experimental proof should be available. Therefore, we tested in vitro, whether B-cell superantigens were capable to induce the formation of oligoclonal IgG bands on isoelectric focussing. In fact, after stimulation of peripheral blood mononuclear cells in vitro with the B-cell superantigen gp120, we detected IgG-bands by isoelectric focussing of the supernatant (Figure 5; Emmer et al., unpublished). This IgG-production

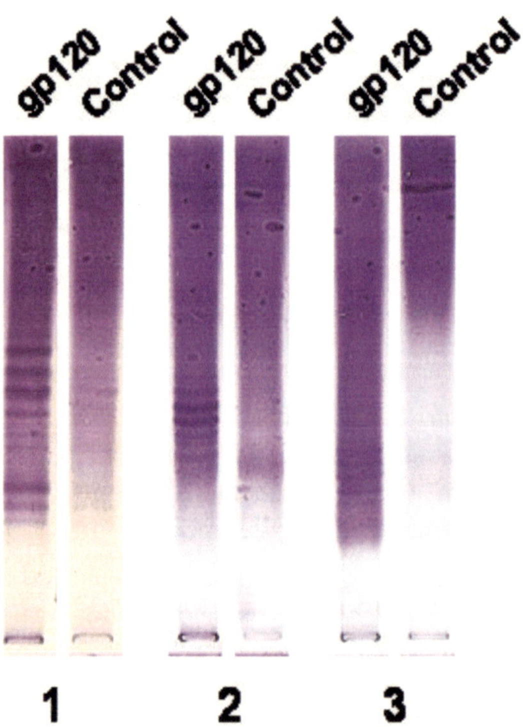

Fig. 5. Representative results obtained by isoelectric focussing after stimulation of peripheral blood mononuclear cells from 3 healthy human donors in vitro with gp120 (8 µg/ml) and without gp120 (control). The numbers underneath the images denote the different subjects.

depended on the concentration of the B-cell superantigen. The detected oligoclonal bands were quite similar to those found by isoelectric focussing in the cerebrospinal fluid of MS-patients. Our results suggest that B-cell superantigens may play a role in the pathogenesis of the inflammatory response of multiple sclerosis.

The expression of oligoclonal IgG in the CSF of MS-patients per se could have a detrimental influence, e.g. by opsonization of central nervous system components and subsequent phagocytosis by macrophages. In fact, the progress of the disease has been reported to be unfavourable if multiple oligoclonal bands are detected in the CSF of MS-patients (Joseph et al., 2009).

7. Conclusion

The present review focusses on the encephalitogenic effects of the intracerebrally expressed T-cell superantigen SEA. It has been demonstrated that SEA is capable to induce a perivascular inflammatory response, which was short lived after a single intracerebral injection. In the context of a pathogen residing within the CNS, a T cell superantigen is, however, expected to be expressed for prolonged periods of time and could, therefore, induce a longer lasting inflammatory response. The latter might add to the noxious response of the pathogen itself. Furthermore it was demonstrated that B-cell superantigens are able to stimulate B-cells to produce IgG which is detected as oligoclonal bands by isoelectric focussing. These oligoclonal bands resemble those found in the CSF of MS-patients.

Beside bacterial infections, the presented findings could be of special relevance for viral encephalitis and possibly for multiple sclerosis.

8. Acknowledgement

A.E. gratefully acknowledges the support obtained within the Wilhelm-Roux-grant (FKZ 21/22) by the Martin-Luther-University of Halle-Wittenberg.

9. References

Antony, JM; Deslauriers, AM; Bhat, RK; Ellestad, KK; Power, C. (2011). Human endogenous retroviruses and multiple sclerosis: innocent bystanders or disease determinants? *Biochim Biophys Acta*, Vol. 1812, No. 2, pp. 162-176

Barnett, MH; Prineas, JW. (2004). Relapsing and remitting multiple sclerosis: pathology of the newly forming lesion. *Annals of Neurolgy*, Vol. 55, No. 4, pp. 458-468

Boven, LA; Montagne, L; Nottet, HS; De Groot, CJ. (2000). Macrophage inflammatory protein-1alpha (MIP-1alpha), MIP-1beta, and RANTES mRNA semiquantification and protein expression in active demyelinating multiple sclerosis (MS) lesions. *Clinical and Experimental Immunology*, Vol. 122, No. 2,pp. 257–263

Carmody, RJ; Hilliard, B; Maguschak, K; Chodosh, LA; Chen, YH. (2006). Genomic scale profiling of autoimmune inflammation in the central nervous system: the nervous response to inflammation. *Journal of Neuroimmunology*, Vol. 133, No. 1, pp. 95–107

Damle, NK; Leytze, G; Klussman, K; Leadbetter, JA. (1993). Activation with superantigens induces programmed death in antigen-primed CD4+ class II major histocompatibility complex T lymphocytes via a CD11a/CD18- dependent mechanism. *European Journal of Immunology*, Vol. 23, No.7, pp. 1513–1522

Dos Santos, AC; Barsante, MM; Arantes, RM; Bernard, CC; Teixeira, MM; Carvalho-Tavares, J. (2005). CCL2 and CCL5 mediate leukocyte adhesion in experimental autoimmune encephalomyelitis - an intravital microscopy study. *Journal of Neuroimmunology*, Vol. 162, No. 1, pp. 122–129

Emmer, A; Gerlach, K; Staege, MS; Kornhuber, ME. (2008). Cerebral gene expression of superantigen encephalitis in the lewis rat induced by Staphylococcal enterotoxin A. *Scandinavian Journal of Immunology*, Vol. 67, No. 5, pp. 464–472

Emmer, A; Gerlach, K; Staege, MS; Kornhuber ME. (2010). T-cell subsets of the encephalitis induced by the superantigen Staphylococcal Enterotoxin A (SEA) in the Lewis rat: an immunohistochemical investigation. *Cellular Immunology*, Vol. 264, No. 1, pp. 93-96

Espejo, C; Penkowa, M; Demestre, M; Montalban, X; Martinez Caceres, EM. (2005). Time course expression of CNS inflammatory, neurodegenerative tissue repair markers and metallothioneins during experimental autoimmune encephalomyelitis. *Neuroscience*, Vol. 32, No. 4, pp. 1135–1149

Espejo, C ; Martinez-Caceres, EM. (2005). The role of metallothioneins in experimental autoimmune encephalomyelitis and multiple sclerosis. *Annals of New York Academy of Science*, Vol. 1051, pp. 88–96

Fainardi, E; Castellazzi, M; Tamborino, C; Seraceni, S; Tola, MR; Granieri, E; Contini, C. (2009). Chlamydia pneumoniae-specific intrathecal oligoclonal antibody response is predominantly detected in a subset of multiple sclerosis patients with progressive forms. *Journal of Neurovirology*, Vol. 15, No.5, pp. 425-433

Fields, BA; Malchiodi, EL; Li, H; Ysern, X; Stauffacher, CV; Schlievert, PM; Karjalainen, K; Mariuzza, RA. (1996). Crystal structure of a T-cell receptor beta-chain complexed with a superantigen. *Nature*, Vol. 384, No. 6605, pp. 188–192

Filippi, M; Rocca, MA; Martino, G; Horsfield, MA; Comi, G. (1998). Magnetization transfer changes in the normal appearing white matter precede the appearance of enhancing lesions in patients with multiple sclerosis. *Annals of Neurology*, Vol. 43, No. 6, pp. 809-814

Ford, ML; Onami, TM; Sperling, AI; Ahmed, R; Evavold, BD. (2003). CD43 modulates severity and onset of experimental autoimmune encephalomyelitis. *Jounal of Immunology*, Vol. 171, No. 12, pp. 6527–6533

Fleischer, B. (1991). Stimulation of the immune system by microbial "superantigens", *Immun Infekt*, Vol. 19, No. 1, pp. 8–11

Franciotta, D; Di Stefano, AL; Jarius, S; Zardini, E; Tavazzi, E; Ballerini, C; Marchioni. E; Bergamaschi, R; Ceroni, M. (2011). Cerebrospinal BAFF and Epstein-Barr virus-specific oligoclonal bands in multiple sclerosis and other inflammatory demyelinating neurological diseases. *Journal of Neuroimmunology*, Vol. 230, No. 1, pp. 160- 163

Fraser, JD. High-affinity binding of staphylococcal enterotoxins A and B to HLA-DR. (1989). *Nature*, Vol. 339, No. 6221, pp. 221–223

Friedl, P; Brocker, EB. (2000). The biology of cell locomotion within threedimensional extracellular matrix. *Cellular and Molecular Life Sciences*, Vol. 57, No. 1, pp. 41–64

Frisullo, G; Angelucci, F; Caggiula, M. (2006). PSTAT1, pSTAT3 and Tbet expression in peripheral blood mononuclear cells from relapsing-remitting multiple sclerosis

patients correlates with disease activity. *Journal of Neuroscience Research*, Vol. 84, No. 5, pp. 1027-1036
Garson, JA; Tuke, PW; Giraud, P; Paranhos-Baccala, G; Perron, H. (1998). Detection of virion-associated MSRV-RNA in serum of patients with multiple sclerosis. *The Lancet*, Vol. 351, No. 9095, pp. 33
Goodyear, CS; Silverman, GJ. (2005). B cell superantigens: a microbe's answer to innate-like B cells and natural antibodies. *Springer Seminars in Immunopathology*, Vol. 26, No. 4, pp. 463-484
Herrman, A; Croteua, G; Sekaly, RP; Kappler, J; Marrack, P. (1990). Effect of isotypes and allelic polymorphism on the binding of staphylococcal exotoxins to MHC class II molecules. *Journal of Experimental Medicine*, Vol. 172, No. 1, pp. 709-717
Hofmann, N; Lachnit, N; Sreppel, M. (2002). Increased expression of ICAM-1, VCAM-1, MCP-1 and MIP-1 alpha by spinal perivascular macrophages during experimental allergic encephalomyelitis in rats. *BMC Immunology*, Vol. 26, pp. 3-11
Jee, Y; Kim, G; Tanuma, N; Matsumoto, Y. (2001). STAT expression and localization in the central nervous system during autoimmune encephalomyelitis in Lewis rats. *Journal of Neuroimmunology*, Vol. 114, No. 1, pp. 40-47
Jelonek, MT; Classon, BJ; Hudson, PJ; Margulies, DH. (1998). Direct binding of the MHC class I molecule H-2Ld to CD8: interaction with the amino terminus of a mature cell surface protein. *Journal of Immunology*, Vol. 160, No. 6, pp. 2809-2814
Jilek, S; Schluep, M; Rossetti, AO. (2007). CSF enrichment of highly differentiated CD8+ T cells in early multiple sclerosis. *Clinical Immunology*, Vol. 123, No. 1, pp. 105-113
Joseph, FG; Hirst, CL; Pickersgill, TP; Ben-Shlomo, Y; Robertson, NP; Scolding, NJ. (2009). CSF oligoclonal band status informs prognosis in multiple sclerosis: a case control study of 100 patients. *Journal of Neurology, Neurosurgery and Psychiatry*, Vol. 80, No. 3, pp. 292-296
Kappler, J; Kotzin, B; Herron, L; Gelfand, EW; Bigler, RD; Boylston, A; Carrel, S; Posnett, DN; Choi, Y; Marrack, P. (1989). V beta-specific stimulation of human T cells by staphylococcal toxins. *Science*. Vol. 244, No. 4906, pp. 811-813
Kim, MD; Cho, HJ; Shin, T. (2004). Expression of osteopontin and its ligand, CD44; in the spinal cords of Lewis rats with experimental autoimmune encephalomyelitis. *Journal of Neuroimmunology*, Vol. 151, No. 1, pp. 78-84
Kornhuber, ME; Ganz, C; Lang, R; Brill, T; Schmahl, W. (2002). Focal encephalitis in the Lewis rat induced by intracerebral enterotoxin superantigen and amplified by activated intravenous splenocytes. *Neuroscience Letters*, Vol. 324, No. 2, pp. 93-96
Kornhuber, ME. (2006). Noninflammatory pathogenesis of lesions in multiple sclerosis. *Nervenarzt*, Vol. 77, No. 8, pp. 989-990
Levine, SM; Chakrabarty, A. (2004). The role of iron in the pathogenesis of experimental allergic encephalomyelitis and multiple sclerosis. *Annals of the New York Academy of Science*, Vol. 1012, pp. 252-266
Lindberg, RLP; De Groot, CJA; Certa, U. (2004). Multiple sclerosis as a generalized CNS disease - comparative microarray analysis of normal appearing white matter and lesions in secondary progressive MS. *Journal of Neuroimmunology*, Vol. 152, No. 1, pp. 154- 167
Liu, GZ; Fang, LB; Hjelmstrom, P; Gao, XG. (2007). Increased CD8+ central memory T cells in patients with multiple sclerosis. *Multiple Sclerosis*, Vol. 13, No. 2, pp. 149-155

Lock, C; Hermans, G; Pedotti, R; Brendolan, A; Schadt, E; Garren, H. (2002). Gene-microrray analysis of multiple sclerosis lesions yields new targets validated in immune encephalomyelitis. *Nature Medicine*, Vol. 8, No. 5, pp. 500–508

Makida, R; Hofer, MF; Takase, K; Cambier, JC; Leung, DY. (1996). Bacterial superantigens induce V beta-specific T cell receptor internalization. *Molecular Immunology*, Vol. 33, No. 10, pp. 891–900

Mattson, DH; Roos, RP; Arnason, BG. (1980). Isoelectric focusing of IgG eluted from multiple sclerosis and subacute sclerosing panencephalitis brains. *Nature*, Vol., 287, No. 5780, pp. 335-337

Müller-Alouf, H; Carnoy, C; Simonet, M; Alouf, JE. (2001). Superantigen bacterial toxins, state of the art. *Toxicon*, Vol. 39, No. 11, pp. 1691–1701

Müller, S; Köhler, H. (1997). B cell superantigens in HIV-1 infection. *International Reviews of Immunology*, Vol. 14, No. 4, pp. 339-349.

Neshat, MN; Goodglick, L; Lim, K; Braun, J. (2000). Mapping the B cell superantigen binding site for HIV-1 gp120 on a V(H)3 Ig. *International Immunology*, Vol. 12, No. 3, pp. 305-312

Niedergang, F; Hémar, A; Hewitt, CR; Owen, MJ; Dautry-Varsat, A; Alcover, A. (1995). The Staphylococcus aureus enterotoxin B superantigen induces specific T cell receptor down-regulation by increasing its internalization. *Journal of Biological Chemistry*, Vol. 270, No. 21, pp. 12839–12845

Owens, GP; Bennett, JL; Lassmann, H; O'Connor, KC; Ritchie, AM; Shearer, A; Lam, C; Yu, X; Birlea, M; DuPree, C; Williamson, RA; Hafler, DA; Burgoon, MP; Gilden, D. (2009). Antibodies produced by clonally expanded plasma cells in multiple sclerosis cerebrospinal fluid. *Annals of Neurology*, Vol. 65, No. 6, pp. 639-649

Pagenstecher, A; Stalder, AK; Kincaid, CL; Shapiro, SD; Campbell, IL. (1998). Differential expression of matrix metalloproteinase and tissue inhibitor of matrix metalloproteinase genes in the mouse central nervous system in normal and inflammatory states. *American Journal of Pathology*, Vol. 152, No. 3, pp. 729–741

Patke, CL; Shearer, WT. (2000). gp120- and TNF-alpha-induced modulation of human B cell function: proliferation, cyclic AMP generation, Ig production, and B-cell receptor expression. *Journal of Allergy and Clinical Immunology*, Vol. 105, No. 5, pp. 975-982

Penkowa, M; Hidalgo, J. (2003). Treatment with metallothionein prevents demyelination and axonal damage and increases oligodendrocyte precursors and tissue repair during experimental autoimmune encephalomyelitis. *Journal of Neurosciene Research*, Vol. 72, No. 5, pp. 574–586

Perron, H; Lang, A. (2010). The human endogenous retrovirus link between genes and environment in multiple sclerosis and in multifactorial diseases associating neuroinflammation. *Clinical Reviews in Allergy and Immunology*, Vol. 39, No. 1, pp. 51-61

Raivich, G; Banati, R. (2004). Brain microglia and blood-derived macrophages: molecular profiles and functional roles in multiple sclerosis and animal models of autoimmune demyelinating disease. *Brain Research Reviews*, Vol. 46, No. 3, pp. 261–281

Redwine, JM; Buchmeier, MJ; Evans, CF. (2001). In vivo expression of major histocompability complex molecules and neurons during viral infection. *American Journal of Pathology*, Vol. 159, No. 4, pp. 1219–1224

Reiber, H; Ungefehr, S; Jacobi, C. (1998). The intrathecal, polyspecific and oligoclonal immune response in multiple sclerosis. *Multiple Sclerosis*, Vol. 4, No. 5, pp. 111-117

Reichert, F; Rotshenker, S. (1999). Galectin-3 / MAC-2 in experimental allergic encephalomyelitis. *Experimental Neurology*, Vol. 160, No. 1, pp. 508–514

Rotshenker, S. (2003). Microglia and macrophage activation and the regulation of complement-receptor-3 (CR3 / MAC-1)-mediated myelin phagocytosis in injury and disease. *Journal of Molecular Neuroscience*, Vol. 21, No. 1, pp. 65–72

Sedgwick, JD; Schwender, S; Gregersen, R; Dörries, R; ter Meulen, V. (1993). Resident macrophages (ramified microglia) of the adult brown Norway rat central nervous system are constitutively major histocompability complex class II positive. *Journal of Experimental Medicine*, Vol. 177, No. 4, pp. 1145–1152

Skorstad G, Vandvik B, Vartdal F, Holmøy T. (2009). MS and clinically isolated syndromes: shared specificity but diverging clonal patterns of virus-specific IgG antibodies produced in vivo and by CSF B cells in vitro. *European Journal of Neurology*, Vol. 16, No. 10, pp. 1124-1129

Staege, MS; Hansen, G; Baersch, G; Burdach S. (2004). Functional and molecular characterization of interleukin-2 transgenic Ewing tumor cells for in vivo immunotherapy. *Pediatric Blood and Cancer*, Vol. 43, No. 1, pp. 23–34

Steinman, L. (1999). Assessment of the utility of animal models for MS and demyelinating disease in the design of rational therapy. *Neuron*, Vol. 24, No. 3, pp. 511–514

Stoll, G. (2002). Inflammatory cytokines in the nervous system. Multifunctional mediators in autoimmunity and cerebral ischemia. *Reviews in Neurology.*, Vol. 158, pp. 887–891

Tajouri, L; Mellick, AS; Ashton, KJ. (2003). Quantitative and qualitative changes in gene expression pattern characterize the activity of plaques in multiple sclerosis. *Molecular Brain Research*, Vol. 119, No. 2, pp. 170–183

Tan, GJ; Zhu, YF; Cao, CF; Zhao, XY; Ma, CS; Yang, TZ. (2004). Dynamic changes of heme oxygenase-1 protein and mRNA in the brains of rats with experimental allergic encephalomyelitis. *Sheng Li Xue Bao*, Vol. 56, No. 5, pp. 579–584

Tani, M; Glabinski, AR; Tuohy, VK; Stoler, MH; Estes, ML; Ransohoff, RM. (1996). In situ hybridization analysis of glial fibrillary acidic protein mRNA reveals evidence of biphasic astrocyte activation during acute experimental autoimmune encephalomyelitis. *American Journal of Pathology*, Vol. 148, No. 3, pp. 889–896

Tanuma, N; Sakuma, H; Sasaki, A; Matsumoto, Y. (2006). Chemokine expression by astrocytes plays a role in microglia/macrophage activation and subsequent neurodegeneration in secondary progressive multiple sclerosis. *Acta Neuropathologica*, Vol. 112, No. 2 ,pp. 195–204

Torkildsen O, Brunborg LA, Myhr KM, Bø L. (2008). The cuprizone model for demyelination. *Acta Neurologca Scandinavica Supplementum*, Vol. 188, pp. 72-76

Tusher, VG; Tibshirani, R; Chu, G. (2001) Significance analysis of microarrays applied to the ionizing radiation response. *Proceedings of the National Academy of Science of the USA*, Vol. 98, No. 9, pp. 5116–5121

Von Essen, M; Menné Bonefeld, C; Siersma, V; Rasmussen, AB; Lauritsen, JPH; Nielsen, BL; Geisle, C. (2004). Constitutive and ligand-induced TCR degradation. *Journal of Immunology*, Vol. 173, No 1, pp. 384–393

Wekerle, H; Linington, C; (1986). Lassmann, H; Meyermann, R. Cellular immunoreactivity within the CNS. *Trends in Neuroscience*, Vol. 9, pp. 271–277

Wilkinson, B; Koenigsknecht-Talboo, J; Grommes, C; Lee, CY; Landreth, G. (2006). Fibrillar beta-amyloid-stimulated intracellular signalling cascades require Vav for induction of respiratory burst and phagocytosis in monocytes and microglia. *Journal of Biological Chemistry*, Vol. 281, No. 30, pp. 20842–20845

Yagi, J; Baron, J; Buxser, S; Janeway Jr., CA. (1990). Bacterial proteins that mediate the association of a defined subset of T cell receptor: CD4 complexes with class II MHC. *Journal of Immunology*, Vol. 3, No. 3, pp. 892–901

Zouali, M. (2007). B cell superantigens subvert innate functions of B cells. *Chemical Immunology and Allergy*, Vol. 93, p. 92-105.

16

Rasmussen's Encephalitis: An Overview

Mayowa Owolabi
University of Ibadan
Nigeria

1. Introduction

Epilepsia partialis continua (EPC) resulting from localized encephalitis was first described by Kozhevnikov and Brun in 1895 in patients suffering from Russian spring-summer encephalitis. (Bien et al., 2005b) In 1958, Rasmussen described a syndrome of focal seizures due to chronic localized encephalitis in three cases. The heterogeneity of this syndrome was demonstrated by Oguni in a description of 48 cases in 1991 among which 80% had focal motor seizures of which 50% were continuous.(Oguni et al., 1991) The syndrome occurred predominantly in children who had hemiparesis and cortical signs.(Oguni et al., 1991) Even though a diagnostic criteria has been proposed(Bien et al., 2005b), the aetio-pathogenesis remains unresolved.

Rasmussen's encephalitis (RE) is a rare neurological disease of childhood characterized by unilateral hemispheric atrophy, focal intractable seizures, and progressive neurological deficits. The affected brain tissue shows a chronic inflammatory histopathology and an autoimmune reaction is suspected. Therapeutic strategies include anticonvulsants, immunomodulation and surgery. (Bien et al., 2005b) This review covers the natural history, aetiopathogenesis, clinical features, diagnosis, and treatment of RE.

2. RE by Theodore Rasmussen

Rasmussen et al presented a clinico-pathologic report of three children suffering from a chronic illness, producing focal seizures and gradually producing severe damage to one cerebral hemisphere.(Rasmussen et al., 1958) Occasional specimens of scarred, atrophic brain removed for the treatment of focal cerebral seizures at the Montreal Neurological Institute showed striking perivascular collections of round cells, particularly in less severely damaged areas of the specimens. Rasmussen observed that in the past this perivascular cuffing was attributed to the effect on the brain of recurring seizures. He inferred, however, that this was a rather unsatisfactory explanation since the great majority of surgical specimens removed from patients with equally frequent focal seizures did not show this change.(Rasmussen et al., 1958) He suggested that this microscopic picture may indicate the presence of an unsuspected, more or less localized, chronic encephalitis that had smoldered along over a period of years.(Rasmussen et al., 1958)

He opined that suggestions for therapy in the active phase of the disease, when it might be possible to prevent destruction of brain tissue, must await determination of etiologic factors. (Rasmussen et al., 1958)

Rasmussen speculated regarding the ability of some dormant viruses in the nervous system to be pertinent to the problem. He reasoned that localization of the lesions and their character are more consistent with viral encephalitis than with postinfectious perivenous encephalitis or with allergic encephalitis. He concluded that the histological appearance in each instance suggested chronic focal encephalitis of unknown cause which manifested with focal epilepsy.(Rasmussen et al., 1958)

3. Aetio-pathogenesis and pathology of RE

RE is a rare disease that should be envisaged as sporadic, since there is no evidence for a genetic component. There is, at present, no conclusive evidence why and how RE starts.

3.1 Is RE an epileptic encephalopathy?

In analogy to other conditions of childhood epilepsies with progressive neurological deterioration, it has been suggested that in RE, the epileptic activity itself may contribute to the functional decline.(Bien et al., 2005b) This is because focal motor deficit usually follows the onset of epilepsy and its severity seems to mirror the intensity of the seizure activity(Bien et al., 2005b; Chinchilla et al., 1994). Steroids given early in the course of the disease are able to reduce the severity of the deficit, when seizure activity is brought under control. The response to steroids may suggest that an inflammatory process underlies the manifestation with seizures and neurological deficit. Because for any inflammatory process, the immune effector cells or antibodies originate from the blood stream, the encephalitis is expected to be bilateral. Thus focal epilepsy has been postulated as the reason for the unilaterality of the encephalitis.(Bien et al., 2005b) It has been suggested that focal seizures may damage the blood brain barrier allowing autoantibodies to cross the it thus causing unilateral brain damage.(Bien et al., 2005b)

However, while seizures may lead to reversible Todd's palsy probably due to neuronal exhaustion, there is no conclusive evidence yet that seizures on their own cause or precede encephalitis.(Rasmussen et al., 1958) Rasmussen reiterated that the great majority of surgical specimens removed from patients with equally frequent focal seizures did not show features of focal encephalitis.(Rasmussen et al., 1958) Furthermore, unilaterality is not a constant finding in RE, and the progressive atrophy and epileptiform processes may progressively involve the other hemisphere.(Bien et al., 2005b) The fact that the seizure is originally focal could not be the basis for focal encephalitis. Rather focal seizures could be a manifestation of focal encephalitis. The effect cannot precede the cause. Therefore asymmetry of the pathogenic process may be responsible for focal seizures and focal neurological deficits. This is corroborated by reports of cases with hemiparesis and focal encephalitis preceding seizures.(Korn-Lubetzki et al., 2004)

The factors responsible for the asymmetry remain unravelled. Nevertheless, the evidence for immunologic mechanisms is growing although the antigenic stimulus remains obscure.

3.2 Role of CD-8 cells

Unilateral encephalitis, an intriguing feature of RE, distinguishes it from any other inflammatory disease of the CNS. Histopathological findings in RE comprise lymphocytic infiltrates, microglial nodules, neuronal and astrocytic loss, and gliosis of the affected hemisphere.(Farrell et al., 1992; Robitaille, 1991) Destruction of neurons and astrocytes by cytotoxic CD8 T cells has been proposed as a pathogenic mechanism underlying RE. (Schwab et al., 2009)

Active brain inflammatory lesions contain large numbers of T lymphocytes, which are recruited early within the lesions suggesting that a T cell dependent immune response contributes to the onset and evolution of the disease(Farrell et al., 1992; Schwab et al., 2009). Moreover, the histopathological observation of granzyme B-containing CD8+ T cells in direct apposition to MHC class I positive neurons raised the hypothesis of a CD8+ T cells-mediated neuronal attack as a key pathogenetic mechanism underlying RE. (Bien et al., 2005b; Bien et al., 2002a; Bien et al., 2002c; Bien et al., 2005a; Schwab et al., 2009) Apart from neuronal cell death, CD8 cells may also be responsible for the degeneration of astrocytes found in RE lesions. (Bauer et al., 2002; Bauer et al., 2007)

The antigens of these brain-infiltrating lymphocytes are still unknown. It is not even clear yet, whether the CNS-directed T-cell response (TCR) is focused towards particular antigens. Experimentally, this could be proven by demonstrating that individual clones are expanded in the tissue.(Bien et al., 2005b)

In a longitudinal analysis of TCR in RE, severe perturbations of the TCR repertoire were found in brain infiltrates from all specimens, while clonal expansions, as evidenced by peripheral blood analysis, belonged to the CD8+ T-cell subset. In line with previous findings, histochemical analysis of the brain lesions showed Vb specific T cells containing the cytotoxic molecule granzyme B and lying in close appositions to NeuN+ neurons and GFAP+ astrocytes.(Bauer et al., 2002; Bauer et al., 2007; Bien et al., 2002b; Bien et al., 2002a; Bien et al., 2005a) Analysis of corresponding CNS/blood specimens revealed overlapping but also CNS-restricted expansions of certain TCR clonotypes suggesting expansions of T cells within the target organ itself. (Bauer et al., 2002; Bauer et al., 2007; Bien et al., 2002b; Bien et al., 2002a; Bien et al., 2005a)

Longitudinal analysis of peripheral blood samples demonstrated dominance but also longitudinal persistence of specific CD8 T-cell clones over time. The Vb/Jb usage, length of the CDR3, and biochemical characteristics of the CDR3 amino acids suggested high similarities putatively related to common driving antigen(s) without shared clones. In conclusion, the data strongly support the hypothesis of an antigen-driven MHC class-I restricted, CD8+ T cell-mediated attack against neurons and astrocytes in the CNS dominating the pathogenesis in RE in contrast to a random attraction of cells as part of a secondary immune response.(Schwab et al., 2009)

This process may persist for at least 1 to 2 years. (Schwab et al., 2009) The long-term persistence (or re-occurrence) of putatively pathogenic T-cell clones despite therapy (or even immunoablation) may indicate an ongoing exposure of the immune system to the antigenic trigger. This trigger (autoantigen or virus) could very well reside within the CNS. The finding of identical TCR clones between the CNS and peripheral blood compartment in patients with matching CNS-blood samples is in line with this assumption. However, because this was a small-scale study, further research is required to validate the hypothesis.

3.3 Glu-R3 autoantibodies

Autoantibodies against glutamate receptors (GluR3 and NR2B), first reported in Rasmussen encephalitis, have been observed in other focal epilepsies, central nervous system ischemic infarcts, transient ischemic attacks, sporadic olivopontocerebellar atrophy, systemic lupus erythematosus, and paraneoplastic encephalopathies.(Pleasure, 2008)

Furthermore, the hypothesis of RE as a primarily antibody-driven attack against neuronal structures [e.g. the glutamate receptor GluR3 could not be confirmed in larger cohorts (Bien et al., 2005b). Thus the detection of glutamate receptor autoantibodies is not useful in the evaluation of Rasmussen encephalitis. (Pleasure, 2008)
This does not exclude that other humoral mechanisms may contribute to the pathogenesis of RE. Future antibody research in RE will probably concentrate on detecting possibly pathogenic antibodies other than glutamate receptor antibodies.(Bien et al., 2005b; Pleasure, 2008)

3.4 Pathological features

The precise nature and sequence of the pathogenetically relevant processes remain controversial. It is unclear if a uniform process exists in all stages of the disease in all RE patients.(Bien et al., 2005b; Pleasure, 2008)
The histopathological properties of RE have been described in several studies.(Bien et al., 2005b; Bien et al., 2002b; Bien et al., 2002c) Using standard histochemical staining techniques, four stages corresponding to disease duration have been proposed. **Group 1** (earliest phase) is characterized by inflammation with numerous microglial nodules, with or without neuronophagia, perivascular round cells and glial scarring. **Group 2** reveals several microglial nodules, cuffs of perivascular round cells, and at least one gyral segment of complete necrosis. **Group 3** shows neuronal loss and gliosis with moderately abundant perivascular round cells and few microglial nodules. Finally, **group 4** (last phase) displays no or few microglial nodules, neuronal loss and mild perivascular inflammation, combined with various degrees of gliosis and glial scarring. (Bien et al., 2005b; Bien et al., 2002b; Bien et al., 2002c; Robitaille, 1991)
The round cell infiltrates in RE brains consist almost exclusively of T lymphocytes. Using a quantitative histopathological immunohistochemical approach, it has been demonstrated that densities of T cells, microglial nodules and activated astrocytes are inversely correlated with disease duration. Furthermore, the immunohistochemical observations showed that the majority of the T cells are CD8+ containing GrB+ granules. A proportion of them laid in apposition to neurons. These neurons were positive for MHC class I. A few neurons were found to die by apoptosis. These findings were interpreted as evidence for a cytotoxic T cell reaction against neurons. (Bien et al., 2005b; Bien et al., 2002b; Bien et al., 2002c; Robitaille, 1991)
Another diagnostically relevant observation was that <5% of the CD68+HLADR + cells had macrophage morphology (the remainder had microglial morphology). In addition, CD20+ cells (B cells) and CD138+ cells (plasma cells) are extremely rare and signs of immunoglobulin deposits or activated complement were not found. (Bien et al., 2005b; Bien et al., 2002b; Bien et al., 2002c)
A viral aetiology was already suggested by Rasmussen based on the constituents of the immune reaction in the brains such as lymphocyte infiltration and microglial nodules (Rasmussen et al., 1958). The similarities of RE and Russian spring summer meningoencephalitis, which is caused by a flavivirus, further supported this hypothesis.(Bien et al., 2005b) However, so far all attempts to identify a pathogenic viral agent have been contradictory and inconclusive. Bien Inclusion bodies suggestive of a viral infection have not been observed in RE.(Bien et al., 2005b)
Available data continue to suggest a T cell-led immune basis to the pathogenesis of RE. However, the antigenic basis is still obscure. Serial examinations in the early phase of the disease might be important in identifying this group of patients, so that more detailed study

of possible etiologic factors might be made before the fire has burned out and only the scarred evidence of earlier damage remains. (Rasmussen et al., 1958)

4. Clinical features

4.1 Natural history and evolution

Although reported cohorts of individuals with RE are not large, three stages have been proposed. (Bien et al., 2005b; Bien et al., 2002c; Bien et al., 2002d). The average age at presentation is 6 years of age. (Bien et al., 2005b; Bien et al., 2002c; Oguni et al., 1991) In about two-thirds of patients, RE may commence in some patients with a non-specific **'prodromal stage'** manifesting with a relatively low seizure frequency and rarely mild hemiparesis with a median duration of 7.1 months (range: 0 months to 8.1 years).(Bien et al., 2005b; Bien et al., 2002c; Bien et al., 2002d; Oguni et al., 1991)

All patients enter an **'acute stage'** of the disease characterized by frequent seizures, mostly simple partial motor seizures often in the form of epilepsia partialis continua (EPC). The neurological deterioration becomes manifest by progressive hemiparesis, hemianopia, cognitive deterioration and, if the dominant dominant hemisphere is affected, aphasia. (Bien et al., 2005b; Bien et al., 2002c; Oguni et al., 1991) The median duration of this stage is 8 months (range 4–8 months).(Bien et al., 2005b; Bien et al., 2002c; Oguni et al., 1991)

The final stage is the **'residual stage'** with permanent and stable neurological deficits and still many seizures, although less frequent than in the acute stage. At this stage, not all the patients are hemiplegic.(Bien et al., 2005b; Bien et al., 2002c; Oguni et al., 1991)

The wide time ranges for the duration of the disease stages indicate the high variability of severity and speed of the destructive process in different patients. For clinical monitoring of the progression, hemiparesis is the most useful marker as this feature is most consistently found, and it allows quantitative evaluation, even in children.(Bien et al., 2005b; Bien et al., 2002c; Oguni et al., 1991) Assessment of degree of hemiparesis is best done in periods with low frequency of seizures, because it can be increased by additional transient postictal paresis in cases with motor seizures. In addition, periodic assessment of neuropsychological performance is recommended in order to detect cognitive decline, especially in cases without overt hemiparesis, such as those of temporal lobe origin. (Bien et al., 2005b; Hennessy et al., 2001)

Monitoring can also be done using the hemispheric ratio on neuroimages.

4.2 Characteristics of the seizures in RE

Epilepsy in RE patients is characterized by the polymorphism of seizures in a given patient; the frequent occurrence of EPC; and the medical intractability of seizures, particularly of EPC.(Bien et al., 2005b) The different semiologies of seizures, often noted on longitudinal evaluation of patient records, is best explained as a 'march (of the epileptic focus) across the hemisphere'. (Oguni et al., 1991) Supportive findings have been made by serial neuroimaging studies. However, apart from the rare cases of bilateral RE, all seizures originate in one hemisphere. (Bien et al., 2005b)

Simple partial motor seizures involving one side of the body are the most common (77% of cases), followed by secondarily generalized tonic clonic seizures (42%), complex partial seizures (19% with automatisms and 31% with subsequent unilateral motor involvement), postural seizures probably originating in the supplementary motor region (24%) and somatosensory seizures (21%) (Oguni et al., 1991). EPC has been reported to occur in 56–92%

of patients at some time during their disease course EPC was originally described in Russian adults suffering from Russian springsummer encephalitis and has subsequently caused extensive discussions regarding its nature and origin. EPC is most commonly viewed as cortical and epileptic.

4.3 Possible variants of RE

In contrast to the classical features mentioned above, certain clinical variants of RE exist.

4.3.1 RE with delayed seizure onset

Patients with progressive hemiparesis and biopsy evidence of RE followed by unilaterally generated seizures only after several months have been reported. (Korn-Lubetzki et al., 2004).

4.3.2 RE with movement disorder

Unilateral basal ganglia involvement (usually the caudate nucleus) has been reported to present with features of hemidystonia and hemiathetosis in addition to EPC. (Bhatjiwale et al., 1998; Bien et al., 2005b)

4.3.3 Localised form

Mild and non-progressive phenotypes of the disease have been reported with childhood or late-onset chronic focal encephalitis, dominated by partial seizures with mild focal motor deficit and choreo-dystonic movements. (Gambardella et al., 2008)

4.3.4 Bilateral cases

The term 'bilateral RE' should be reserved for cases with inflammatory lesions in both hemispheres. Although several clinical and electrophysiological features have suggested bilateral cerebral invlovelment in many cases (e.g. secondary spread of focal seizures to the contralateral side, interictal epileptiform abnormalities on the contralateral side, or mild contralateral atrophy). (Andermann et al., 2006; Bien et al., 2005b; Hart, 2004) True bilateral RE is very rare.

There is no evidence for an inherent tendency of RE to spread to the contralateral side after longstanding disease. Furthermore with over 10 years follow-up: no case of RE initially cured by surgery from the epilepsy point of view exhibited delayed relapse on the contralateral side, even when the affected hemisphere was not removed but purely disconnected.(Bien et al., 2005b; Delalande et al., 2004)

4.3.5 Late-onset RE

Although RE is generally considered as a childhood disease, adolescent and adult patients have been described and may account for about 10% of all RE cases. (Bien et al., 2005b) The oldest patient reported so far was 58-years-old. (Hunter et al., 2006)

While adult-onset Rasmussen's syndrome may mimic the early-onset form, symptoms often progress more slowly and the neurological defect is more variable. They appear to have a more protracted and milder clinical course with less residual functional deficits and lower degrees of hemiatrophy and more frequent occipital lobe seizure onset (Bien et al., 2005b; Hart et al., 1997), but identical histopathological as well as clinical, electrophysiological and neuroimaging findings.(Bien et al., 2005b)

Some atypical features may be noted such as bilateral hemispheric involvement or a picture of temporal lobe epilepsy or the presence of movement disorders at the beginning of the disease. Surgical hemispheric disconnection that appears the most effective treatment in children to improve seizure control is not indicated in adults for evident functional reasons. Based on recent pathogenic concepts, different medical treatments may be proposed. Large multicentre controlled studies are mandatory to define a clear medical therapeutic strategy in these cases of adult-onset.(Jaillon-Riviere et al., 2007)

4.3.6 RE with unilateral brainstem encephalitis

The case of an adult woman with Rasmussen encephalitis with brainstem involvement responsive to immunosupression is reported. (Quesada et al., 2007)

4.3.7 RE with neurological comorbidity

Cases with double cranial pathology (RE plus low grade tumour, cortical dysplasia, tuberous sclerosis, vascular abnormalities or old ischaemic lesions) have been described.(Bien et al., 2005b; Hart et al., 1998) In the Montreal series, about 10% of cases had double pathology. (Bien et al., 2005b; Hart et al., 1998) The diagnosis of dual pathology was suspected based on MRI findings and confirmed by histopathology (biopsy or resective epilepsy surgery).

5. Investigations

5.1 EEG features

As early as 4 months after disease onset, EEG shows polymorphic delta waves over the affected hemisphere, mainly in a temporal and central location (Figure 1).(Bien et al., 2005b; Hart et al., 1998; Owolabi et al., 2008) This may be accompanied by epileptiform abnormalities, which may evolve into (subclinical) ictal EEG patterns. During the disease course, in most cases, contralateral asynchronous slow waves and epileptiform discharges occur. However, ictal patterns are rarely recorded from contralateral electrodes. As in other conditions, EPC in RE is not always accompanied by rhythmic EEG discharges on surface EEG.(Bien et al., 2005b)

Thus EEG may contribute to the tentative diagnosis of RE already in early disease stages. The following unihemispheric findings strongly suggest RE: impairment of background activity and sleep spindles; focal slow activity; multifocal ictal discharges; and subclinical ictal discharges. In cases with the secure diagnosis of RE, the documentation of an independent contralateral seizure onset may raise the suspicion of bilateral disease.(Bien et al., 2005b)

5.2 Radiological features

5.2.1 CT and MRI

Rarely, CT and MRI may be normal on very early scans. (Bien et al., 2005b; Bien et al., 2002c; Bien et al., 2002d) Within the first 4 months after disease onset, the majority of patients exhibit unilateral enlargement of the inner and outer CSF compartments, most accentuated in the insular and periinsular regions, with increased cortical or subcortical (or both) T2 (and FLAIR) signal (Figures 2 and 3). In addition, in most cases, there is atrophy of the ipsilateral head of the caudate nucleus.

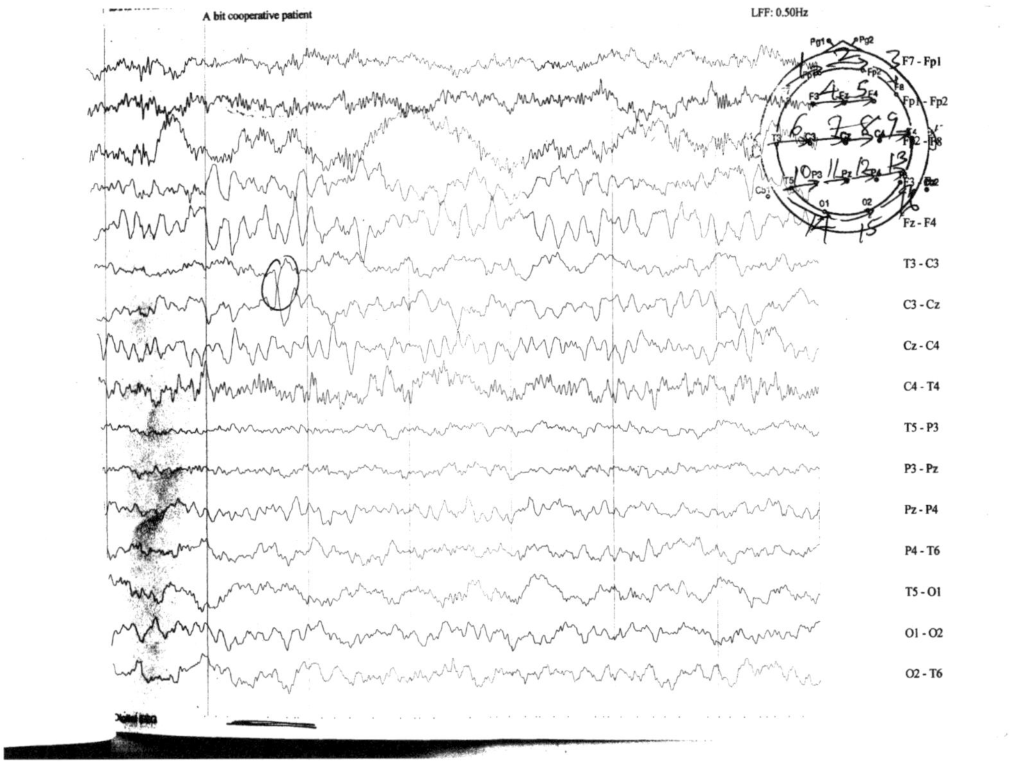

Fig. 1. EEG features in a young girl with RE (Owolabi et al., 2008)
Theta and delta waves on the left hemisphere with epileptiform sharp and slow wave complexes and phase reversal pattern. These features predominated in the temporo-central region. No evidence of secondary generalization.

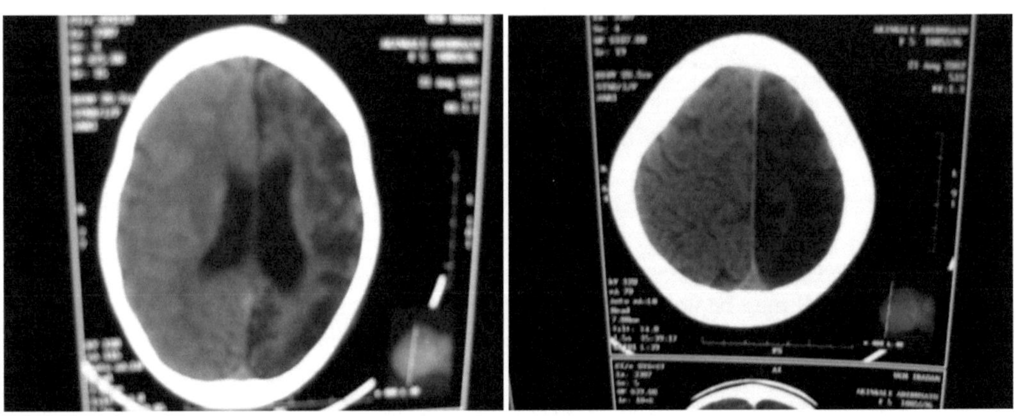

Fig. 2. Cranial CT scan
Isolated left hemispheric atrophy with non-enhancing hypodense lesions.

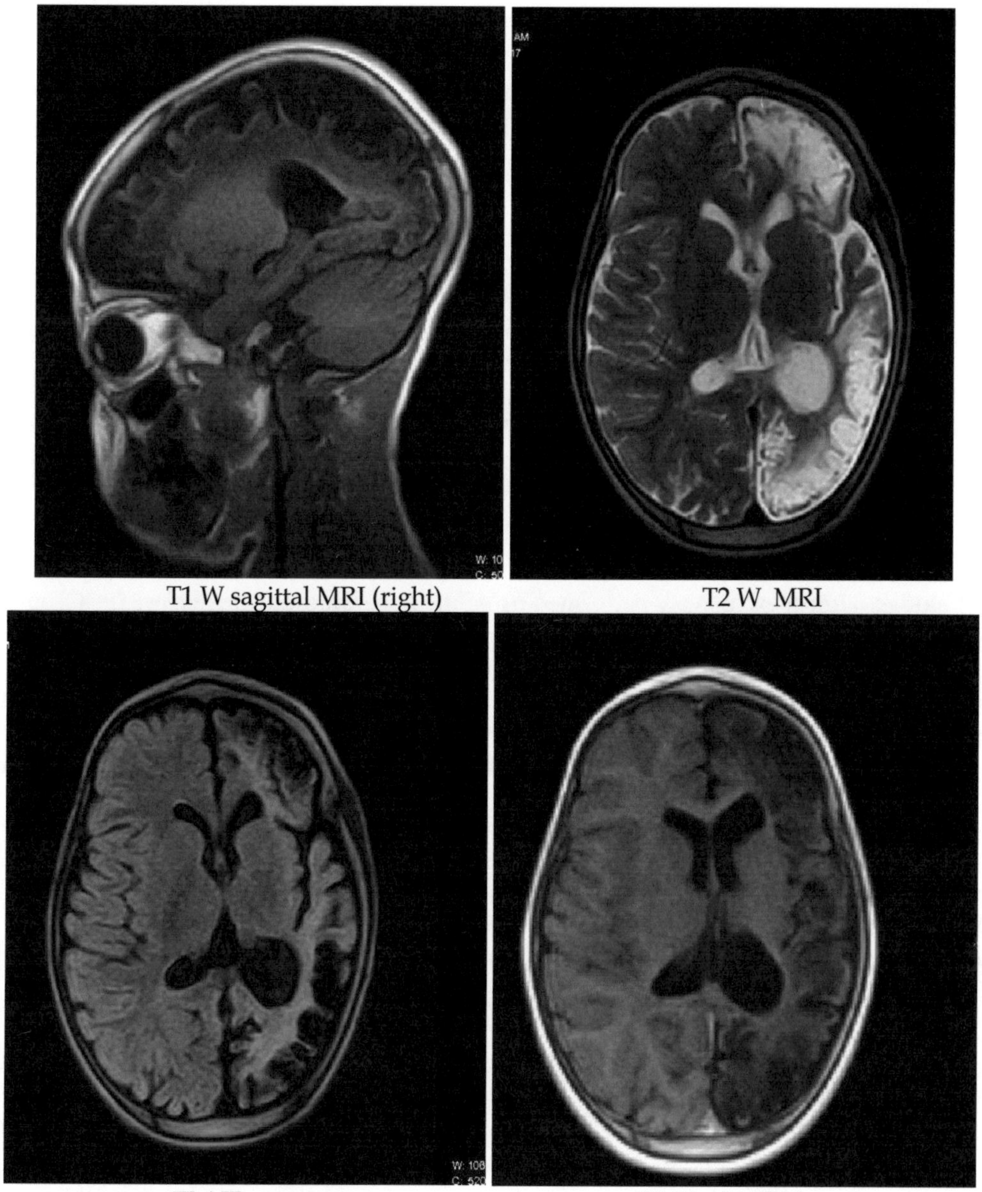

Fig. 3. Brain MRI T1W and T2W transverse and sagittal images as well as FLAIR transverse and coronal images were obtained. The images show left unilateral cerebral atrophy worse at the frontal occipital and perisinsular regions. There is associated ipsilateral dilatation of the lateral ventricle and widening of the cerebral sulci. The T2W images show diffuse increased signal intensity in the cortical and subcortical white matter which are of decreased signal on T1W images. The FLAIR images also show increased signal changes in the frontal and occipital white matter on the left.
The right cerebral hemisphere, brainstem and cerebellum are all within normal limits.
The post gadolinium images show no evidence of enhancement.

A few patients transiently show focal cortical swelling on early scans. Subsequently, a spread of signal changes and atrophy within the affected hemispheres is observed.
In areas with increased MRI signal, the intensity of inflammation as measured by number of T cells, microglial nodules and GFAP+ astrocytes is increased compared with more chronically affected areas with advanced atrophy and no more signal increase.(Bien et al., 2005b; Bien et al., 2002c; Bien et al., 2002d) Using a quantitative approach (calculation of the 'hemispheric ratio', i.e. the ratio affected/unaffected hemisphere on planimetry of axial and coronal slices including the Sylvian fissure) to assess the temporal evolution of hemiatrophy, most of the tissue loss occurs during the first 12 months after onset of the acute disease stage.(Bien et al., 2005b; Bien et al., 2002c; Bien et al., 2002d) However, it may, in some cases, go on for several years.(Bien et al., 2005b; Bien et al., 2002c; Bien et al., 2002d)
In a series of immunotreated RE patients, volumetric assessment of serial MRIs during early disease stages revealed a median tissue loss of 29.9 cm^3 per year in the affected and of 6.8 cm^3 in the unaffected hemispheres.(Larionov et al., 2005) Gadolinium enhancement is very rare in RE.(Bien et al., 2005b; Bien et al., 2002c)

5.2.2 PET studies

PET studies, almost exclusively performed using the tracer fluorodeoxyglucose (FDG), show abnormalities confined to the affected hemisphere. In most cases, large areas of hypometabolism are observed; in the remainder (mostly 'ictal' studies in patients with ongoing EPC), additional areas of focal hypermetabolism are found.(Bien et al., 2005b) FDG-PET changes in early stages (disease duration up to 1 year) are confined to frontotemporal areas. In later stages, abnormalities also affect posterior cortical regions. (Bien et al., 2005b)
One case study suggested that FDG-PET-hypermetabolism correlates with ongoing electrical seizure activity whereas methionin- PET-hypermetabolism indicates areas of inflammation, but this needs to be confirmed in larger patients group.(Bien et al., 2005b) It has been proposed that PET might guide brain biopsy in cases with inconclusive or normal MRI findings, especially in early stages.

5.2.3 Single photon emission computed tomography (SPECT)

With interictal and ictal SPECT, the same type of results and conclusions have been reached as with PET (Bien et al., 2005b)

5.2.4 Magnetic resonance spectroscopy (MRS)

Magnetic resonance spectroscopy (MRS) studies consistently showed decreased N-acetyl-aspartate (NAA) levels and increased (or normal) choline (cho) peaks resulting in a decreased NAA/cho-ratio suggestive of neuronal loss or dysfunction.(Bien et al., 2005b) Partly observed increased lactate peaks seemed to be associated with the presence of EPC. The present studies do not provide evidence for RE-specific MRS abnormalities.
In conclusion, PET, SPECT and MRS techniques are not suitable for defining the inflammatory nature of the condition. They may, however, help in confirming the unihemispheric nature in suspected early RE findings. (Bien et al., 2005b) Simultaneous *fMRI* and EEG recording may be useful in planning surgery. (Cuspineda Bravo et al., 2010)

5.3 Laboratory features

No laboratory test is available to positively support the diagnosis of RE. The largest series of CSF tests has been reported by the Montreal group. In about half of the examinations, cell counts and protein levels were in the normal range. In the remainder, elevated cell counts (16–70 cells/ml, predominantly lymphocytes), and increased protein content (50–100 mg/dl) or a first or midzone elevation of the colloidal gold curve were observed. In only 15% of the abnormal CSF tests, were all three parameters were abnormal.(Bien et al., 2005b) Oligoclonal bands are an inconsistent finding ranging from 0 to 67% in some small series.(Bien et al., 2005b)

GluR3 antibodies in serum (and CSF alike) do not discriminate between RE and noninflammatory epilepsy.(Bien et al., 2005b) Moreover, the presence or absence of GluR3 antibodies does not allow specific pathogenic clues in a given patient and should not be used to select or exclude a specific treatment.

Therefore, CSF standard tests are not suitable to exclude or confirm the diagnosis of RE. Serological CSF tests are usually applied to rule out a CNS infection by known neurotropic agents.

5.4 Brain biopsy

Brain biopsy is not required in all RE cases because other criteria can be sufficient to diagnose the condition. In 'burnt out' cases, brain biopsy may give nonspecific results and not lead to initiation of immunomodulatory treatment.(Bien et al., 2005b) In cases not fulfilling the noninvasive diagnostic criteria as well as in less common RE forms, brain biopsy can contribute considerably to diagnostic certainty.(Bien et al., 2005b)

However, false negative results may be obtained in a small stereotactic needle biopsy because normal and abnormal tissue elements may be located in very close apposition.(Bien et al., 2005b) Therefore, if there are no contraindications, an open biopsy comprising meninges, grey and white matter is preferable. If, in suspicious cases, histology does not clearly show lymphocytic inflammation and microglial (nodular) activation, evaluation of serial sections may be necessary. Biopsy should be taken from a non-eloquent area where there is increased T2/FLAIR signal on MRI or abnormal findings in PET or SPECT. (Bien et al., 2005b)

A gradient of inflammatory intensity from frontotemporal to occipital areas, especially in early cases, has been observed. Therefore, frontal or temporal biopsies are generally preferable. Cases with predominant parietal or occipital involvement, however, exist.(Bien et al., 2005b)

True histopathological differential diagnoses to RE are not as numerous as sometimes assumed. Chronic viral encephalitides, paraneoplastic encephalitis and nonparaneoplastic limbic encephalitis(Bien et al., 2005b) need to be considered. If the results of brain biopsy are inconclusive, further clinical and MRI follow-up studies (e.g. every 6 months) are required to clarify the nature of the disease.

6. Diagnostic criteria

A diagnostic criteria is proposed by the European Consensus statement (Table 1). RE can be diagnosed if either all three criteria of Part A or two out of three criteria of Part B are present.(Bien et al., 2005b)

RE can be diagnosed if either all three criteria of Part A or two out of three criteria of Part B are present. Check first for the features of Part A. Then, if these are not fulfilled, of Part B. In addition: If no biopsy is performed, MRI with administration of gadolinium and cranial CT needs to be performed to document the absence of gadolinium enhancement and calcifications to exclude the differential diagnosis of a unihemispheric vasculitis .
Part A:
1. Clinical Focal seizures (with or without Epilepsia partialis continua) and Unilateral cortical deficit(s)
2. EEG Unihemispheric slowing with or without epileptiform activity and Unilateral seizure onset
3. MRI Unihemispheric focal cortical atrophy and at least one of the following:
Grey or white matter T2/FLAIR hyperintense signal
Hyperintense signal or atrophy of the ipsilateral caudate head
Part B:
1. Clinical Epilepsia partialis continua or Progressive* unilateral cortical deficit(s)
2. MRI Progressive* unihemispheric focal cortical atrophy
3. Histopathology T cell dominated encephalitis with activated microglial cells (typically, but not necessarily forming nodules) and reactive astrogliosis. Numerous parenchymal macrophages, B cells or plasma cells or viral inclusion bodies exclude the diagnosis of RE.
*'Progressive' means that at least two sequential clinical examinations or MRI studies are required to meet the respective criteria. To indicate clinical progression, each of these examinations must document a neurological deficit, and this must increase over time. To indicate progressive hemiatrophy, each of these MRIs must show hemiatrophy, and this must increase over time.

Table 1. European Consensus Diagnostic Criteria for RE (2005)(Bien et al., 2005b)

7. Differential diagnoses

Differential diagnoses include unihemispheric epileptic syndromes, inflammatory diseases, metabolic or degenerative disorders. Unihemispheral epileptic syndromes include cortical dysplasia, hemimegalencephaly, tuberous sclerosis,
Sturge-Weber-syndrome, stroke, and hemiconvulsion-hemiplegia-epilepsy-syndrome. (Bien et al., 2005b)
Inflammatory diseases such as cerebral vasculitis in systemic connective tissue disease and unihemispheric cerebral vasculitis usually present with typical serological features, calcification on brain CT and gadolinium enhacement on MRI. Subacute sclerosing panencephalitis presents with period discharges on EEG.
Epilepsia partialis continua (EPC) due to metabolic disorders such as DM and hepatic encephalopathy can be diagnosed with blood tests. Metabolic or degenerative progressive neurological diseases such as MELAS and other can be diagnosed by mitochondrial DNA genetic testing for mutations and muscle biopsy.

8. Treatment

The goals of treatment are to reduce inflammation, control seizures and reverse functional deficits (motor, sensory, cognitive, etc). Pharmacologic, immunotherapeutic, surgical and rehabilitative techniques are used to achieve these goals. Rarity of the condition makes it difficult to conduct RCTs to compare treatment options.

8.1 Pharmacological control of seizures

Classical AEDs are more effective in the control of complex partial seizures and secondarily generalized seizures than EPC. (Bien et al., 2009a) No anticonvulsive mono- or combination-therapy has been described to be superior to other regimens. There is no evidence that the new AEDs have higher efficacy than older AEDs. However, their improved tolerability and reduced potential for pharmacokinetic interactions may be of particular importance if long-term immune-treatment is applied. (Bien et al., 2009a)

Enzyme-inducing drugs reduce blood-levels of corticosteroids and tacrolimus; enzyme-inhibiting drugs, on the other hand, confer the risk of tacrolimus intoxication and encephalopathy. Substances with high albumin bound fraction may be difficult to keep at a constant blood level if in parallel with plasma exchange. As a general rule, number and dose of AEDs should be kept as low as possible, i.e., one should try to abolish secondarily generalized tonic clonic and, possibly, complex partial seizures; EPC, however, is almost never suppressed by AEDs and it provides little benefit to the patients if one tries to suppress this focal motor status epilepticus. In cases of localised EPC, botulinum toxin has been successfully injected. (Bien et al., 2009a) Epilepsy surgery and immunotherapy are also helpful in seizure control.

8.2 Immunotherapy

Immunotherapeutic interventions include corticosteroids, immunoglobulin, plasmapheresis, interferon, rituximab, and tacrolimus.

8.2.1 Corticosteroids

Prednisolone/prednisone started at high doses and slowly tapered down have been reported to have beneficial effects on seizures and neurological functions in several series, particularly when started early in the course of the disease.(Bien et al., 2009a) However, serious side effects partly necessitating steroid withdrawal have been noticed. These include fluid retention/Cushing's syndrome in all patients and, in single cases, psychosis, behavioural abnormalities, septicaemia, osteoporosis, hypertension and candidiasis.(Bien et al., 2009a) Therefore, for long-term steroid therapy, it has been recommended to start with boluses of intravenous methylprednisolone (e.g. 400 mg/m^2/day) or, in children, 20 mg/kg/day and then to introduce 1–2 mg/kg/day oral prednisolone or prednisone. This dose should be slowly reduced, ideally to a dose below the threshold of Cushing's syndrome. Short-term steroid bolus administration (dosing as above) has been found to be effective in blocking status epilepticus.(Bien et al., 2009a)

8.2.2 Intravenous Immunoglobulin (IVIG)

Good effects of IVIG on seizures and neurological functions were reported in some case studies and seriess where IVIG is recommended as the first-line immunotherapy. Furthermore, favourable responses of adult cases have lead to the proposal IVIG as first-line treatment especially in late-onset cases.(Bien et al., 2009a) The recommended dosing scheme is to start with three to five consecutive infusions of 0.4 g/kg/day and to proceed with a monthly dose of 0.4–2.0 g/kg distributed over 1–5 consecutive days. Side effects of IVIG treatment are rare.

8.2.3 IVIG plus steroid

In case of insufficient effect of IVIG, a combination of 0.4 g/kg/month IVIG plus corticosteroids (dosing as above) is recommended. (Bien et al., 2009a)

8.2.4 Plasma exchange/plasmapharesis

Plasma exchange cycles have been performed at a frequency of three to six single volume exchanges on consecutive or alternate days, repeated every 2 to 8 weeks. Selective periodic immuno-adsorption with protein A has been used as a long-term management with positive results in adolescent-adult onset patients. Both measures improved neurological function and seizure frequency in some patients during the weeks following the intervention that could be reinstituted by repeat treatment. However there is very limited experience with long term treatment in RE. (Bien et al., 2009a) Long-term immunotherapy is usually ineffective against seizures.

8.2.5 Tacrolimus

Tacrolimus is a T cell inhibiting immunosuppressant. In a small controlled trial, the tacrolimus patients had a superior outcome regarding neurological function and progression rate of cerebral hemiatrophy on MRI, but no better seizure outcome. Their cognitive outcome was good.(Bien et al., 2004; Bien et al., 2009a) The results of a randomized prospective trial, comparing tacrolimus and IVIG are still being awaited.(Bien et al., 2004; Bien et al., 2009a)

8.2.6 IFN-alpha

Report of seizure control with the use of intraventicular interferon-alpha has been made.(Bien et al., 2009a; Dabbagh et al., 1997) However it is an invasive measure and further trials are required to verify its efficacy and determine its role in RE therapy.

8.2.7 Rituximab

Rituximab is a chimeric monoclonal antibody against the protein CD20. Although CD20+ cells (B cells) are extremely rare, rituximab may in single cases be a viable treatment alternative; a formal trial is underway. (Bien et al., 2005b)

8.3 Surgical treatment

Surgical treatment is indicated in medically-refractory seizures. Options include anatomic hemispherectomy, functional hemispherectomy, perisylvian hemispherotomy, trans-sylvian hemispherotomy and central/vertical hemispherotomy.(Bien et al., 2005b; Bien et al., 2009b; Bien et al., 2009a; Terra-Bustamante et al., 2009) However, only hemispherectomy (anatomical or functional) is effective in RE.(Bien et al., 2005b; Bien et al., 2009b; Bien et al., 2009a; Terra-Bustamante et al., 2009)

The basic principle of the modern techniques is to replace resection by disconnection.

Presurgical evaluation for hemispherectomy should be performed in all patients with pharmacoresistant and handicapping seizures due to RE. Some special considerations during this presurgical assessment arise from the fact that RE represents the rare case of an epilepsy due to acquired hemispheric brain damage. In RE, patients with disease onset >4 years of age (when secondary language transfer is no longer highly likely) need to be

investigated with particular scrutiny to predict the post-HE functioning. (Bien et al., 2005b; Bien et al., 2009b; Bien et al., 2009a; Terra-Bustamante et al., 2009)
The following steps are recommended in the pre-op work-up of RE patients: brain MRI and video-EEG-monitoring for registration of interictal and ictal activity and prediction of postoperative functional outcome by assessment of the actual language, motor, visual function (visual field) and language dominance lateralization, usually by means of Wada testing.(Bien et al., 2005b; Bien et al., 2009b; Bien et al., 2009a; Terra-Bustamante et al., 2009) However, it is imperative to determine cerebral dominance by Wada test prior to surgery.(Bien et al., 2005b; Bien et al., 2009b; Bien et al., 2009a; Terra-Bustamante et al., 2009) Language functional MRI alone has not been shown to be sufficient due to limited comparability of the two hemispheres as well as the restricted ability of the patients to follow instructions.(Bien et al., 2005b; Bien et al., 2009b; Bien et al., 2009a; Terra-Bustamante et al., 2009)

8.4 Rehabilitation

Depending on the type of neurological deficits, different modalities of rehabilitation are employed to improve the health-related quality of life of the patient. This includes physiotherapy, vocational therapy, occupational therapy, speech and language therapy, and cognitive rehabilitation. Botulinum toxin A is useful in the management of localized refractory EPC.

8.5 Choice of therapy for individual patients

Anti-seizure effect of anti-epilepsy drugs is usually limited to secondarily generalized seizures and complex partial seizures whereas EPC is usually refractory. (Bien et al., 2005b; Bien et al., 2009a) Hemispherectomy in one of its modern variants offers a very high chance of seizure freedom, however at the price of irreversible loss of functions located in the affected hemisphere.(Bien et al., 2005b; Bien et al., 2009a; Terra-Bustamante et al., 2009) In a proportion of patients, long-term immunotherapy is able to prevent or slow down hemispheric tissue loss and the associated functional decline. It does, however, mostly not improve the epilepsy. Whereas for many patients unequivocal treatment proposals can be readily made, a dilemma may emerge in those with severe epilepsy but still preserved hemispheric function.(Bien et al., 2005b; Bien et al., 2009a; Terra-Bustamante et al., 2009)
In the European consensus statement on RE, a therapeutic protocol(Bien et al., 2005b; Bien et al., 2009a) for any patient with the diagnosis of RE has been suggested.

8.5.1 Mild or absent epilepsy, with progressed functional deficit

A low dose AED therapy will usually suffice in these cases. If complete seizure freedom cannot be achieved but is a major goal of the patient, surgery can be offered.(Bien et al., 2005b; Bien et al., 2009a)

8.5.2 Handicapping epilepsy, and no findings predicting a relevant post-op deterioration

Here, surgery is clearly the treatment of choice. The patient and his family needs to be informed about the general risks of the procedure.(Bien et al., 2005b; Bien et al., 2009a; Terra-Bustamante et al., 2009)

8.5.3 Mild or absent epilepsy with limited neurological deficit

If the patient is still in the acute disease stage, i.e., has recently experienced a functional decline, this is certainly the ideal situation for long-term immunotherapy. The epilepsy is no or only a minor problem, and the functional decline may be stopped or at least slowed down by the immunotherapy. If, however, the patient is already in the residual stage (i.e., no functional decline within the previous 6 months or so), initiation of immunotherapy is no longer recommended.(Bien et al., 2005b; Bien et al., 2009a)

8.5.4 Handicapping epilepsy, but prediction of significant functional deterioration after surgery

This is certainly the most problematic situation.(Bien et al., 2005b; Bien et al., 2009b; Bien et al., 2009a; Terra-Bustamante et al., 2009) Early institution of long-term immunotherapy is recommended to prevent functional decline. If seizures remain severe and disabling, additional "short-term/intense" immunotherapy should be tried (e.g., an i.v. pulse of several days of methylprednisolone at 20 mg/(kg day) in children or 500–1000 mg/day in adults, or plasma exchange, or IVIG). If no satisfying effect is achieved, this add-on immunotherapy should be discontinued, and the option of HE should be considered as discussed above. (Bien et al., 2005b; Bien et al., 2009a)

The severity of each of the expected deficits after surgery should be weighed in relation to the severity of epilepsy.(Bien et al., 2005b; Bien et al., 2009a; Terra-Bustamante et al., 2009; Terra-Bustamante et al., 2007) This requires extensive and in-depth discussions with the patient and his family. Whereas the prediction of postoperative aphasia in a still communicable child (RE of the language dominant hemisphere) will usually preclude surgery, the perspective of a fixed dense hemiparesis with preserved walking abilities may be an acceptable price for seizure freedom. This is particularly clear in cases, in which continuous or near-continuous motor seizures impair hand and leg function anyway. (Bien et al., 2005b; Bien et al., 2009a; Terra-Bustamante et al., 2009; Terra-Bustamante et al., 2007)

Regardless of the affected side, the probably least relevant consequence of surgery is hemianopia, which is usually well compensated in everyday life. In conclusion, especially in patients with impairing seizures and affection of the non-dominant hemisphere, surgery will often emerge as the superior long-term option compared to ongoing conservative treatment.(Bien et al., 2005b; Bien et al., 2009a; Terra-Bustamante et al., 2009; Terra-Bustamante et al., 2007)

9. Conclusions and future prospects

Rasmussen's encephalitis (RE) is a very rare disease of the brain, usually in children, characterized by focal seizures, ipsilateral cortical deficits and hemiparesis, as well as hemiatrophy of the contralateral cerebral hemisphere. Even though the European Consensus criteria has been proposed for its diagnosis, the aetio-pathogenesis remains enigmatic.

The affected brain tissue shows a chronic T-cell mediated inflammatory histopathology and an autoimmune reaction is suspected. Four groups of histopathological changes have been described with variable densities of microglial nodules, gyral necrosis, neuronal loss, glial scarring and gliosis. Following the natural history of the disease, three stages have been proposed: the *prodromal stage* with a relatively low seizure frequency and mild hemiparesis; the *acute stage* with frequent seizures, and the *residual stage*. Focal epilepsy can be demonstrated by EEG while neuroimaging by CT scan or MRI demonstrates cerebral hemiatrophy.

Anti-epileptic drugs have limited efficacy particularly in the control of EPC. Several immunomodulatory therapies have been tried. However being an orphan disease, no randomized clinical trials have demonstrated the long-term outcome of steroids, tacrolimus, plasmapharesis and immunoglobulin therapy. Whereas epileptic surgery is effective for seizure control, it is at the price of inducing severe neurological deficit.

It is hoped that in the nearest future early diagnosis and extensive study of new cases in the prodromal phase may help unravel the antigenic stimulus for the T-cell-mediated response as well as the basis for the unilaterality of hemispheric damage. This may lead to specific immunotherapeutic techniques which can then be tested in multicenter randomized control trials.

Better understanding of epilepsy therapeutics with combination of new and older antiepileptic drugs may result in better seizure control. (Owolabi et al., 2008) However, successes of non-surgical approaches have to be proven in the context of the natural evolution of the disease to a non-progressive phase. The decision to undergo surgery has to be individualized and predicated on the full information about the risks and benefits for the index patient. Novel and holistic approach to rehabilitation may result in improved quality of life for RE patients who can then march on to achieve their goals in life despite the fire of inflammation in the brain.

10. References

Andermann,F., and Farrell,K. (2006). Early onset Rasmussen's syndrome: a malignant, often bilateral form of the disorder. Epilepsy Res. 70 Suppl 1, S259-S262.

Bauer,J., Bien,C.G., and Lassmann,H. (2002). Rasmussen's encephalitis: a role for autoimmune cytotoxic T lymphocytes. Curr. Opin. Neurol 15, 197-200.

Bauer,J., Elger,C.E., Hans,V.H., Schramm,J., Urbach,H., Lassmann,H., and Bien,C.G. (2007). Astrocytes are a specific immunological target in Rasmussen's encephalitis. Ann. Neurol 62, 67-80.

Bhatjiwale,M.G., Polkey,C., Cox,T.C., Dean,A., and Deasy,N. (1998). Rasmussen's encephalitis: neuroimaging findings in 21 patients with a closer look at the basal ganglia. Pediatr. Neurosurg. 29, 142-148.

Bien,C.G., and Bauer,J. (2005a). T-cells in human encephalitis 22. Neuromolecular. Med 7, 243-253.

Bien,C.G., Bauer,J., Deckwerth,T.L., Wiendl,H., Deckert,M., Wiestler,O.D., Schramm,J., Elger,C.E., and Lassmann,H. (2002a). Destruction of neurons by cytotoxic T cells: a new pathogenic mechanism in Rasmussen's encephalitis. Ann. Neurol 51, 311-318.

Bien,C.G., Elger,C.E., and Wiendl,H. (2002b). Advances in pathogenic concepts and therapeutic agents in Rasmussen's encephalitis. Expert. Opin. Investig. Drugs 11, 981-989.

Bien,C.G., Gleissner,U., Sassen,R., Widman,G., Urbach,H., and Elger,C.E. (2004). An open study of tacrolimus therapy in Rasmussen encephalitis 33. Neurology 62, 2106-2109.

Bien,C.G., Granata,T., Antozzi,C., Cross,J.H., Dulac,O., Kurthen,M., Lassmann,H., Mantegazza,R., Villemure,J.G., Spreafico,R., and Elger,C.E. (2005b). Pathogenesis, diagnosis and treatment of Rasmussen encephalitis: a European consensus statement 28. Brain 128, 454-471.

Bien,C.G., and Schramm,J. (2009a). Treatment of Rasmussen encephalitis half a century after its initial description: promising prospects and a dilemma. Epilepsy Res 86, 101-112.

Bien,C.G., Szinay,M., Wagner,J., Clusmann,H., Becker,A.J., and Urbach,H. (2009b). Characteristics and surgical outcomes of patients with refractory magnetic resonance imaging-negative epilepsies. Arch. Neurol. 66, 1491-1499.

Bien,C.G., Urbach,H., Deckert,M., Schramm,J., Wiestler,O.D., Lassmann,H., and Elger,C.E. (2002c). Diagnosis and staging of Rasmussen's encephalitis by serial MRI and histopathology. Neurology 58, 250-257.

Bien,C.G., Widman,G., Urbach,H., Sassen,R., Kuczaty,S., Wiestler,O.D., Schramm,J., and Elger,C.E. (2002d). The natural history of Rasmussen's encephalitis. Brain 125, 1751-1759.

Chinchilla,D., Dulac,O., Robain,O., Plouin,P., Ponsot,G., Pinel,J.F., and Graber,D. (1994). Reappraisal of Rasmussen's syndrome with special emphasis on treatment with high doses of steroids. J Neurol Neurosurg. Psychiatry 57, 1325-1333.

Cuspineda Bravo,E.R., Iturria,Y., Praderes,J.C., Melie,L., Valdes,P.A., Virues,T., Machado,C., and Valdes,U.L. (2010). Noninvasive multimodal neuroimaging for Rasmussen encephalopathy surgery: simultaneous EEG-fMRI recording. Clin EEG. Neurosci. 41, 159-165.

Dabbagh,O., Gascon,G., Crowell,J., and Bamoggadam,F. (1997). Intraventricular interferon-alpha stops seizures in Rasmussen's encephalitis: a case report. Epilepsia 38, 1045-1049.

Delalande,O., Fohlen,M., Bulteau,C., and Jalin,C. (2004). [Surgery for intractable focal epilepsy in children]. Rev. Neurol (Paris) 160 Spec No 1, 5S195-5S202.

Farrell,M.A., DeRosa,M.J., Curran,J.G., Secor,D.L., Cornford,M.E., Comair,Y.G., Peacock,W.J., Shields,W.D., and Vinters,H.V. (1992). Neuropathologic findings in cortical resections (including hemispherectomies) performed for the treatment of intractable childhood epilepsy. Acta Neuropathol. 83, 246-259.

Gambardella,A., Andermann,F., Shorvon,S., Le,P.E., and Aguglia,U. (2008). Limited chronic focal encephalitis: another variant of Rasmussen syndrome? Neurology 70, 374-377.

Hart,Y. (2004). Rasmussen's encephalitis. Epileptic. Disord. 6, 133-144.

Hart,Y.M., Andermann,F., Fish,D.R., Dubeau,F., Robitaille,Y., Rasmussen,T., Berkovic,S., Marino,R., Yakoubian,E.M., Spillane,K., and Scaravilli,F. (1997). Chronic encephalitis and epilepsy in adults and adolescents: a variant of Rasmussen's syndrome? Neurology 48, 418-424.

Hart,Y.M., Andermann,F., Robitaille,Y., Laxer,K.D., Rasmussen,T., and Davis,R. (1998). Double pathology in Rasmussen's syndrome: a window on the etiology? Neurology 50, 731-735.

Hennessy,M.J., Koutroumanidis,M., Dean,A.F., Jarosz,J., Elwes,R.D., Binnie,C.D., and Polkey,C.E. (2001). Chronic encephalitis and temporal lobe epilepsy: a variant of Rasmussen's syndrome? Neurology 56, 678-681.

Hunter,G.R., Donat,J., Pryse-Phillips,W., Harder,S., and Robinson,C.A. (2006). Rasmussen's encephalitis in a 58-year-old female: still a variant? Can. J Neurol Sci. 33, 302-305.

Jaillon-Riviere,V., Dupont,S., Bertran,F., De,L.S., V, Beuvon,F., Baulac,M., and Defer,G. (2007). [Late onset Rasmussen's syndrome: clinical and therapeutic characteristics]. Rev. Neurol (Paris) 163, 573-580.

Korn-Lubetzki,I., Bien,C.G., Bauer,J., Gomori,M., Wiendl,H., Trajo,L., Ovadia,H., Wilken, B., Hans,V.H., Elger,C.E., Hurvitz,H., and Steiner,I. (2004). Rasmussen encephalitis with active inflammation and delayed seizures onset 37. Neurology 62, 984-986.

Larionov,S., Konig,R., Urbach,H., Sassen,R., Elger,C.E., and Bien,C.G. (2005). MRI brain volumetry in Rasmussen encephalitis: the fate of affected and "unaffected" hemispheres 27. Neurology 64, 885-887.

Oguni,H., Andermann,F., and Rasmussen,T.B. (1991). The natural history of the syndrome of chronic encephalitis and epilepsy: a study of the MRI series of fortyeight cases. In Chronic encephalitis and epilepsy. Rasmussen's syndrome., F.Andermann, ed. (Boston: Butterworth-Heinemann) pp. 7-35.

Owolabi,M.O., Ogbole,G., and Lagunju,I. (2008). Conservative management of Rasmussen's encephalitis in a Nigerian girl. Journal of Pediatric Neurology 6, 389-394.

Pleasure,D. (2008). Diagnostic and pathogenic significance of glutamate receptor autoantibodies. Arch. Neurol. 65, 589-592.

Quesada,C.M., Urbach,H., Elger,C.E., and Bien,C.G. (2007). Rasmussen encephalitis with ipsilateral brain stem involvement in an adult patient 10. J Neurol Neurosurg. Psychiatry 78, 200-201.

Rasmussen,T., Olszewski,J., and LLOYDSMITH,D. (1958). Focal seizures due to chronic localized encephalitis. Neurology 8, 435-445.

Robitaille,Y. (1991). Neuropathologic aspects of chronic encephalitis. In Chronic encephalitis and epilepsy. Rasmussen's syndrome, F.Andermann, ed. (Boston: Butterworth-Heinemann) pp. 79-110.

Schwab,N., Bien,C.G., Waschbisch,A., Becker,A., Vince,G.H., Dornmair,K., and Wiendl,H. (2009). CD8+ T-cell clones dominate brain infiltrates in Rasmussen encephalitis and persist in the periphery. Brain 132, 1236-1246.

Terra-Bustamante,V.C., Inuzuka,L.M., Fernandes,R.M., Escorsi-Rosset,S., Wichert-Ana, L., Alexandre,V., Jr., Bianchin,M.M., Araujo,D., Santos,A.C., Oliveira dos, S.R., Machado,H.R., and Sakamoto,A.C. (2007). Outcome of hemispheric surgeries for refractory epilepsy in pediatric patients 11. Childs Nerv. Syst. 23, 321-326.

Terra-Bustamante,V.C., Machado,H.R., dos Santos,O.R., Serafini,L.N., Souza-Oliveira,C., Escorsi-Rosset, S., Yacubian, E. M., Naffah-Mazzacoratti, M. G., Scorza, C. A., Cavalheiro, E.A., Scorza,F.A., and Sakamoto,A.C. (2009). Rasmussen encephalitis: long-term outcome after surgery. Childs Nerv. Syst. 25, 583-589.

17

Clinical Aspects of Anti-NMDA Receptor Encephalitis

Haruo Shimazaki
Division of Neurology, Department of Internal Medicine, Jichi Medical University, Tochigi Japan

1. Introduction

Paraneoplastic limbic encephalitis (PLE) is a rare neurological syndrome characterized by short-term memory impairment, seizures and various psychiatric disturbances. It is often associated with small-cell lung cancer, germ-cell tumors of the testis and breast cancer, but rarely with ovarian teratomas (Gultekin et al., 2000). Several cases of PLE with ovarian teratomas had been reported in Japan (Okamura, Oomori, and Uchitomi, 1997; Nokura et al., 1997), but the autoantigens in this disease remained unknown. In 2005, Dalmau et al. reported an antibody to the membranes of neurons of the hippocampus (antigens colocalized with exchange factor for ADP-ribosylation factor 6 A (EFA6A)) in association with PLE and ovarian teratomas (Ances et al., 2005; Vitaliani et al., 2005).

We sent samples from a patient suffering from limbic encephalitis with an ovarian teratoma to Prof. Dalmau's Laboratory in November 2005. They identified antibodies to the antigens colocalized with EFA6A in our patient's samples (Figure 1) (Shimazaki et al., 2007), and in another Japanese one (Koide et al., 2007).

Their further analysis of the antibodies disclosed that were ones against NR1/NR2 heteromers of N-methyl-D-aspartate (NMDA) receptors. They diagnosed and reported twelve women (including our case) as having 'paraneoplastic anti-NMDA receptor encephalitis associated with an ovarian teratoma', the cases developing prominent psychiatric symptoms, amnesia, seizures, frequent dyskinesias, autonomic dysfunction, and a decreased level of consciousness often requiring ventilatory support (Dalmau et al., 2007). After this publication, several reports about anti-NMDA receptor encephalitis have appeared in Japan (Iizuka et al., 2008; Seki et al., 2008; Kataoka, Dalmau, and Ueno, 2008; Ishiura et al., 2008; Shindo et al., 2009). Analysis of a worldwide one hundred anti-NMDA receptor encephalitis case series revealed that about 60% of them had associated tumors such as ovarian teratomas (Dalmau et al., 2008).

Meanwhile, Kamei et al. proposed 'acute juvenile female non-herpetic encephalitis (AJFNHE)' (Kamei et al., 2009). The clinical symptoms and course of AJFNHE are similar to those of anti-NMDA receptor encephalitis. These two diseases are considered to be the same clinical entity, anti-NMDA receptor antibodies being detected in samples from some AJFNHE cases.

We herein describe five young Japanese cases who had fever, psychiatric symptoms and orofacial dyskinesias, and whose sera and cerebrospinal fluids (CSF) contained antibodies against NMDA receptors.

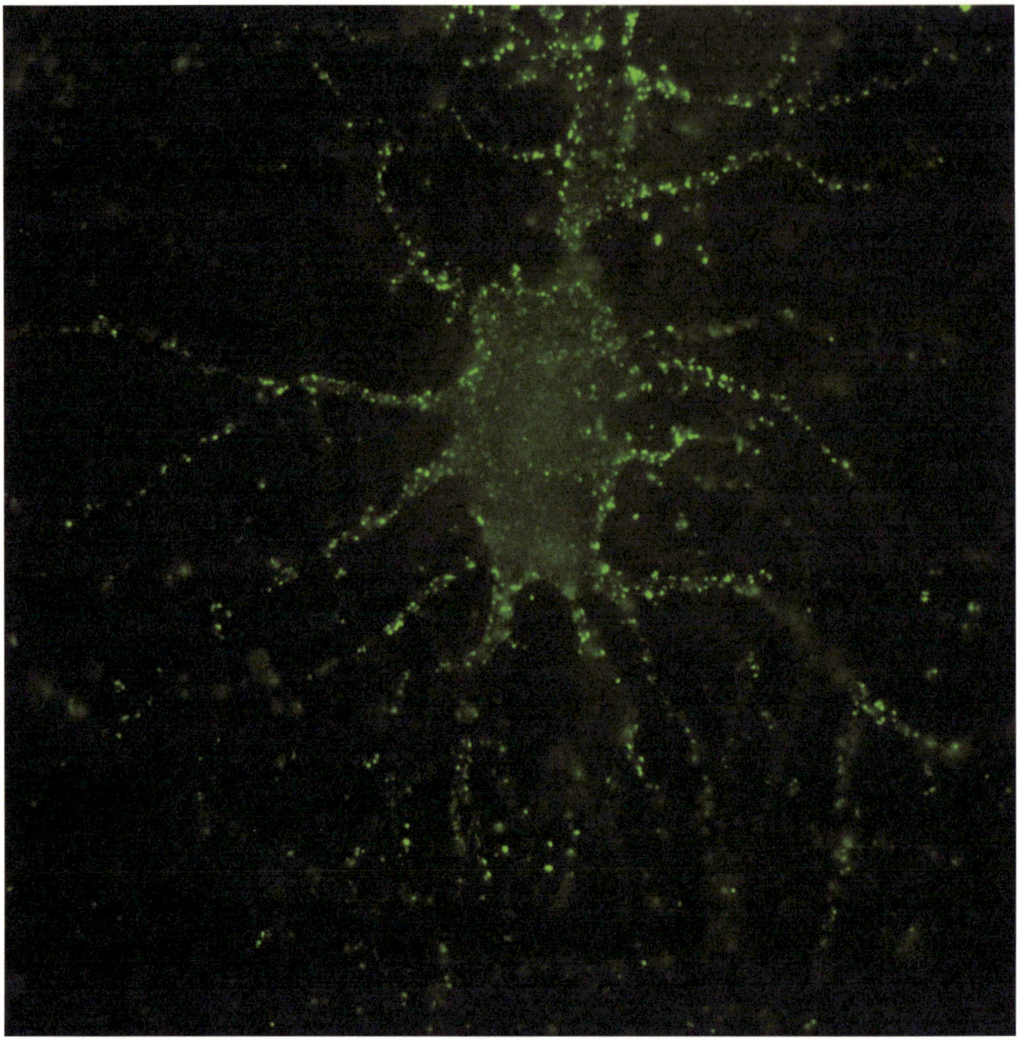

Fig. 1. Detection of anti-NMDA receptor antibodies in cerebrospinal fluid of case 3. Antibodies for the NR1/NR2 heteromers of NMDA receptors caused intense immunolabelling of cultured rat neuronal cell membranes and processes.

2. Characteristic clinical features of anti-NMDA receptor encephalitis

The clinical symptoms of 100 cases of anti-NMDA receptor encephalitis have been reported in detail (Dalmau et al., 2008). According to this report, the median age of patients was 23 years (range, 5-76 years), and 91 out of the 100 cases were women.

In our cases (Table 1), the time of disease onset ranged from 17 to 30 of age. Four cases were female and one was male. Headache, fever and flu-like symptoms preceded other encephalitis features in our cases and about 90% of the above 100 cases (Dalmau et al., 2008). To our knowledge, antecedent infection has not been described for this disease, but case 5 had suffered from influenza B infection before his psychiatric symptoms emerged.

2.1 Psychiatric symptoms

Seventy-seven of 100 anti-NMDA receptor encephalitis cases developed marked schizophrenia-like psychiatric symptoms at onset (Dalmau et al., 2008), and they tended to have visited a psychiatric clinic initially. The psychiatric symptoms were as follows: anxiety, agitation, bizarre behavior, delirium, visual and auditory hallucination, and short-term memory disturbance. Catatonia-like symptoms have been reported (Lee, Glick, and Dinwiddie, 2006; Iizuka et al., 2008; Kleinig et al., 2008; Schimmel et al., 2009). Emotional incontinence and disorientation were observed in our series.

Notably, our case 5 showed prominent psychiatric symptoms such as abnormal behavior, hallucination and agitation with mild orofacial dyskinesia, although convulsions, abnormal eye movements, autonomic instability, hypoventilation and CSF pleocytosis were not observed. Modified electroconvulsive therapy was effective for his psychiatric symptoms that were uncontrolled with medications due to their side effects (Ando et al., 2011).

Recently, anti-NMDA receptor antibodies were detected in a small percentage of patients with a first episode of psychosis (Zandi et al., 2011), and in cases with a pure neuropsychiatric disorder (De Nayer, Myant, and Sindic, 2009). A good response to electroconvulsive therapy has been reported for anti-NMDA receptor encephalitis (Braakman et al., 2010).

2.2 Involuntary movements

Involuntary movements are one of the most characteristic symptoms of anti-NMDA receptor encephalitis. They were seen in 85 of 100 anti-NMDA receptor encephalitis cases. The most frequent types were orofacial dyskinesia including grimacing, masticatory-like movements, and forceful jaw opening and closing (Dalmau et al., 2008). Other types of involuntary movement were also observed, as follows: choreiform movement, dystonic posture and myoclonus. It is suggested that interruption of forebrain corticostriatal inputs by anti-NMDA receptor antibodies removes tonic inhibition of brainstem pattern generators releasing primitive patterns of bulbar and limb movement (Kleinig et al., 2008).

In our cases, we observed blinking and grimacing, to and fro dyskinesia of the tongue, tremorous movements of the extremities, and increasing paroxysmal muscle tonus throughout the whole body. In patients 1 and 3, the orofacial dyskinesia was too severe to break their teeth, whereas that in case 5 was mild and of short duration.

2.3 Oculomotor symptoms

Oculogyric crisis has been reported as the most frequent oculomotor finding in anti-NMDA receptor encephalitis (Ko, Dalmau, and Galetta, 2008). Moreover, nystagmus and deviation of the ocular position have been observed in some cases (Dalmau et al., 2008).

In our cases, we observed oculogyric crisis in case 1, disconjugation in case 2, and skew deviation and inverse ocular bobbing in case 3 (Shimazaki et al., 2008) (Fig. 2)(Table 1). Inverse ocular bobbing, referred to as ocular dipping, consists of a slow, spontaneous downward eye movement with fast return to midposition. It may be observed in anoxic coma (Ropper, 1981) or following prolonged status epileptics (Mehler, 1988), and is thought to be a marker of diffuse brain damage (Stark, Masucci, and Kurtzke, 1984). This case had not only signs of brainstem involvement such as skew deviation and hypoventilation, but also of diffuse encephalopathy, causing the inverse ocular bobbing.

Patient No.	1	2	3	4	5
Onset age, Gender	22, F	19, F	30, F	16, F	18, M
Initial symptoms (Prodromes)	emotional incontinence, restlessness, fever, headache	disorientation, emotional incontinence, fever, headache, nausea	disorientation, fever, headache, nausea	abnormal behavior, convulsions, fever, headache	fever (influenza B), abnormal behavior, hallucination, agitation
Seizures	clonic	clonic	tonic	tonic	-
Orofacial & limb dyskinesia	++	+++	++	+	+-
Duration of dyskinesia	9 weeks	> 5 weeks	2 weeks	4 weeks	2 days
Eye position, movement	oculogyric crisis	disconjugation	skew deviation, inverse ocular bobbing	horizontal nystagmus like	-
Autonomic instability	++	++	++	+	-
Hypersalivation	++	+++	+++	+-	-
Ventilatory assistance	12 weeks	> 6 weeks	6 weeks	-	-
Hospital stay (months)	5.5	2	3.5	2	4
CSF cells (/μl)	104	242	40	10	1
CSF protein (mg/dl)	26	55	67	32	20
CSF glucose (mg/dl)	70	48	67	72	70
MRI (FLAIR) high intensity	unremarkable	unremarkable	medial temporal, hippocampus	right pontine base, right cerebellum	unremarkable
EEG	δ	δ	θ-δ	θ-δ	normal
Ovarian teratoma	mature cystic (dermoid cyst)	(not detected)	immature, rapid enlargement	(not detected)	(not detected)
Tumor markers (CA19-9, CA125)	CA19-9 <1 CA125 18	(not examined)	CA19-9 138 CA125 65	CA19-9 52 CA125 19	CA19-9 2
Time to tumor diagnosis	47 months	-	0.5 months	-	-
NR1 antibody titer in CSF (rfu, normal < 5000)	444556	2197200	31360	NR1/NR2 antibody +	NR1/NR2 antibody +
Therapy	CS, tumor resection	CS, PP, IVIg	CS, PP, IVIg, tumor resection	IVIg, CS	electroconvulsive therapy
Outcome	recovery (1 year 8 months) w/epilepsy	death (2 months)	full recovery (1 year)	full recovery (11 months)	full recovery (1 year)

Table 1. Clinical and laboratory findings in five cases of anti-NMDA receptor encephalitis. rfu: relative fluorescence units.

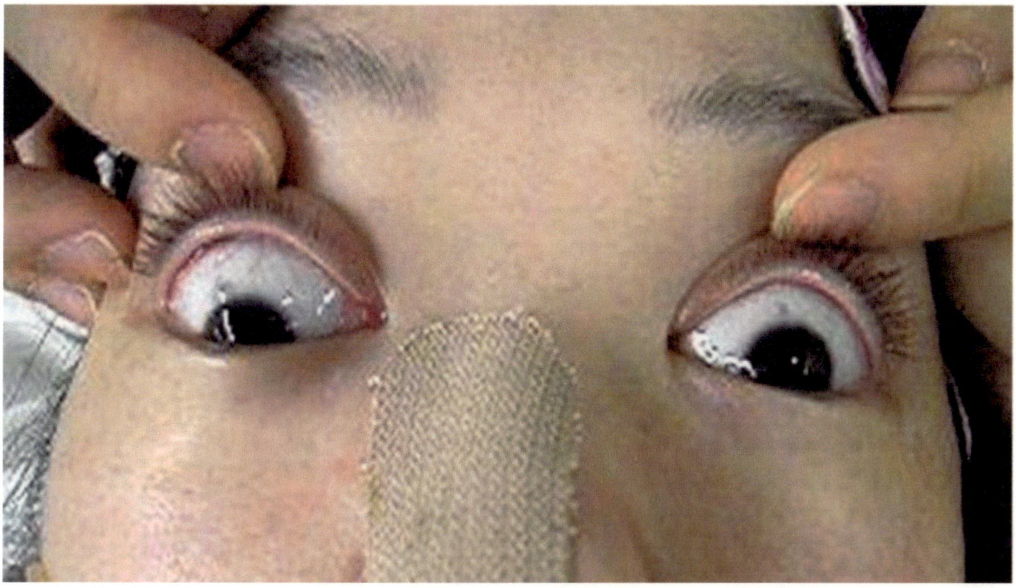

Fig. 2. The position of the eyes in case 3 showed skew deviation when the inverse ocular bobbing resolved.

2.4 Autonomic symptoms

Anti-NMDA receptor encephalitis is complicated by autonomic instability, which is indicated by an unstable blood pressure level or pulse rate, hypersalivation, central hypoventilation, etc.

We found excess salivary excretion of up to 1400ml/day in all cases except for patients 4 and 5. Case 3 suffered from sudden hypotension and bradycardia. Three of the five cases were intubated and required mechanical ventilatory support due to the central hypoventilation, the other two cases not needing assisted ventilation.

2.5 Ovarian teratomas

Fifty-eight of 98 anti-NMDA receptor encephalitis patients had a neoplasm, the most frequent one being an ovarian teratoma (Dalmau et al., 2008). Analysis of 400 patients confirmed that the younger the patient, the less likely that a tumor will be detected (Dalmau et al., 2011), and that in female patients older than 18 years, the frequency of an underlying teratoma is much the same as they previously reported (Dalmau et al., 2008).

Of our cases, two (22 and 30 years old) had ovarian teratomas, the other three (16, 18 and 19 years old) had no associated tumor. The mature teratoma of an ovary in case 1 was not discovered in hospital with encephalitis symptoms, but was diagnosed four years after onset (Figure 3A-a, b). The immature teratoma of an ovary in case 3 was detected at two weeks after onset (Figure 3B-a). Pelvic MRI showed her enlarged teratoma, double in diameter, at two months after onset (Figure 3B-b) (Shimazaki et al., 2007). Both teratomas were resected, but the tumors in the other three cases were not identified until now.

2.6 Brain MRI findings

Brain MRI showed abnormal findings in 55 of 100 cases with anti-NMDA receptor encephalitis (Dalmau et al., 2008).

Of our cases, cases 1, 2 and 5 exhibited no remarkable findings on the brain MRI. FLAIR images of case 3 disclosed areas of high intensity in the bilateral medial temporal and hippocampal areas (Figure 4A-a), which disappeared after two months (Figure 4A-b)(Shimazaki et al., 2007). FLAIR images of case 4 showed areas of high intensity in the right ventral pons (Figure 4B-a) and the right cerebellum (Figure 4B-b).

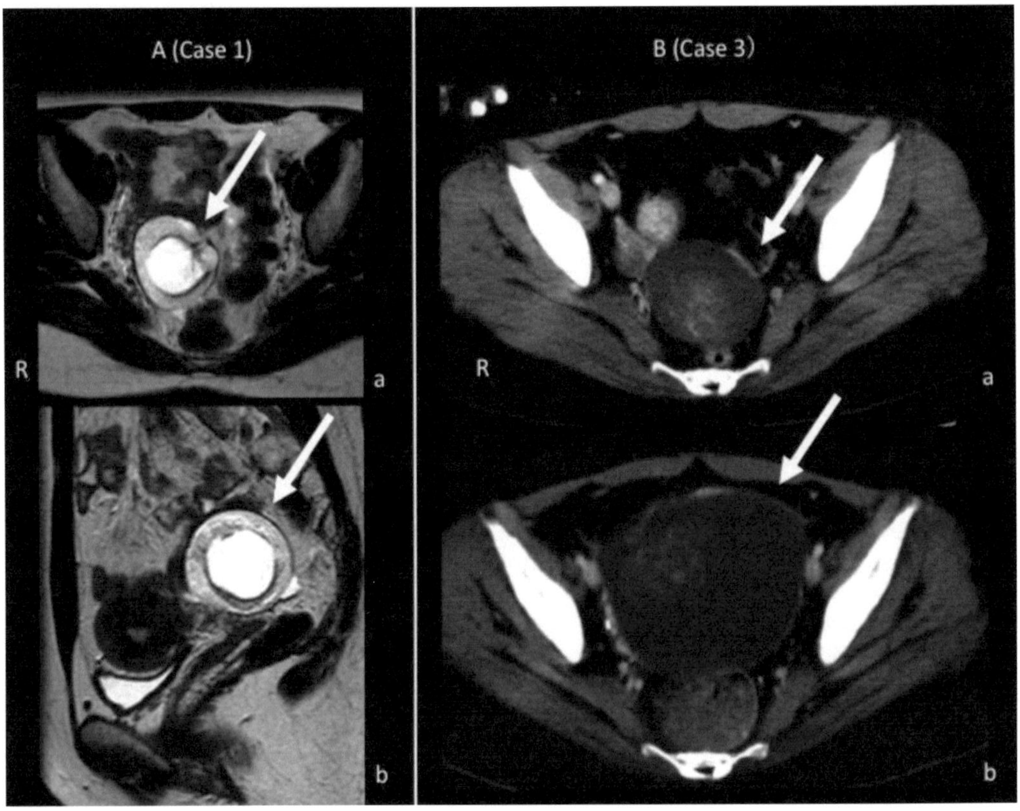

A. Pelvic T2-weighted MRI (a: axial, b: sagittal image) in case 1 at four years after onset. It revealed a right ovarian teratoma with a diameter of 5 cm. It was resected and the pathological diagnosis was a mature teratoma (dermoid cyst).

B. Pelvic enhanced CT in case 3. CT at two weeks after onset (a) revealed a 5 cm tumor in the right ovary, which was considered to be a benign cyst unrelated to the neurological disorder. At two months after onset, the patient developed progressive constipation and a bulging appearance of the lower abdomen. Follow-up abdominal computed tomography (b) and MRI showed an enlarged ovarian tumor, with a transverse diameter of 10 cm. Resection of the tumor revealed an immature teratoma that contained hair follicles, cartilage tissue, glandular structures and cerebral cortex-like tissue with normal appearing neurons. No inflammatory infiltrates were evident in the tumor.

Fig. 3. Ovarian teratomas in cases 1 and 3.

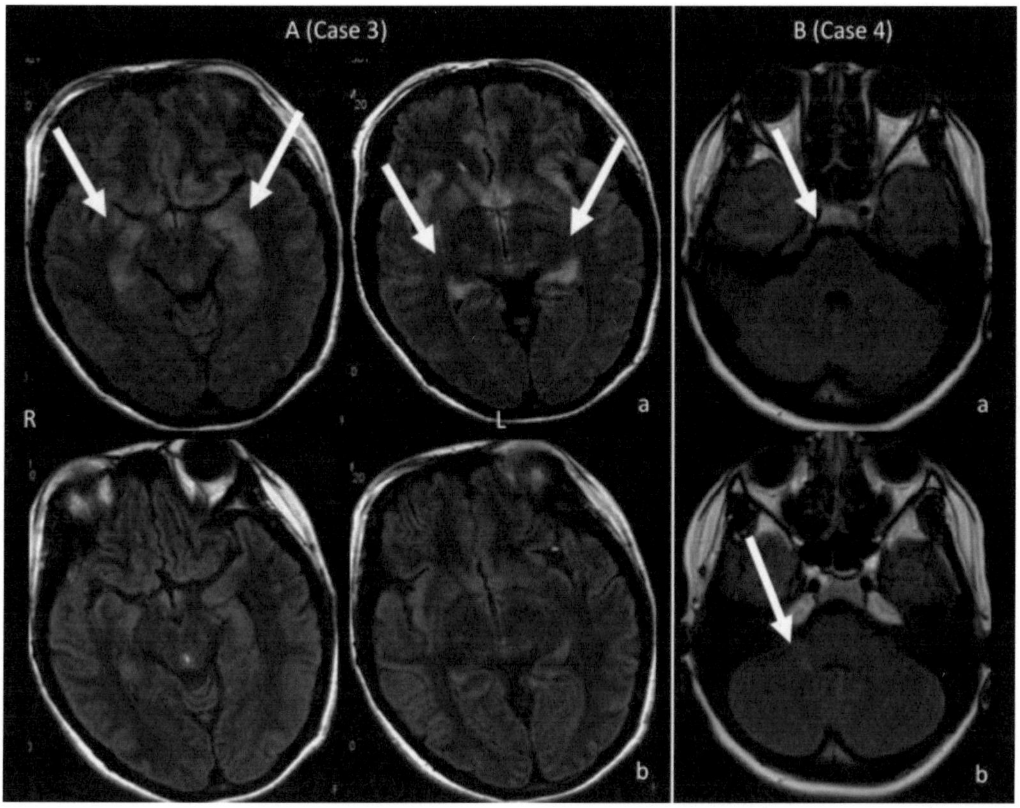

A. Brain MRI in case 3. Axial plane and Gadolinium-enhanced T1-weighted MRI were unremarkable, but MRI fluid-attenuated inversion recovery images of the brain showed areas of hyperintensity in the medial temporal lobes and hippocampus on admission (A-a). These abnormalities had resolved by two months after admission (A-b).
B. Brain MRI in case 4. Axial plane and Gadolinium-enhanced T1-weighted MRI were unremarkable, but T2-weighted and FLAIR images showed areas of slightly high intensity in the right ventral pons (a) and cerebellum (b).

Fig. 4. Brain MRI (FLAIR) findings in two patients (cases 3 and 4).

2.7 Electroencephalography (EEG)

Generalized or frontotemporal slow waves were observed in 71 of 100 cases with anti-NMDA receptor encephalitis. Epileptic discharges were only recorded in 22 of the 100 cases (Dalmau et al., 2008). The EEG records for all our cases except for case 5 mainly showed slow waves in the theta to delta ranges.

2.8 Cerebrospinal fluid findings

Cerebrospinal fluid (CSF) examination disclosed abnormal findings in 95 of 100 cases (Dalmau et al., 2008). Lymphocytic pleocytosis was found in 91 cases, and increased protein concentrations in 32 of the 100 cases.
In our cases, mild to moderate pleocytosis was found in all patients except for patient 5. CSF protein elevation was only observed in two cases (patients 2 and 3).

3. Treatment and prognosis

Several effective treatments have been reported for anti-NMDA receptor encephalitis other than the administration of steroids, immunoglobulin, and plasmapheresis. Ovarian tumor removal in the acute phase (Sansing et al., 2007; Seki et al., 2008), chemotherapy for the tumors (Eker et al., 2008), cyclophosphamide (Sansing et al., 2007; Wilder-Smith and Ng, 2008), and rituximab (Ishiura et al., 2008) were also effective treatments for a small number of cases.
In our cases (Table 1), corticosteroids were administered to four cases, and high-dose intravenous gammaglobulin to three cases. We performed plasmapheresis for two cases. Two women underwent resection of ovarian teratomas. Modified electroconvulsive therapy was found to be dramatically effective for the psychiatric symptoms in case 5.
The severity of anti-NMDA receptor encephalitis is incompletely correlated with the titer of anti-NMDA receptor antibodies in the acute phase. (Prof. Dalmau, written communication Jul 2008).
In our cases, we did know the titers in three (Table 1). Case 3 exhibited the lowest titer with a full recovery, whereas case 2 exhibited the highest titer with severe involuntary movements and poor prognosis.
The prognosis of anti-NMDA receptor encephalitis had relatively good compared to that of herpes simplex encephalitis. Of 100 cases, 47 exhibited full recovery, 28 mild stable deficits, 18 severe deficits, and seven died as a result of the neurological disorder (Dalmau et al., 2008). Our three cases exhibited a complete recovery, one had mild sequelae with epilepsy, and one died.

4. Conclusions

We have discussed five cases of anti-NMDA receptor encephalitis compared to the other numerous reported cases. From the clinical aspect, our cases and the reported ones had some symptoms in common, for example, preceding psychiatric symptoms, and characteristic orofacial dyskinesia.
Meanwhile, the clinical manifestations in our cases included a peculiar ocular symptom (ocular dipping) in case 3 and an atypical clinical presentation (predominant schizophrenic

psychiatric symptoms) in case 5. In particular, case 5 was initially misdiagnosed as having schizophrenia by a psychiatrist because of no findings of encephalitis (no CSF pleocytosis, normal brain MRI and EEG). Ovarian teratomas were found in two patients, one became rapidly enlarged in hospital, and the other was found at four years after onset. Therefore, we should carefully follow up patients even if the tumors are not identified during hospitalization. In our experience, anti-NMDA receptor encephalitis exhibits severe symptoms such as convulsions and hypoventilation in the acute phase, but this disease could be curable. Characteristic symptoms and antibody measurement can be useful for prompt diagnosis of this disease, and early immunosuppressive treatment and tumor resection are important as well as general care of critically ill patients.

5. Acknowledgements

We thank Professor Josep Dalmau (Department of Neuro-oncology, University of Pennsylvania) and Professor Keiko Tanaka (Department of Neurology, Kanazawa Medical University) for measurement of the anti-NMDA receptor antibodies. We also thank Professor Imaharu Nakano (Division of Neurology, Department of Internal Medicine, Jichi Medical University) for supervision.
This work was supported by a Grant-in-Aid for Scientific Research (C) (23591253 to Dr Shimazaki) from The Ministry of Education, Culture, Sports, Science and Technology of Japan.

6. References

Ances, B. M., R. Vitaliani, R. A. Taylor, D. S. Liebeskind, A. Voloschin, D. J. Houghton, S. L. Galetta, M. Dichter, A. Alavi, M. R. Rosenfeld, and J. Dalmau. (2005). Treatment-responsive limbic encephalitis identified by neuropil antibodies: MRI and PET correlates. *Brain*, Vol.128, No.Pt 8, (Aug 2005), pp. 1764-1777, ISSN 1460-2156

Ando, Y., M. Sawada, H. Shimazaki, K. Yoshida, S. Sakamoto, K. Tanaka, and I. Nakano. (2011). Modified electroconvulsive therapy is effective for psychiatric symptoms in a man with anti-NMDAR encephalitis. *Rinsho Shinkeigaku*, Vol.51, No.1, (Jan 2011), pp. 73, ISSN 0009-918X

Braakman, H. M., V. M. Moers-Hornikx, B. M. Arts, R. M. Hupperts, and J. Nicolai. (2010). Pearls & Oy-sters: electroconvulsive therapy in anti-NMDA receptor encephalitis. *Neurology*, Vol.75, No.10, (Sep 7 2010), pp. e44-46, ISSN 0028-3878

Dalmau, J., A. J. Gleichman, E. G. Hughes, J. E. Rossi, X. Peng, M. Lai, S. K. Dessain, M. R. Rosenfeld, R. Balice-Gordon, and D. R. Lynch. (2008). Anti-NMDA-receptor encephalitis: case series and analysis of the effects of antibodies. *Lancet Neurol*, Vol.7, No.12, (Dec 2008), pp. 1091-1098, ISSN 1474-4422

Dalmau, J., E. Lancaster, E. Martinez-Hernandez, M. R. Rosenfeld, and R. Balice-Gordon. (2011). Clinical experience and laboratory investigations in patients with anti-NMDAR encephalitis. *Lancet Neurol*, Vol.10, No.1, (Jan 2011), pp. 63-74, ISSN 1474-4465

Dalmau, J., E. Tuzun, H. Y. Wu, J. Masjuan, J. E. Rossi, A. Voloschin, J. M. Baehring, H. Shimazaki, R. Koide, D. King, W. Mason, L. H. Sansing, M. A. Dichter, M. R. Rosenfeld, and D. R. Lynch. (2007). Paraneoplastic anti-N-methyl-D-aspartate receptor encephalitis associated with ovarian teratoma. *Ann Neurol*, Vol.61, No.1, (Jan 2007), pp. 25-36, ISSN 0364-5134

De Nayer, A. R., N. Myant, and C. J. Sindic. (2009). A subacute behavioral disorder in a female adolescent. Autoimmune anti-N-methyl-D-aspartate receptor encephalitis associated with ovarian teratoma. *Biological psychiatry*, Vol.66, No.6, (Sep 15 2009), pp. e13-14, ISSN 0006-3223

Eker, A., E. Saka, J. Dalmau, A. Kurne, C. Bilen, H. Ozen, D. Ertoy, K. K. Oguz, and B. Elibol. (2008). Testicular teratoma and anti-N-methyl-D-aspartate receptor-associated encephalitis. *J Neurol Neurosurg Psychiatry*, Vol.79, No.9, (Sep 2008), pp. 1082-1083, ISSN 0022-3050

Gultekin, S. H., M. R. Rosenfeld, R. Voltz, J. Eichen, J. B. Posner, and J. Dalmau. (2000). Paraneoplastic limbic encephalitis: neurological symptoms, immunological findings and tumour association in 50 patients. *Brain*, Vol.123 (Pt 7), (Jul 2000), pp. 1481-1494, ISSN 0006-8950

Iizuka, T., F. Sakai, T. Ide, T. Monzen, S. Yoshii, M. Iigaya, K. Suzuki, D. R. Lynch, N. Suzuki, T. Hata, and J. Dalmau. (2008). Anti-NMDA receptor encephalitis in Japan: long-term outcome without tumor removal. *Neurology*, Vol.70, No.7, (Feb 12 2008), pp. 504-511, ISSN 1526-632X

Ishiura, H., S. Matsuda, M. Higashihara, M. Hasegawa, A. Hida, R. Hanajima, T. Yamamoto, J. Shimizu, J. Dalmau, and S. Tsuji. (2008). Response of anti-NMDA receptor encephalitis without tumor to immunotherapy including rituximab. *Neurology*, Vol.71, No.23, (Dec 2 2008), pp. 1921-1923, ISSN 1526-632X

Kamei, S., S. Kuzuhara, M. Ishihara, A. Morita, N. Taira, M. Togo, M. Matsui, M. Ogawa, K. Hisanaga, T. Mizutani, and S. Kuno. (2009). Nationwide survey of acute juvenile female non-herpetic encephalitis in Japan: relationship to anti-N-methyl-D-aspartate receptor encephalitis. *Internal Medicine*, Vol.48, No.9, 2009), pp. 673-679, ISSN 1349-7235

Kataoka, H., J. Dalmau, and S. Ueno. (2008). Paraneoplastic encephalitis associated with ovarian teratoma and N-methyl-D-aspartate receptor antibodies. *Eur J Neurol*, Vol.15, No.1, (Jan 2008), pp. e5-6, ISSN 1468-1331

Kleinig, T. J., P. D. Thompson, W. Matar, A. Duggins, T. E. Kimber, J. G. Morris, C. S. Kneebone, and P. C. Blumbergs. (2008). The distinctive movement disorder of ovarian teratoma-associated encephalitis. *Movement Disorders*, Vol.23, No.9, (Jul 15 2008), pp. 1256-1261, ISSN 1531-8257

Ko, M. W., J. Dalmau, and S. L. Galetta. (2008). Neuro-ophthalmologic manifestations of paraneoplastic syndromes. *J Neuroophthalmol*, Vol.28, No.1, (Mar 2008), pp. 58-68, ISSN 1536-5166

Koide, R., T. Shimizu, K. Koike, and J. Dalmau. (2007). EFA6A-like antibodies in paraneoplastic encephalitis associated with immature ovarian teratoma: a case report. *J Neurooncol*, Vol.81, No.1, (Jan 2007), pp. 71-74, ISSN 0167-594X

Lee, A., D. B. Glick, and S. H. Dinwiddie. (2006). Electroconvulsive therapy in a pediatric patient with malignant catatonia and paraneoplastic limbic encephalitis. *J ECT*, Vol.22, No.4, (Dec 2006), pp. 267-270, ISSN 1095-0680

Mehler, M. F. (1988). The clinical spectrum of ocular bobbing and ocular dipping *J Neurol Neurosurg Psychiatry*, Vol.51, No.5, (May 1988), pp. 725-727, ISSN 0022-3050

Nokura, K., H. Yamamoto, Y. Okawara, H. Koga, H. Osawa, and K. Sakai. (1997). Reversible limbic encephalitis caused by ovarian teratoma. *Acta Neurol Scand*, Vol.95, No.6, (Jun 1997), pp. 367-373, ISSN 0001-6314

Okamura, H., N. Oomori, and Y. Uchitomi. (1997). An acutely confused 15-year-old girl. *Lancet*, Vol.350, No.9076, (Aug 16 1997), pp. 488, ISSN 0140-6736

Ropper, A. H. (1981). Ocular dipping in anoxic coma. *Arch Neurol*, Vol.38, No.5, (May 1981), pp. 297-299, ISSN 0003-9942

Sansing, L. H., E. Tuzun, M. W. Ko, J. Baccon, D. R. Lynch, and J. Dalmau. (2007). A patient with encephalitis associated with NMDA receptor antibodies. *Nat Clin Pract Neurol*, Vol.3, No.5, (May 2007), pp. 291-296, ISSN 1745-834X

Schimmel, M., C. G. Bien, A. Vincent, W. Schenk, and J. Penzien. (2009). Successful treatment of anti-N-methyl-D-aspartate receptor encephalitis presenting with catatonia. *Arch Dis Child*, Vol.94, No.4, (Apr 2009), pp. 314-316, ISSN 1468-2044

Seki, M., S. Suzuki, T. Iizuka, T. Shimizu, Y. Nihei, N. Suzuki, and J. Dalmau. (2008). Neurological response to early removal of ovarian teratoma in anti-NMDAR encephalitis. *J Neurol Neurosurg Psychiatry*, Vol.79, No.3, (Mar 2008), pp. 324-326, ISSN 1468-330X

Shimazaki, H., Y. Ando, I. Nakano, and J. Dalmau. (2007). Reversible limbic encephalitis with antibodies against the membranes of neurones of the hippocampus. *J Neurol Neurosurg Psychiatry*, Vol.78, No.3, (Mar 2007), pp. 324-325, ISSN 1468-330X

Shimazaki, H., M. Morita, I. Nakano, and J. Dalmau. (2008). Inverse ocular bobbing in a patient with encephalitis associated with antibodies to the N-methyl -D-aspartate receptor. *Arch Neurol*, Vol.65, No.9, (Sep 2008), pp. 1251, ISSN 0003-9942

Shindo, A., K. Kagawa, Y. Ii, R. Sasaki, Y. Kokubo, and S. Kuzuhara. (2009). Anti-N-methyl-D-aspartate receptor-related grave but reversible encephalitis with ovarian teratoma in 2 Japanese women presenting with excellent recovery without tumor resection. *Eur Neurol*, Vol.61, No.1, 2009), pp. 50-51, ISSN 1421-9913

Stark, S. R., E. F. Masucci, and J. F. Kurtzke. (1984). Ocular dipping. *Neurology*, Vol.34, No.3, (Mar 1984), pp. 391-393, ISSN 0028-3878

Vitaliani, R., W. Mason, B. Ances, T. Zwerdling, Z. Jiang, and J. Dalmau. (2005). Paraneoplastic encephalitis, psychiatric symptoms, and hypoventilation in ovarian teratoma. *Ann Neurol*, Vol.58, No.4, (Oct 2005), pp. 594-604, ISSN 0364-5134

Wilder-Smith, E. P., and E. S. Ng. (2008). The writing on the wall. *Lancet*, Vol.372, No.9635, (Jul 26 2008), pp. 344, ISSN 0140-6736

Zandi, M. S., S. R. Irani, B. Lang, P. Waters, P. B. Jones, P. McKenna, A. J. Coles, A. Vincent, and B. R. Lennox. (2011). Disease-relevant autoantibodies in first episode schizophrenia. *J Neurol*, Vol.258, No.4, (Apr 2011), pp. 686-688, ISSN 0340-5354

18

Non-Herpetic Acute Limbic Encephalitis: A New Subgroup of Limbic Encephalitis?

Hiroshi Shoji[1], Noriyuki Kimura[2], Toshihide Kumamoto[2], Takashi Ichiyama[3] and Yukitoshi Takahashi[4]
[1]Division of Neurology, St. Mary Hospital, Fukuoka 830-8543,
[2]Department of Internal Medicine III, Faculty of Medicine, Oita University, Oita,
[3]Department of Pediatrics, Yamaguchi University Graduate School of Medicine, Yamaguchi,
[4]National Epilepsy Center, Shizuoka Institute of Epilepsy and Neurological Disorders, Shizuoka
Japan

1. Introduction

Non-herpetic acute limbic encephalitis (NHALE) was found at 1994 during the survey of herpes simplex encephalitis (HSE) in the Kyushu district, Japan. NHALE is characterized by a lack of evidence of the herpes simplex virus (HSV) genome or HSV antibody, non-paraneoplastic limbic encephalitis, and magnetic resonance imaging (MRI) abnormalities in bilateral medial temporal lobes such as the hippocampi and amygdalae (Kusuhara et al., 1994; Kaji et al., 1996; Shoji et al., 2004). Etiologies of NHALE consist of various causes, including viral origins, autoimmune disorders, and several anti-neural antibodies. Since Urgent Conference on Non-Herpetic Limbic Encephalitis, at Ichikawa City, Japan, November 2002, many cases have been accumulated as viral related acute limbic encephalitis, autoantibody-mediated acute limbic encephalitis, paraneoplastic limbic encephalitis or encephalopathy (Yuasa et al, 2003). Cerebrospinal fluid (CSF) shows a mild pleocytosis with increase of pressure, mild increase of protein, and sometimes, a lack of the pleocytosis. The CSF level of interferon-γ (IFN-γ) is unchanged with an increase of interleukin (IL)-6 (Asaoka et al., 2004; Ichiyama et al., 2008a). Among them, NHALE patient group with the onset symptoms of abnormal behavior and incoherence, and the detection of anti-glutamate receptor (GluRε2 NR2B) antibodies is gaining attention (Nemoto et al., 2005; Hayashi et al. 2005; Takahashi et al., 2007). This NHALE type is indicated to form a new subgroup of acute limbic encephalitis or encephalopathy. GluRε2 is a subunit of the N-methyl-D-asparate (NMDA) glutamate receptor. NHALE overlaps clinically to anti-NMDA receptor (NR1+2A) encephalitis, but the NMDA encephalitis is usually associated with ovarian teratoma (Dalmau et al., 2007; Iizuka et al., 2008).

In this review, two NHALE patients with positive anti-GluRε2 antibody are briefly described, and the pathogenesis of NHALE, clinical features, differential diagnosis, prognosis, and sequelae are discussed.

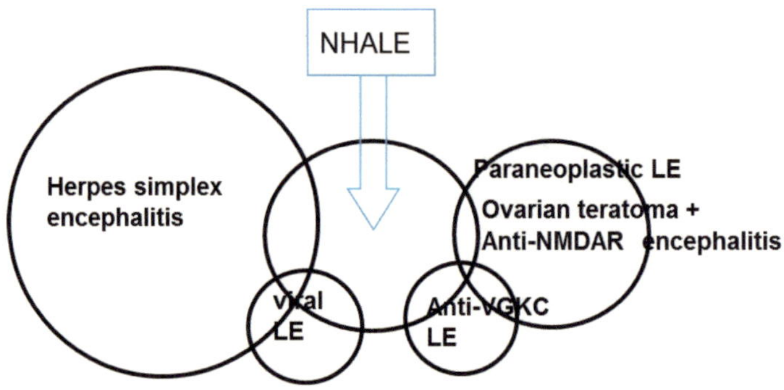

Fig. 1. Possible relationships of NHALE and related disorders.
NHALE=non-herpetic acute limbic encephalitis, NMDAR=N-methyl-D-asparate receptor
VGKC =voltage-gated potassium channel, LE=limbic encephalitis

2. Case presentation

Here, we present two representative patients with NHALE who were evaluated at A rehabilitation hospital 3 months to 2 years after the onset (Noto et al., 2008; Shoji et al., 2009).
Patient 1: A 50 year-old man was restless and became talkative with a fever and palpitation in the end of July 200x. Several days later, he was admitted with collapsed state to a nearby hospital. On admission, he showed a fever of 38.4°C, coma state, and generalized myoclonus without nuchal stiffness, then paroxysmal atrial fibrillation, status epileptics, and needed an artificial respirator for 3 months. The CSF exhibited no abnormalities in the cell count, protein and glucose contents, and polymerase chain reaction (PCR) for HSV and human herpesvirus (HHV)-6 was negative. The serum antibodies were negative for herpesvirus groups (HSV, HHV-6, varicella-zoster virus and cytomegalovirus). The MRI revealed hyperintensity lesions bilaterally in the hippocampi, amygdalae and claustrum. His CSF at the 5th illness day was positive for anti-GluRε2 IgG and IgM antibodies. Acyclovir (ACV) administration, thereafter methylprednisolone pulse therapy was performed with sodium valproate and clonazepam. Amnestic syndrome and partial seizure remained. Three months after the onset he was transferred to A rehabilitation hospital which was near to his home town. Neuropsychological tests such as the Wechsler adult intelligence scale-revised (Japanese edition, WAIS-R), Wechsler memory scale-revised (Japanese edition, WMS-R), and functional independence measure (FIM) were conducted to assess the sequelae for 2 years after the onset. WMS-R showed severe impairment of recent memory with normal total WAIS IQ and FIM points. The MRI at the recovery stage showed bilateral atrophic changes in the hyppocampi and amygdalae with hyperintensity lesions in the rectus gyri (Fig 2a). Thereafter, he moved to an another rehabilitation hospital. At 2 years after the onset, moderate amnestic syndrome and focal seizure remained, and he is still unable to return to his previous job.
Patient 2: A 36 year-old man had diarrhea for several days, and he then developed a fever of 40℃ for one week, but he did not stop his job of rescue party. Convulsive seizures and delirium appeared, and he was admitted to a nearby hospital. His consciousness level was stupor state without nuchal stiffness and pathologic reflexes. The CSF contained 6 mononuclear cells per mm^3 and protein content of 46 mg/dl, and HSV PCR was negative in

the CSF. Serum enzyme immunosorbent assay (EIA) tests for herpesvirus groups, rubella, measles and mumps were all negative. His CSF showed positive for anti-GluRε2 IgG and IgM antibodies. Electroencephalogram (EEG) revealed periodic lateralized epileptiform discharges (PLEDs). The MRI exhibited hyperintensity lesions in the bilaterally medial temporal lobes including hippocampi and amygdalae. Patient 2 was diagnosed as having NHALE with positive anti-GluRε2 antibodies. Anticonvulsant drugs and ACV were administered, but he developed status epileptics, and put on a respirator, and methylpredonisolone pulse and immunoglobulin therapies were conducted. Three months after the onset, he was transferred to A rehabilitation hospital. He showed a fever of 37°C, attention impairment, nystagmus, myoclonus at the left face and upper extremity, and weakness and atrophy of the both legs as a disuse syndrome. MRI revealed bilaterally atrophy of the hippocampi and amygdalae with hyperintensity lesions (Fig.2b). WAIS-R showed 69 of total IQ, and 44/126 at FIM. Intensive rehabilitation was performed, and 6 months later he was discharged with improvement of scores of WAIS-R, WMS-R and FIM. At 2 years after the onset, mild dysarthria, attention impairment, and gait disturbance have remained, and he is now trying to return to his previous job.

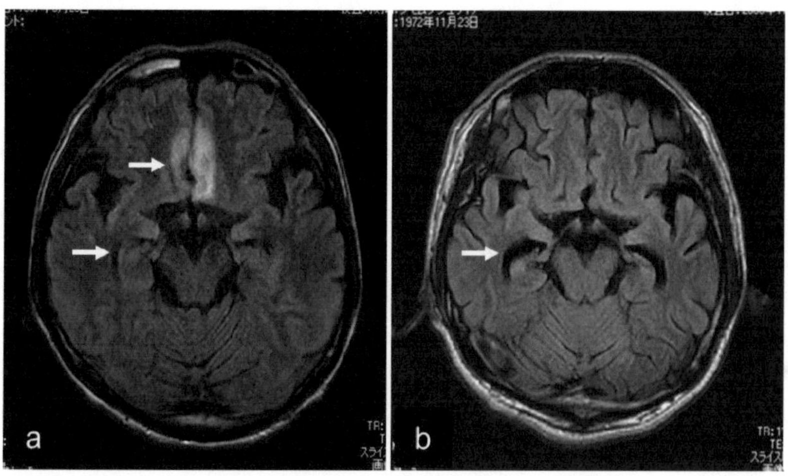

Fig. 2. a,b: MRIs of Patients 1 & 2 with NHALE at the recovery stage; a: an axial fluid attenuated inversion recovery (FLAIR) MRI of Patient 1 reveals hyperintensity lesions in the rectus gyri, and mild dilatation of the inferior horn. b: an axial FLAIR MRI of Patient 2 shows moderate dilatation of the inferior horn.

3. Pathogenesis

In the CSF cytokines of NHALE patients, the IFN-γ value is not elevated with an increase of IL-6 (Asaoka et al., 2004; Ichiyama et al., 2008a; Fig.3). CSF IFN-γ levels were elevated in the central nervous system (CNS) disorders due to direct viral invasion, such as viral meningitis and HSE (Matsubara et al., 2000; Ichiyama et al., 2005; Ichiyama et al., 2008a), but not in immune-mediated CNS disorders, such as acute disseminated encephalomyelitis, influenza-associated encephalopathy, and acute encephalopathy following prolonged febrile seizures, and hemolytic uremic syndrome with encephalopathy (Ichiyama et al., 2002; Ichiyama et al., 2004; Ichiyama et al., 2008b; Shiraishi et al., 2008). IFN-γ, which is produced by NK cells,

CD8+ and Th1 type CD4+ T lymphocytes, plays an important role in host defense against viral infection, and inhibits viral replication (Samuel., 1991). Therefore, IFN-γ elevating in the CSF may exert an inhibitory effect against viruses invading the CNS. With respect to CSF IFN-γ levels, we suggest that the main pathogenesis of NHALE is not caused by the direct invasion of virus into the CNS.

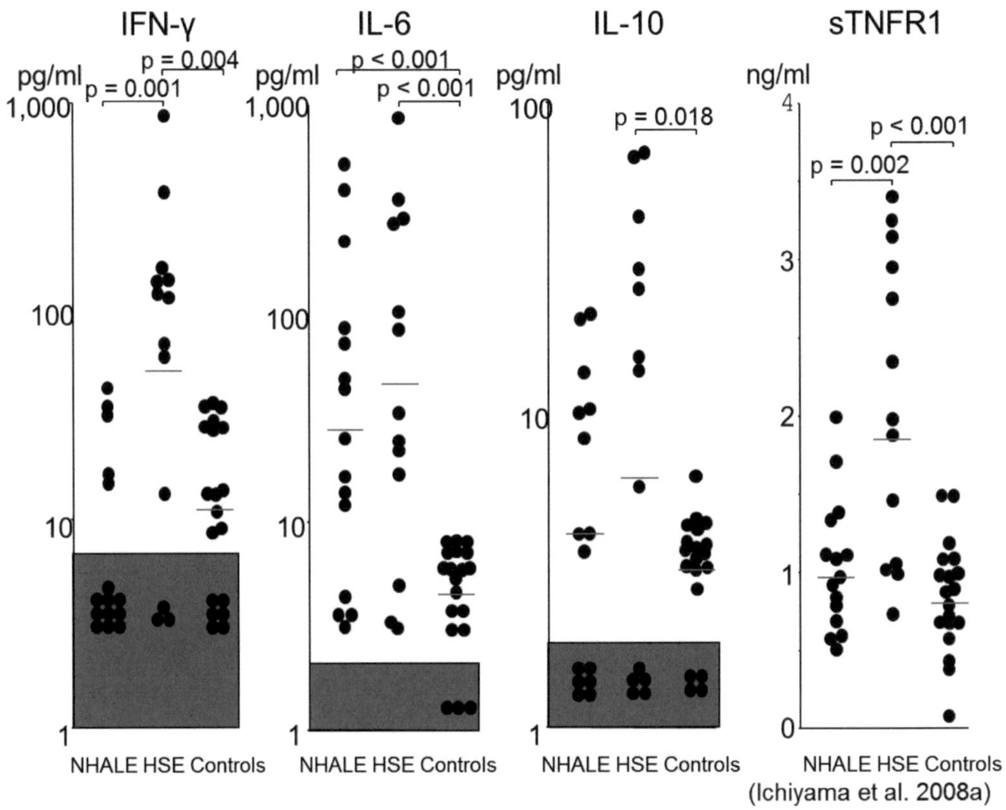

Fig. 3. The CSF concentrations of IFN-γ, IL-6, IL-10, and sTNFR1 in patients with NHALE, HSE, and controls. Horizontal lines indicate geometric means. Shaded areas indicate values below the detection limits. IFN-γ=interferon-γ, IL=interleukin, sTNFR1=soluble tumor necrosis factor receptor-1

In a major subgroup of NHALE patients presenting psychiatric symptoms such as abnormal behavior or incoherence, a subunit of NMDA glutamate receptor antibody (GluRε2 NR2B) was detected in the sera and CSF. In Japan, many similar cases have been accumulated (Nemoto et al., 2005; Hayashi et al., 2005; Noto et al., 2008). Patients 1 & 2 here described are regarded as anti-GluRε2 positive NHALE. Mochizuki et al. (2006) reported an autopsy case of NHALE with positive Anti-GluRε2 NR2B antibody, and a few autopsy cases followed (Okamoto et al., 2008; Maki et al., 2008). Thus, this NHALE type should be regarded as belonging to a new subgroup of acute limbic encephalitis. Anti-NMDA type GluR antibodies categorized into NMDA glutamate receptor complex antibodies {GluRζ1 (NR1) + GluRε1 (NR2A) or GluRε2 (NR2B)} and antibodies to each subunits composing of the complex antibodies. Antibodies to GluRε2 (NR2B) subunit are antibodies to a whole molecules of GluRε2 (NR2B) subunit (Takahashi et al., 2008, Fig.4). Takahashi et al. (2008) reported 60% positive rate of Anti-GluRε2 antibodies in the serum of NHALE patients from the acute to convalescent stage, whereas these Anti-GluRε2 antibodies in the CSF of NHALE patients were detected in 50% at the acute stage, and 40% at the recovery stage; anti-GluRε2 antibodies is indicated to invade from serum to CNS with injury of the blood-brain barrier, and may involve the pathogenesis of acute limbic encephalitis or encephalopathy (Takahashi et al., 2007; 2010). Ichiyama et al. (2009) reported that high matrix metalloproteinase-9/tissue inhibitor of metalloproteinase 1 (MMP-9/TIMP-1) ratio which indicates to injure the blood-brain barrier continues from the acute to convalescent stages (Fig. 5).

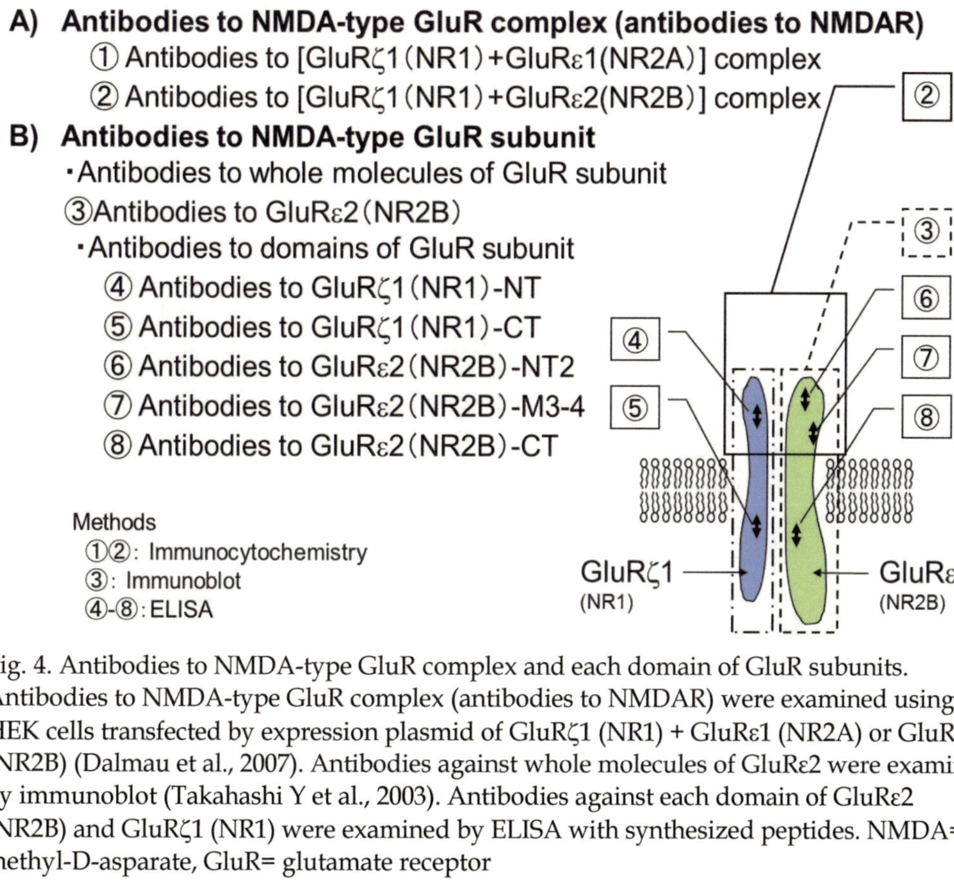

Fig. 4. Antibodies to NMDA-type GluR complex and each domain of GluR subunits. Antibodies to NMDA-type GluR complex (antibodies to NMDAR) were examined using HEK cells transfected by expression plasmid of GluRζ1 (NR1) + GluRε1 (NR2A) or GluRε2 (NR2B) (Dalmau et al., 2007). Antibodies against whole molecules of GluRε2 were examined by immunoblot (Takahashi Y et al., 2003). Antibodies against each domain of GluRε2 (NR2B) and GluRζ1 (NR1) were examined by ELISA with synthesized peptides. NMDA=N-methyl-D-asparate, GluR= glutamate receptor

On the other hand, the anti-GluR ε2 antibodies are also detected in Rasmussen encephalitis, acute encephalitis with refractory repetitive partial seizures (AERRPS), mild encephalopathy with a reversible splenial lesion (MERS), or HSE (Takahashi et al., 2003; 2005; Sakuma et al., 2009; Kai et al., 2009). Anti-GluRε2 antibody encephalitis may form a wider spectrum of encephalitis and encephalopathy. The antibody reacts cross to anti-NMDA-type GluR complex antibodies, and the clinical significance and specificity to NHALE of anti-GluRε2 antibodies is not established. In near future, the specificity, or further pathological mechanism of GluRε2 NR2B for NHALE should be investigated.

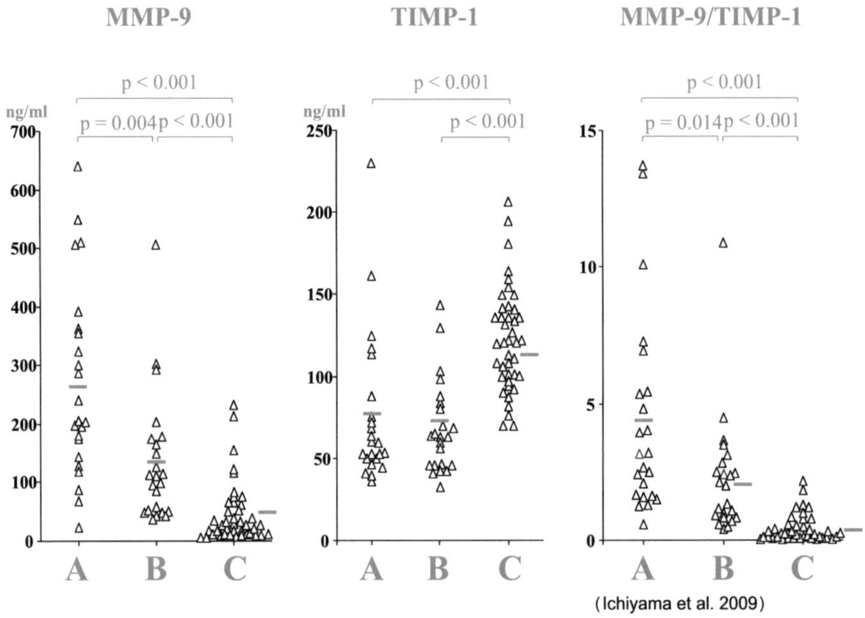

Fig. 5. Serum concentrations of MMP-9 and TIMP-1 and the ratio of MMP-9/TIMP-1 in patients with NHALE and in controls. The high ratio of MMP-9/TIMP-1 continues from the acute to convalescent stages. A: Patients with NHALE in the acute stage, B: patients with NHALE in the convalescent stage, and C: controls. The horizontal lines indicate median values. MMP-9=matrix metalloproteinase-9 , TIMP-1=tissue inhibitor of metalloproteinase 1

4. Clinical characteristics

4.1 Clinical findings

Incidence rate is 4.7 persons per million person-year. Mean onset ages of NHALE show 44.8 years in male and 31.6 years in female, respectively (Wada-Isoe et al., 2008).
In response to the limbic system disorder, various symptoms such as changeable disorientation, memory impairment, catalepsy, schizophrenic-like delusions, anger, hallucinations, convulsive seizures, autonomic seizures, pulse rate or respiratory abnormalities, and hyponatremia can appear (Yuasa, 2003). Our Patients 1 & 2 showed restlessness, palpitation and delirious state as initial symptoms. In the acute stage of NHALE, schizophrenic-like symptoms consisting of abnormal behavior, incoherence, delusions, and hallucination are frequently observed, and then convulsive seizures, status epileptics, and autonomic seizures are follows. Meningeal irritation signs appear mildly. Takahashi et al. (2008) analyzed 53 cases of non-paraneoplastic non-herpetic acute limbic encephalitis compared with 16 negative anti-GluRε2 antibody cases; abnormal behavior, delusions, and hallucination are more frequently observed including autonomic seizures, pyramidal and extrapyramidal signs, and cerebellar symptoms. Status epileptics appeared at 56.5% of the adult cases, and the other complexes partial seizures without convulsive seizure are also described. Prognostic outcome is comparative favorable, and several limited autopsy cases have been reported (Mochizuki et al., 2006). As the complications of NHALE, hypertrophic pachymeningitis or Vogt-Koyanagi-Harada disease has been reported (Usui et al., 2007; Masuda et al., 2009).

4.2 Laboratory findings

PCR and antibody tests including sensitive enzyme-linked immunosorbent assay for herpesvirus groups result in all negative. However, in the serum tests of the adults or elderly patients we may sometimes encounter carrier having HSV positive antibody (Shoji et al., 2004).

CSF shows a mild pleocytosis with increase of pressure, mild increase of protein, and sometimes, a lack of the pleocytosis. The CSF level of IFN-γ is unchanged with an increase of IL-6 (Asaoka et al., 2004; Ichiyama et al., 2008a). Ichiyama et al. (2008a) reported the comparison of CSF cytokines between NHALE and HSE; increases of IFN-γ, IL-6, IL-10, and sTNFR were observed in HSE, whereas only increase of IL-6 was found in NHALE. Brain MRI exhibits often bilateral abnormalities in the limbic areas; abnormal signals distribute in the bilateral hippocampi, amygdalae, rectus, cingulated gyri, and insula. Diffusion weighted images (DWI) is most sensitive to detect the lesions, and the hyperintensity lesions decreased by apparent diffusion coefficient (ADC) (Fig.6). Brain CT is difficult to detect the medial temporal lesions. Also, it should be evaluated that the hyperintensity lesions are apt to appear by DWI as similar lesions after status epilepticus. At the acute stage the inferior horn narrowing is often observed by MRI or CT probably reflecting the brain edema, and at the recovery stage the inferior horn is dilated suggesting the brain atrophy. ^{99m}Tc-ECD using easy z-score imaging system (eZIS) analysis single photon emission CT (SPECT) may reveal wider hypo- or hyper-perfusion lesions than the corresponding MRI lesions in the limbic areas (Fig. 7). Moreover, the hyperintensity lesions on DWI may show relatively increased regional cerebral blood flow (rCBF) on eZIS analysis. EEG reveals whole moderate slowness, and PLEDs or periodic synchronous discharges (PSD) are observed at approximately 20-30% for the acute stage.

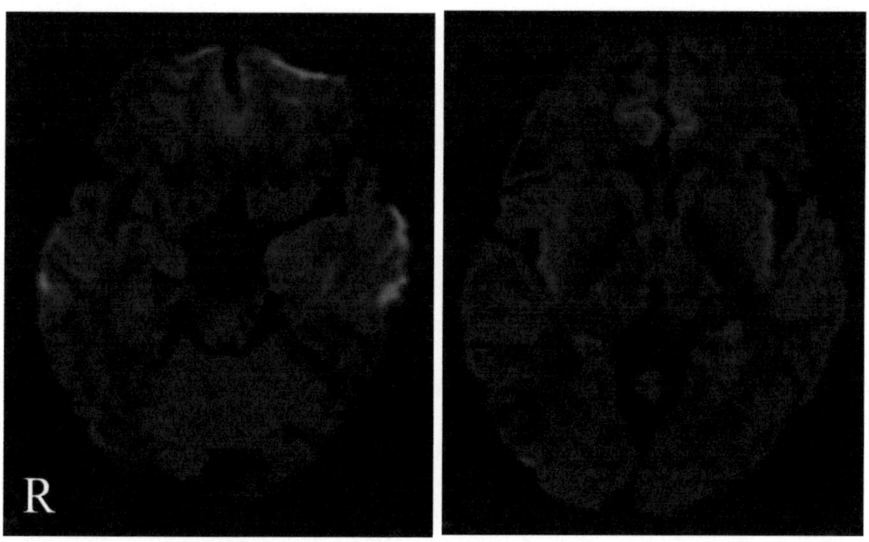

Fig. 6. MRIs of patient with NHALE at the acute stage.
Diffusion-weighted MR images showed hyperintensity lesions in the bilateral medial temporal lobes, cingulate gyri, and insulas.
NHALE=non-herpetic acute limbic encephalitis

4.3 Treatment

There is no standard therapy for NHALE. Most treatment approaches have employed some form of nonspecific immunosuppressant therapy similar to that used for other encephalitis/encephalopathy and autoimmune diseases, including corticosteroid, intravenous immunoglobulin (IVIg), plasmapheresis, or a combination of these therapies. High-dose intravenous steroids are widely accepted as first-line therapy. Most of the data describing treatment for NHALE are derived from case reports and small series. To date, there have been no randomized, controlled trials for the treatment of NHALE. On the other hand, ACV therapy is usually conducted at the acute stage due to difficulty to exclude HSE.

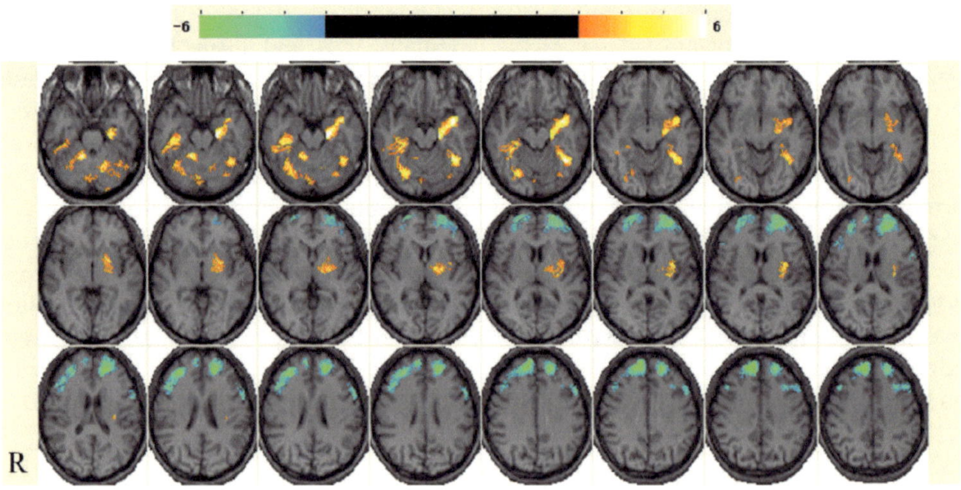

Fig. 7. eZIS images in (axial view) patients with NHALE at acute stage.

The eZIS analysis detected a significantly increased rCBF in the bilateral medial temporal lobes, left insula, and left putamen, and a significantly decreased rCBF in the bilateral frontal lobes. The color images represent the statistical significance (Z-score) of the increase (red) or decrease (blue) in rCBF.
eZIS =easy z-score imaging system, NHALE=non-herpetic acute limbic encephalitis, rCBF=regional cerebral blood flow

4.4 Differential diagnosis

Differential diagnosis with HSE is important in the choice of anti-viral drug starting or immunological therapy. HSE presents a fever, meningeal irritation signs, consciousness impairment, convulsive seizures, and memory impairment, while NHALE shows the onset symptoms with abnormal behavior or talk, and meningeal signs appear mildly. Neuroimaging of HSE often involves predominantly unilateral temporal lobe, but NHALE tends to localize bilateral medial temporal lobes. The CSF findings of NHALE are apt to reveal mild changes. Differentiation between NHALE and NMDAR encephalitis at the initial stage may be difficult, because 25% of NMDAR encephalitis exhibits localized limbic encephalitis form (Iizuka et al., 2008). Therefore, particularly in juvenile female patients with acute encephalitis, ovarian teratoma should be checked rapidly (Kamei S., 2004, 2008). On the other hand, anti-voltage-gated potassium channel (VGKC) antibody limbic encephalitis shows often encephalopathy type with hyponatremia, and overlaps Morvan syndrome with neuromyotonia. Hashimoto encephalopathy should be noticed to present limbic encephalopathy type, although this encephalopathy usually shows whole encephalitis type.

5. Sequelae

As sequelae, memory impairment, and personality or emotional changes have been most frequently described. Regards with the sequelae of our Patients 1 & 2 at 2 years after the onset, Patient 1 shows prominent impairment for recent memory with intact intelligence and immediate memory. Another Patient 2 presents memory and intelligence impairments, involuntary movement, and paresis in both legs as disuse syndrome. They are still unable to return their previous jobs.

Next, we analyzed the sequelae evaluated in questionnaires from 19 cases of NHALE and 13 cases of anti- NMDAR encephalitis, which was registered for an encephalitis research group of Japanese Ministry of Health & Welfare (Shoji et al., 2010). The Barthel score contains activity of daily living (ADL 0-20), epilepsy (0-4), psychosis (0-2), intelligence (0-4), memory impairment (0-2), and motor function (0-3) were assessed at 3 months and 1 year after the onset. Average ages of the NHALE and anti-NMDAR encephalitis groups were mean ± SD=37.5 ± 17.5 and 29.4 ± 3.2 years, respectively. Male and female ratio was all women in the NMDAR encephalitis. The statistical significance was evaluated using the Wilcoxon test. P values less than 0.10 were considered significant, because of the small case study for both groups.

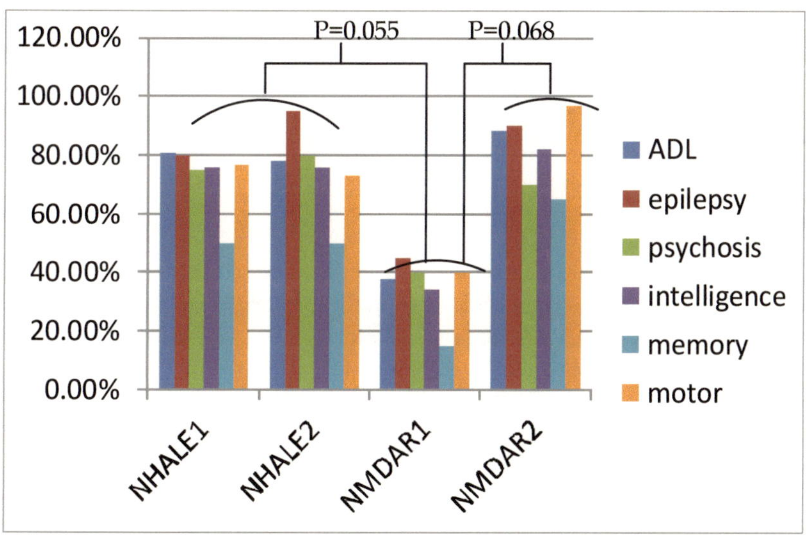

Fig. 8. The comparison of sequelae between NHALE and anti-NMDAR encephalitis (average/full score%).
NHALE1= non-herpetic acute limbic encephalitis; 3 months after the onset, NHALE2=1 year after the onset, NMDAR1=anti- N-methyl-D-asparate receptor encephalitis; 3 months after the onset, NMDAR2=1 year after the onset, ADL=activity of daily living.

In the comparison between NHALE and NMDAR groups at 3 months after onset, in NHALE group memory impairment most frequently involved, while in NMDAR group ADL, intelligence and memory impairments severely disturbed (Fig. 8, p=0.055 by Wilcoxon test). These results may suggest that NHALE has a localized limbic lesion with comparative good prognosis, and NMDAR may represent whole brain encephalitis. However, the comparison between 3 months and 1 year after onset in both groups showed significant improvement in NMDAR than NHALE group (p=0.068 by Wilcoxon test).
Prognostic outcome of NHALE is relatively favorable compared with HSE. However, many patients with NHALE are unable to return to their jobs because of memory impairments, and personality or emotional changes. Further collaborative investigation for the sequelae of NHALE and related disorders are expected.

6. Conclusion

Etiologies of NHALE consist of various causes, including viral origins, collagen disorders, and several anti-neural antibodies. Among them, anti- GluRε2 NR2B antibodies were detected. This NHALE type is indicated to form a new subgroup of acute limbic encephalitis or encephalopathy. The NHALE type may be characterized by the onset of abnormal behavior or incoherence, positive anti-GluRε2 NR2B antibodies, a lack of evidence of the HSV genome or HSV antibody, non-paraneoplastic limbic encephalitis, and MRI abnormalities predominantly in bilateral limbic systems, including hippocampi and amygdalae. CSF shows a mild pleocytosis, and sometimes, a lack of the pleocytosis. The CSF level of IFN-γ is not elevated with an increase of IL-6. The CSF cytokines' profile suggests that the main pathogenesis of NHALE is not caused by the direct invasion of virus into the CNS.
Prognostic outcome is relatively favorable, and differential diagnosis with HSE is important in the choice of anti-viral drug starting or immunological therapy. Furthermore, the specificity and pathological role of GluRε2 NR2B antibodies for NHALE should be investigated.

7. References

Asaoka, K.; Shoji, H., Nishizaka, S., Ayabe, M., Abe, T., Ohhori, N., Ichiyama, T. & Eizuru, Y. (2004). Non-herpetic acute limbic encephalitis. *Intern Med* 43. 42-48.

Dalmau, J.; Turzen. E., Wu, H.Y., Masjuan, J., Voloschin, A., Baehring, J.M., Shimazaki, H., Koide, R., King,D., Mason, W., Sansing, L.H., Dichter, M.A., Rosenfeld, M.R. & , D.R. (2007). Paraneoplastic anti-N-methyl-D-asparate receptor encephalitis associated with ovarian teratoma. *Ann Neurol* 61. 25-36.

Hayashi, Y.; Matsuyama, Z., Takahashi, Y., Wakida, K., Hashizume, T., Kimura, A., Hozumi, I., Murase, M. & Inuzuka, T. (2005). A case of non-herpetic acute encephalitis with autoantibodies for ionotropic glutamate receptor delta2 and epsilon2. *Rinshou Shinkeigaku* 45. 657-662.

Ichiyama, T.; Shoji, H., Kato, M., Sawaishi, Y., Ozawa, H., Matsubara, T. & Furukawa, S. (2002) . Cerebrospinal fluid levels of cytokines and soluble tumor necrosis factor receptor in acute disseminated encephalomyelitis. *Eur J Pediatr* 161. 133-137.

Ichiyama, T.; Morishima, T., Isumi, H., Matsufuji, H., Matubara, T. & Furukawa, S. (2004). Analysis of cytokine levels and NF-κB activation in peripheral blood mononuclear cells in influenza virus-associated encephalopathy. *Cytokine* 27. 31-37.

Ichiyama, T.; Maeba, S., Suenaga, N., Saito, K., Matsubara, T. & Furukawa, S. (2005). Analysis of cytokine levels in cerebrospinal fluid in mumps meningitis: comparison with echovirus type 30 meningitis. *Cytokine* 30. 243-247.

Ichiyama, T.; Shoji, H., Takahashi, Y., Matsushige, T., Kajimoto, M., Inuzuka, T. & Furukawa, S. (2008a). Cerebrospinal fluid levels of cytokines in non-herpetic acute limbic encephalitis: comparison with herpes simplex encephalitis. *Cytokine* 44.149-153.

Ichiyama, T.; Suenaga, N., Kajimoto, M., Tohyama, J., Isumi, H., Kubota, M. & Mori, M. & Furukawa, S. (2008b). Serum and CSF levels of cytokines in acute encephalopathy following prolonged febrile seizures. *Brain Dev* 30. 47-52.

Ichiyama, T.; Takahashi, Y., Matsushige, T., Kajimoto, M., Fukunaga, S. & Furukawa, S. (2009). Serum matrix metalloproteinase-9 and tissue inhibitor of metalloproteinase-1 levels in non-herpetic acute limbic encephalitis. *J Neurol* 256. 1846-1850.

Iizuka, T.; Sakai, F., Ide, T., Monzen, T., Yoshii, S., Iigaya, M., Suzuki, K., Lynch, D.R., Suzuki, N., Hata, T. & Dalmau, J. (2008). Anti-NMDA receptor encephalitis in Japan:long-term outcome without tumor removal. *Neurology* 70. 504-511.

Iizuka, T. (2008). Pathophysiology of anti-NMDAR antibody positive limbic encephalitis. *Clin Neurosci* 26. 516-522.

Kai, T.; Wada-Isoe, K., Nakashima, K. & Takahashi, Y. (2009). Clinically mild encephalitis/encephalopathy with a reversible splenial lesion(MERS) with anti-glutamate receptor antibody. A case report. *Shinkeinaika* 71. 397-401.

Kaji, M.; Kusuhara, T., Ayabe, M., Hino, H., Shoji, H. & Nagao, T. (1996). Survey of herpes simplex virus infections of the central nervous system, including acute disseminated encephalomyelitis, in the Kyushu and Okinawa regions of Japan. *Mult Scler* 2. 83-87.

Kamei, S. (2004). Acute juvenile female non-herpetic encephalitis. *Adv neurol Sci* 48. 827-836.

Kamei, S.; Kuzuhara, S., Ishihara, M., Morita, A., Taira, N., Togo, M., Matsui, M., Ogawa, M., Hisanaga, K., Mizutani, T. & Kuno, S. (2009). Nationwide survey of acute juvenile female non-herpetic encephalitis in Japan: relationship to anti-N-methyl-D-aspartate receptor encephalitis. *Intern Med* 48. 673-679.

Kusuhara, T.; Shoji, H., Kaji, M., Ayabe, M. & Hino, H. (1994). Non-herpetic acute limbic encephalitis. *Rinshou Shinkeigaku* 34. 1083-1088.

Maki, T.; Kokubo, Y., Nishida, S., Suzuki, H. & Kuzuhara, S. (2008). An autopsy case with non-herpetic acute limbic encephalitis (NHALE). *Neuropathlogy* 28. 521-525.

Masuda, T., Kimura, N., Ishibashi, M., Ito, M., Takahashi, Y. & Kumamoto, T. (2009). A case of Vogt-Koyanagi-Harada disease associated with non-herpetic acute limbic encephalitis with autoantibodies against glutamate receptor epsilon2 in the cerebrospinal fluid. *Rinshou Shinkeigaku* 49. 483-487.

Matsubara, T.; Matsuoka, T., Katayama, K., Yoshitomi, T., Nishikawa, M., Ichiyama, T. & Furukawa, S. (2000) Mononuclear cells and cytokines in the cerebrospinal fluid of echovirus 30 meningitis patients. *Scand J Infect Dis* 32. 471-474.

Mochizuki, Y.; Mizutani, T., Isozaki, E., Ohtake, T. & Takahashi, Y. (2006). Acute limbic encephalitis: a new entity? *Neurosci Lett* 394. 5-8.

Nemoto, H.; Takahahsi, Y. & Yuasa, T. (2005). Autoantibody mediated acute reversible Limbic encephalitis (AMED-ARLE). *Neuroinfection* 1. 44-46.

Noto, Y.; Mori, S., Kawakami, O., Yamada, K. & Takahashi, Y. (2008). A patient with non-herpetic limbic encephalitis followed-up using MRI. *Shinkeinaika* 68. 378-382.

Okamoto, K.; Yamazaki, T., Banno, H., Sobue, G., Yoshida, M. & Takatama, M. (2008). Neuropathological studies of patients with possible non-herpetic acute limbic encephalitis and so-called acute juvenile female non-herpetic encephalitis. *Intern Med* 47. 231-236.

Sakuma, H.; (2009). Acute encephalitis with refractory, repetitive partial seizures. *Brain Dev* 31. 510-514.

Samuel, C.E.; (1991). Antiviral actions of interferon. Interferon-regulated cellular proteins and their surprisingly selective antiviral activities. *Virology* 183. 1-11.

Shiraishi, M.; Ichiyama, T., Matsushige, T., Iwaki, T., Iyoda, K., Fukuda, K., Makata, H., Matsubara, T. & Furukawa, S. (2008) Soluble tumor necrosis factor receptor 1 and tissue inhibitor of metalloproteinase-1 in hemolytic uremic syndrome with encephalopathy. *J Neuroimmunol* 196. 147-152.

Shoji, H.; Asaoka, K., Ayabe, M., Ichiyama, T. & Sakai, K. (2004). Non-herpetic acute limbic encephalitis: a new subgroup of limbic encephalitis? *Intern Med* 43. 348.

Shoji, H.; Hazama, K., Tanaka, R., Koike, F., Nakahara, K., Utsunomia, H., Tabata, E., Eriguchi, M. & Takahashi, Y. (2009). A study of sequelae in non-herpetic acute limbic encephalitis. *Bulletin of the Fukuoka School of Rehabilitation Sciences & Fukuoka School of Nursing International University of Health & Welfare* 6. 7-12.

Shoji, H.; Tamekazu., T., Kaneko, M., Muraoka, N., Koike, F., Tabata, E. & Takahashi, Y. (2010). A study of sequelae in non-herpetic acute limbic encephalitis and related disorders. *Bulletin of the Fukuoka School of Rehabilitation Sciences & Fukuoka School of Nursing International University of Health & Welfare* 6. 7-12.

Takahashi, Y., Mori, H., Mishima, M., Watanabe, M., Fujiwara, T., Shimomura, J., Aiba, H., Miyajima, T., Saito Y, Nezu A, Nishida H, Imai K, Sakaguchi, N. & Kondo N. (2003). Autoantibodies to NMDA receptor in patients with chronic forms of epilepsia partialis continua. *Neurology* 61.891-896.

Takahashi Y., Mori, H., Mishima, M., Watanabe, M., Kondo, N., Watanabe, M., Kondo, N., Shimomura, J., Kubota, Y., Matsuda, K., Fukushima, K., Shiroma, N., Akasaka, N., Nishida, H., Imamura, A., Watanabe, H., Sugiyama, N., Ikezawa, M. & Fujiwara, T. (2005):Autoantibodies and cell-mediated autoimmunity to NMDA-type GluR $\varepsilon 2$ in patients with Rasmussen's encephalitis and chronic progressive epilepsia partialis continua. *Epilepsia* 46 (Suppl 5). 152-158.

Takahashi, Y., Yamasaki, E., Kubota, Y., Nishimura, S., Tsunogae, H., Ikeda, H., Takahashi, H., Mine, J., Otani, S. & Fujiwara, T. (2007). Autoantibodies against glutamate receptors in patients with encephalitis. *Rinshou Shinkeigaku* 47. 848-851.

Takahashi, Y., Mogami, Y., Takayama, R., Ikeda, H. & Imai, K. (2010). Antibodies to glutamate receptorin limbic encephalitis. *Brain Nerve* 62. 827-837.

Usui, T., Nishizawa, E. & Tei, H. (2007). Nonherpetic acute limbic encephalitis with hypertrophic pachymeningitis. A case report. *Shinkeinaika* 66. 464-468.

Wada-Isoe, K., Kusumi, M., Kai, T., Awaki, E., Shimoda, M.,Yano, H., Suzuki, K., Nakayasu, H., Oota, K., Kowa, H. & Nakashima, K. (2008). Epidemiological study of acute encephalitis in Tottori Prefecture, Japan. *Eur J Neurol* 15. 1075-1079.

Part 4

Experimental Model of Encephalitis

19

Experimental Model Systems to Define Mechanisms of Immune-Mediated Blood Brain Barrier Disruption in Acute Disseminated Encephalomyelitis (ADEM) and Acute Hemorrhagic Leukoencephalitis (AHLE)

Holly L. Johnson, Istvan Pirko and Aaron J. Johnson
Mayo Clinic
USA

1. Introduction

Blood brain barrier (BBB) disruption is an integral feature of numerous neurological diseases with infectious, inflammatory, neoplastic and vascular components. It is of particular interest in the immune mediated neurological diseases multiple sclerosis (MS), acute disseminated encephalomyelitis (ADEM), and acute hemorrhagic leukoencephalitis (AHLE). In particular, AHLE is associated with very high mortality. A fundamental question in these diseases is the extent inflammatory immune cells contribute to CNS vascular permeability. This lack of understanding currently undermines therapeutic approaches to ameliorate uncontrolled BBB disruption. In this review, we highlight the current experimental model systems available to address the contribution of inflammatory cells in BBB disruption. The contribution of T cells and other immune cell subsets in altering blood brain barrier tight junctions in the experimental autoimmune encephalomyelitis (EAE), lipopolysaccharide (LPS), and virus induced CNS vascular permeability model systems is also addressed. Results obtained from the use of these model systems have put forward a defined role for neutrophils, CD4 and CD8 T cells and vascular endothelial growth factor (VEGF) in BBB disruption. Based on these findings, we describe models in which immune cells engage and alter CNS cell types of the neurovascular unit and define future avenues of research.

Acute disseminating encephalomyelitis (ADEM) and acute hemorrhagic leukoencephalitis (AHLE) are demyelinating diseases that usually present shortly after infections or vaccination (Callen et al., 2009; Gibbs et al., 2005). ADEM typically has an overall favorable prognosis, with 60-80% of patients showing a complete recovery (Dale et al., 2000; Gibbs et al., 2005; Rust, 2000; Tenembaum et al., 2002). AHLE, which is also known as Hurst's disease, has been considered a severe form of ADEM and has a very poor prognosis, usually resulting in death in 2-14 days (Geerts et al., 1991; Hart & Earle 1975; Pinto et al., 2011; Posey et al., 1994; Suchowersky et al., 1983). This disease is characterized by extensive BBB disruption and microhemorrhage formation. Typical acute symptoms of AHLE include fever, malaise, and headache, followed by a rapid progression of multifocal neurologic signs

(Posey et al., 1994). The MRIs of AHLE patients present with edema, white matter lesions, and petechial hemorrhage (Gibbs et al., 2005; Fugate et al., 2010; Pinto et al., 2011). Neutrophilic leukocytosis in the CSF has also been shown in cases of AHLE. (Pinto et al., 2011). Usually, the patient's level of consciousness progressively declines, resulting in coma (Posey et al., 1994). AHLE progresses rapidly, causing an accelerated deterioration of the patient. This coupled with its close resemblance to herpes simplex encephalitis (HSVE) may cause this disease to be under diagnosed in addition to demonstrating a probably viral etiology to AHLE (Gibbs et al., 2005). Furthermore, recent clinical cases have shown that this commonly fatal disease may also result from severe H1N1 influenza infection (Fugate et al., 2010; Wang, G., et al., 2010) and Epstein-Barr virus (Befort et al., 2010).

There are currently no standard treatments for ADEM or AHLE, and the etiology of these two disorders is still not well understood. Several studies have demonstrated that the neurovascular unit (NVU), which is composed of cerebral endothelial cells (CECs) surrounded by astrocytes, pericytes, axonal endings, and microglia (Begley, 2004), may ultimately control permeability of the BBB through tight junctions between CECs of the vasculature. These tight junctions are composed of the proteins occludin and claudin, which seem to provide the primary seal of the tight junction, JAMs, which may play a role in monocyte and leukocyte adhesion, (Ballabh et al., 2004; Hawkins & Davis 2005) and the zona-occludin proteins, which provide the stability for the formation of tight junctions (Lai et al., 2005). However, the extent inflammatory immune cells contribute to the alteration of the NVU to a permeable state remains largely undefined. This relative lack of knowledge currently undermines effective therapies to treat diseases characterized by uncontrolled disruption of the BBB. Therefore, it is essential for the role of immune cells to be investigated in experimental mouse models, including experimental autoimmune encephalomyelitis (EAE), lipopolysaccharide (LPS), and virus induced CNS vascular permeability model systems, including the lymphocytic choriomeningitis virus (LCMV) and the peptide induced fatal syndrome (PIFS) models. These models may lead to the development of effective therapeutic approaches for these devastating diseases.

2. The Concept of the Blood Brain Barrier (BBB)

Before delving into how the BBB can be altered by immune cells, contributing to a variety of neurological diseases, it is important to understand the basic concept of the BBB and how different molecules gain access to it. The BBB is a highly specialized brain endothelial structure that plays a role in separating components of the circulating blood from neurons (Zlokovic, 2008). It is important to note that diffusion of soluble factors in the blood is controlled by capillaries, which contain specialized tight junctions. Meanwhile, recruitment of immune cells takes place at postcapillary venules (Bechmann et al., 2007). While an intact BBB is essential, it is also important that certain blood derived factors, such as nutrients, be able to cross this barrier. This is achieved through transcellular transport systems, including carrier-mediated, ion, active efflux, receptor-mediated, and caveolae-mediated transport. Carrier-mediated transport allows the transport of essential nutrients such as glucose to meet the metabolic needs of the brain. Ion transporters such as the sodium pump are important in order to meet energy demands. Active efflux of molecules from the brain endothelium is important for rapid removal of harmful substances such as ingested toxic lipophilic metabolites. Receptor-mediated transport systems have played an important role as targets for drug delivery to the brain. Caveolae, a special type of lipid raft, contributes to transcellular permeability by regulating endocytosis and transcytosis (Zlokovic, 2008). Therefore, the BBB has multiple mechanisms by which blood derived agents could enter the CNS. In this review, we will focus on the role of immune-mediated alterations of the neurovascular unit and the subsequent alterations in vascular endothelial cell tight junctions.

3. Organization of the Neurovascular Unit

The vascular permeability observed in ADEM and AHLE has generated a central question of how inflammation promotes alteration of the BBB. The BBB has unique features that enable it to create a solute impermeable barrier (Begley 2004). Based on electron microscopy data, the current model of the BBB is composed of CNS vasculature consisting of interlocking cerebral endothelial cells (CECs). Surrounding CECs are astrocytes, pericytes, axonal endings, and microglia (Begley 2004). Collectively, this group of cells is referred to as the neurovascular unit (NVU). Several recent models of BBB disruption place the NVU as a dynamic interacting multicellular network that ultimately controls permeability of the BBB (Begley, 2004; Minagar & Alexander, 2003; Zlokovic, 2008). Specific properties of each NVU cell type in maintaining BBB integrity are described below and depicted in Figure 1.

3.1 Cerebral Endothelial Cells (CECs)

CECs form tight junctions with one another, creating microvasculature that serves as a seal between the blood and CNS tissue (Fanning et al., 1999; Itoh et al., 1999; Tsukita et al., 1999; Wolburg & Lippoldt 2002). While these tight junctions are considered the actual gate of the BBB, it is thought that CECs alter tight junctions following signaling from other cells of the NVU (Demeuse et al., 2002; Marchi et al., 2009). Numerous *in vitro* and *in vivo* studies have demonstrated that CECs only form blood brain barrier properties if they are in the presence of astrocytes or astrocyte-derived factors (Hayashi et al., 1997; Janzer & Raff, 1987; Maxwell et al., 1987; Neuhaus et al., 1991; Sobue et al. 1999).

3.2 Astrocytes

Greater than 90% of the albuminal surface of CECs are in direct contact with astrocytes (Abbott, 2002; Demeuse, et al., 2002). Astrocytes have been shown *in vitro* to promote the opening and maintenance of CEC tight junctions upon stimulation (Schroeter et al., 2001; Siddharthan et al., 2007; Smith, 2007). For this reason, it is hypothesized that astrocytes play a critical role in maintaining CEC integrity through direct contact and chemical messengers *in vivo* (Abbott, 2005; Abbott et al., 2006; Haseloff et al., 2005). In addition, astrocytes form complex networks with vasculature, potentially communicating through endfeet and Ca^{2+} waves (Koehler et al., 2006). Their close association with CECs and their role in BBB formation make astrocytes a potential candidate NVU cell type involved in altering vascular permeability.

3.3 Pericytes

Pericytes have been found to promote tighter BBB formation and reduced transendothelial resistance *in vitro* (Dohgu et al., 2005; Ramsauer, et al., 2002). Pericytes are also an important source of TGF-β in CEC microvessel formation (Dohgu et al., 2005). Transgenic approaches to inhibit migration of pericytes to vasculature through selective disruption of PDGF-β in CECs results in susceptibility to vascular permeability and edema (Hellstrom et al., 2001).

This evidence, while indirect, suggests a potential role for pericytes in maintaining CEC BBB stability *in vivo*.

3.4 Neurons

Neurons have been implicated in CNS vascular permeability due to the close proximity of axonal endings with astrocyte endfeet and CECs (Hamel, 2006). Neuronal activity could therefore communicate with astrocytes which are in direct contact with CECs. Specific subpopulations of cortical GABAergic interneurons have been demonstrated to promote vasodilation through close association with astrocyte endfeet (Cauli et al., 2004). Furthermore, neurons express high levels of nitric oxide and COX-2, implying a potential mechanism to signal alteration of smooth muscle near vasculature (Vidensky et al., 2003). These observations suggest a potential mechanism for neurons to regulate CEC function in a process dependent or independent of astrocytes.

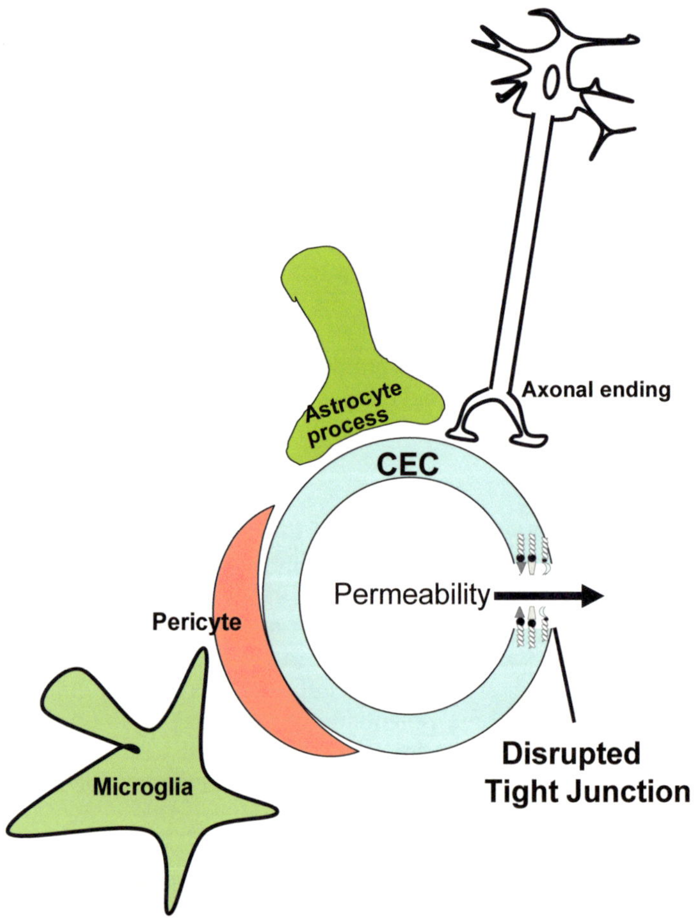

Fig. 1. A model depicting the organization of the neurovascular unit (NVU). The NVU is composed of cerebral endothelial cells (CECs) surrounded by astrocytes, pericytes, axonal endings, and microglia. The NVU may ultimately control permeability of the BBB through tight junctions between CECs of the vasculature.

3.5 Microglia

Microglia have been implicated as mediators of CNS vascular permeability due to their expression of proinflammatory cytokines that promote BBB disruption *in vitro*, the most notable being TNF-α (Zhao et al., 2007). Microglia are potent antigen-presenting cells of the CNS that express both class I and class II molecules. *Ex vivo* isolated microglia have also been demonstrated to activate T cells *in vitro* (Mack et al., 2003). Therefore, microglia have the capacity to both interact with T cells and express proinflammatory factors that could alter the NVU resulting in BBB disruption.

4. Cerebral endothelial cell tight junctions and CNS vascular permeability

The NVU has been implicated in controlling entry of blood derived products across the BBB through tight junctions between CECs of the vasculature. Tight junctions are composed of both cytoplasmic and transmembrane proteins. These proteins are linked to an actin-based cytoskeleton allowing for a tight seal among cerebral endothelial cells of CNS vasculature (Petty & Lo, 2002). Cytoplasmic proteins collectively referred to as the Membrane-Associated Guanylate Kinase-Like homolog family provide structural support and play an organizational role for CECs (Hawkins & Davis, 2005). The current model of how the transmembrane proteins occludin, claudin and junctional adhesion molecules (JAMs) present in tight junctions interact is shown in Figure 2. Among these proteins, occludin and claudin appear to form the primary seal of the tight junction, whereas JAMs are proposed to

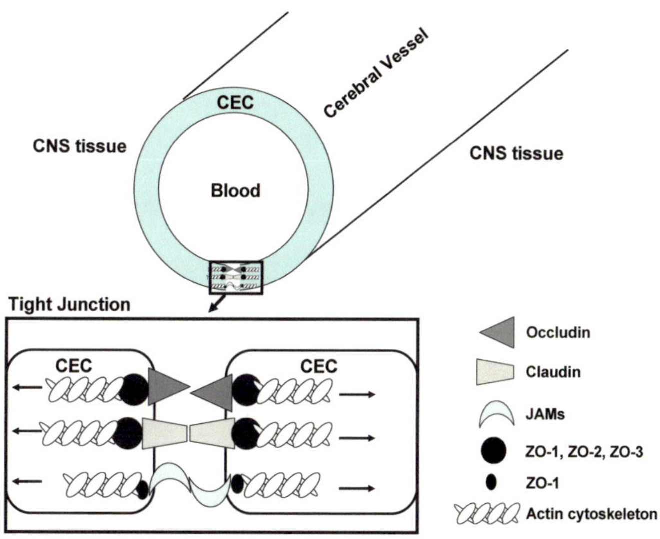

Fig. 2. Molecular model of tight junctions between cerebral endothelial cells (CECs). Occludins, claudins and junctional adhesion molecules (JAMs) regulate adhesion of CECs. Occludins and claudins adhere to the zona occludin complex which consists of an interaction of ZO-1, ZO-2, and ZO-3 proteins. In contrast JAMs adhere only to zona occludin-1 (ZO-1). The zona occludin proteins in turn adhere to actin cytoskeleton proteins. Opening of tight junctions during inflammation appears to be an orchestrated event of degradation and expression of occludins and claudins, respectively and contraction of actin cytoskeleton. Model is modified from (Minagar & Alexander, 2003).

be involved in monocyte and leukocyte adhesion and transmigration through the BBB (Ballabh et al., 2004; Brooks et al., 2005). The zona-occludin proteins, ZO-1, ZO-2 and ZO-3, have been shown to connect the transmembrane proteins to actin, providing stability for tight junction formation (Lai, 2005). Expression of occludin is much higher in neural endothelial cells when compared to peripheral endothelial cells whereas claudins are found in both (Ballabh et al., 2004). Occludin could therefore contribute to structural differences in BBB tight junctions as compared to tight junctions found in peripheral tissue.

Following insult to the CNS, inflammatory immune cells home to the CNS tissue. Despite the ability of immune cells to enter the CNS, the BBB remains relatively impermeable to other blood derived products. This is potentially due to immune cells entering the CNS without opening tight junctions between CECs via post capillary venules (Bechmann et al., 2007; Burns et al., 2000; Wolburg et al., 2005). However, tight junctions do not remain closed in all cases of CNS inflammation. Some instances of CNS inflammation promote opening of tight junctions and increased permeability of blood derived products through the BBB. Why tight junctions and the BBB open under some inflammatory circumstances but not others remains unknown. Current models suggest inflammatory immune cells promote opening of tight junctions between CECs through the activation of cells that line the BBB (Minagar & Alexander, 2003; Zlokovic, 2008). Chemokine and cytokine emission from immune cells have been implicated in this process with some examples being VEGF, IFN-γ, TNF-α, IL-1β and IL-6 (Argaw et al., 2009; Blamire et al., 2000; Didier et al., 2003; Ferrari et al., 2004; Krizanac-Bengez, et al., 2003; Laflamme, 1999; Paul et al., 2003; Stoll et al., 2000; Suidan et al., 2010; Wong et al., 2004). Chemokines enable adhesion of immune cells by mediating the activation of integrins on these cells. Additional signals lead to cytoskeletal reorganization, permitting transmigration of immune cells across the BBB, which is directed by matrix metalloproteinases (MMPs). Current therapies focus on blocking the integrins, which have resulted in reductions of BBB breakdown in patients with active multiple sclerosis. Targeting MMPs may also serve to stabilize BBB dysfunction (Zlokovic, 2008).

5. Importance of vascular endothelial growth factor (VEGF) in promoting CNS vascular permeability

Clinical observations and current experimental model systems used to address the contribution of inflammatory cells in BBB disruption have put forth a potential role for VEGF, a cytokine that has an instrumental role in vascular development and angiogenesis (Deininger et al., 2003; Karamysheva, 2008; Olsson et al., 2006; Su et al., 2006). However, VEGF was originally defined as "vascular permeability factor" which was found to be secreted by tumor cells (Senger et al., 1983). VEGF is over 50,000 fold more potent than histamine in promoting vascular permeability in *in vitro* assays, demonstrating the potency of this cytokine to promote deregulation of the vasculature (Shulman et al., 1996). VEGF mediated permeability occurs through modification of endothelial cells to develop (a) vesiculo-vacuolar organelles, (b) increased caveolae formation, (c) fenestrations in membranes, and (d) alteration of tight junctions (Antonetti et al., 1999; Esser et al., 1998; Feng et al., 1999; Roberts & Palade, 1995). These modifications in endothelial cells could result in different levels of vascular permeability that range from the entry of small particles up to whole erythrocytes (Weis & Cheresh, 2005). The prevailing hypothesis is that VEGF's effects on endothelial cells of vasculature result in local edema, hemorrhage and tissue damage (Chi et al., 2005). However, the specific interactions between inflammatory cells that result in VEGF-mediated vascular permeability remain a developing area of research.

The role of VEGF in the CNS is further complicated by the dual role of this cytokine in both angiogenesis and development, as well as in mediating vascular permeability. VEGF-deficient mice are an embryonic lethal phenotype which fail to develop normal vasculature (Carmeliet et al., 1996; Ferrara et al., 1996). Adding to the complexity of VEGF in the CNS is the rather ubiquitous nature of VEGF expression. During the onset of neuropathology, several CNS cell types including astrocytes, neurons and microglia have been reported to upregulate VEGF expression (Hayashi et al., 1997; Issa et al., 1999; Marti & Risau, 1998; Plate et al., 1999). Meanwhile, the CNS cell types that express the VEGF receptors, Flt-1 and Flk-1, include endothelial cells, smooth muscles and neurons (Carmeliet & Storkebaum, 2002; Ishida et al., 2001). VEGF is expressed in the CNS within 6 hours following a stroke and this cytokine has also been localized to MS lesions (Marti et al., 2000; Proescholdt et al., 2002). In experimental rodent models of hypoxia, VEGF expression in the CNS increases with the incidence of vascular permeability. Blocking VEGF in this model resulted in reduced vascular permeability (Schoch et al., 2002). Therefore, there is significant evidence in the literature that VEGF may be a viable target to treat neurological diseases characterized by vascular permeability and hemorrhage.

6. Tight junction alterations in the Experimental Autoimmune Encephalomyelitis (EAE) model

Experimental autoimmune encephalomyelitis (EAE) is an animal model used to study brain inflammation, and its clinical and pathological characteristics closely resemble those of ADEM. Induction of EAE produces neurological deficits, inflammatory CNS lesions, and disruption of the BBB (Morgan, Shah et al. 2007). This demyelinating disease of the CNS is induced by immunizing mice with well characterized myelin peptides, such as PLP, MAG, or myelin oligodendrocyte glycoprotein $(MOG)_{35\text{-}55}$ peptide in complete Freund's adjuvant (CFA), which causes inflammatory responses to the protein/peptide. It is also common to co-inject the mice with pertussis toxin to break down the blood brain barrier (BBB), allowing immune cells to gain access to the CNS tissue (Chen & Brosnan, 2006; Gurfein et al., 2009). The use of this mouse model has revealed the role that VEGF, CD4 T cells, astrocytes, tight junction proteins, and certain cytokines, such as IL-17, IL-22, and IFN-γ, have in the breakdown of the BBB.

Although IFN-γ was originally believed to play a pathogenic role in EAE, evidence has emerged that this cytokine may actually play a suppressive role. Since EAE in general is mediated by CD4 T cells, the proliferation and apoptosis of these cells in IFN-γ-deficient mice was investigated in order to define the role of IFN-γ in EAE. It was discovered that in the absence of IFN-γ, activated CD4 T cells exhibited a more extensive proliferation as well as decreased apoptosis when compared to wild-type mice. Therefore, it appears that IFN-γ is essential to limit the extent of EAE by serving to suppress the expansion of activated CD4 T cells (Chen & Brosnan, 2006).

Argaw et al (2009) have employed the MOG peptide induced EAE model to investigate the potential links between the reactivity of astrocytes and BBB disruption. Through the use of confocal imaging, they have shown that astrocyte-derived VEGF-A causes down-regulation and disruption of the tight junction proteins claudin-5 and occludin, promoting breakdown of the BBB, as shown in Figure 3 (Argaw et al., 2009).

Morgan et al took a closer look at occludin and the signaling events that occur during EAE through analysis of spinal cord tissue of naïve and EAE animals. Neurological impairment

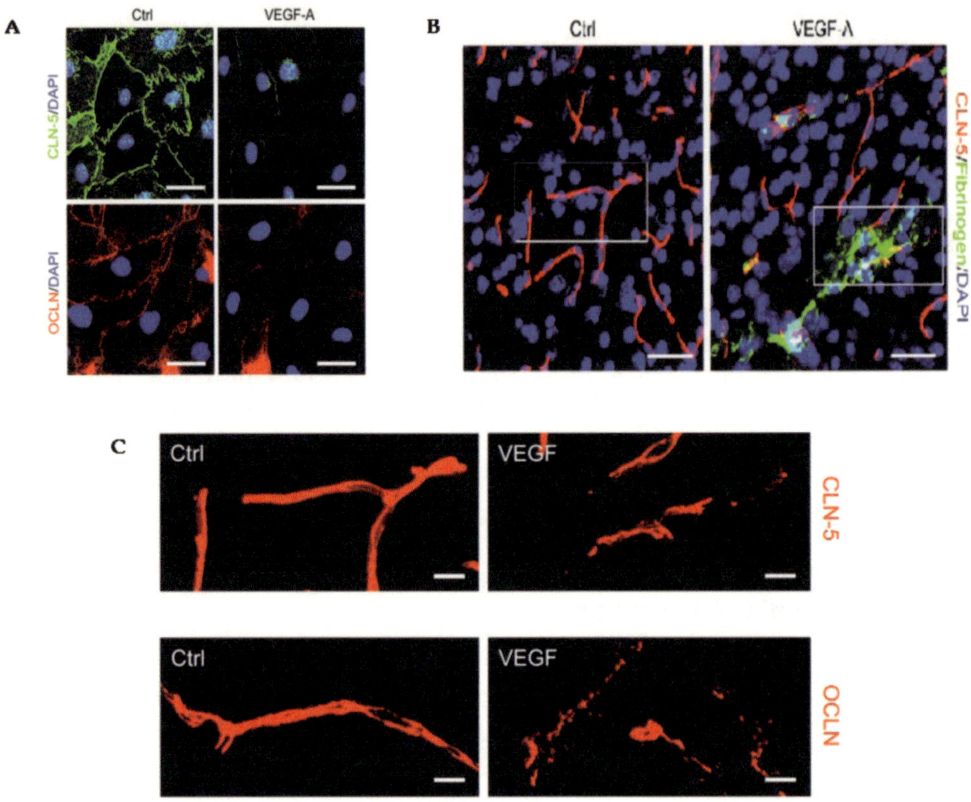

Fig. 3. (A) VEGF down-regulates claudin-5 and occludin in human BMVECs. Confocal imaging of human BMVEC treated with 100 ng/mL VEGF-A for 24 hours and immunostained for claudin-5 and occludin. In controls, both proteins localize to the plasma membrane in areas of cell-cell contact. Note that claudin-5 and occludin are both down-regulated by VEGF-A. Data are representative of at least 3 separate experiments on 3 distinct cultures. (B) Sections of cerebral cortex from 12-week adult C57BL/6 mice 24 h following stereotactic microinjection of murine $VEGF_{165}$ (60 ng in 3 µl PBS/BSA) or vehicle control. Sections are immunostained for claudin-5 (red channel) plus fibrinogen (green channel). Note that BBB permeability is observed around vessels in VEGF-injected areas. (C) Immunoreactivity for claudin-5 and occludin appears patchy and discontinuous in VEGF-injected areas. (Scale bars: A, 20 µm; B, 75 µm; C, 20 µm.) Data shown in B and C are representative of findings from at least 4 mice per time point per condition. (This figure was reproduced from Argaw, A. T., B. T. Gurfein, et al. (2009). VEGF-mediated disruption of endothelial CLN-5 promotes blood-brain barrier breakdown. *Proceedings of the National Academy of Sciences of the United States of America* 106(6): 1977-1982. Permission was granted by PNAS).

was observed in the animals undergoing EAE, which demonstrated a progressive development of tail and hind limb weakness and eventually became paraplegic. Immunohistochemical analysis of tissue revealed an increase in the number of nuclei through Hoechst staining and the presence of infiltrated macrophages and activated microglia through ED1 labeling in animals treated with EAE, thus confirming the inflammatory nature of the disease. Additionally, an increase in the abundance of the plasma proteins albumin and transferrin was observed in EAE tissue, which is also consistent with inflammation leading to BBB breakdown. Immunoprecipitation revealed increased electrophoretic mobility of occludin in EAE animals which was found to be a result of occludin dephosphorylation. This was confirmed through the use of phosphatase treatment, which caused a further increase in electrophoretic mobility, while phosphatase inhibitors blocked this effect. These changes in occludin phosphorylation may signal changes in permeability of tight junctions. Furthermore, localization of occludin was analyzed via immunohistochemistry and was observed at intercellular junctions in naïve tissue, which is consistent with previous findings. However, localization of occludin to intercellular junctions in EAE tissue was often not apparent. Junctionally-localized claudin-5 was also disrupted in EAE tissue, indicating that the structure of tight junctions is disrupted in EAE. These findings reveal a potential role for occludin in BBB disruption (Morgan et al., 2007). Therefore, further investigation of this tight junction protein, along with its phosphorylation changes and signaling pathways, may open the door to new potential therapeutics for diseases involving breakdown of the BBB.

In addition to claudin-5 and occludin, the tight junction adaptor protein ZO-1 has also been analyzed using the EAE model. CNS tissue from naïve and EAE animals was analyzed for expression of ZO-1. Immunohistochemistry and confocal microscopy revealed disrupted expression of ZO-1 in lesion areas of EAE animals when compared to naïve animals. In order to correlate this disruption with clinical symptoms, time-course studies of ZO-1 distribution were performed. It was found that disruption of ZO-1 preceded clinical disease in EAE in lesion areas and correlated with symptomatic clinical signs in non-lesion areas. Additionally, vascular permeability was analyzed through the use of Evans blue dye, and an increase in permeability was found at the peak of EAE. Taken together, it is evident that a complete understanding of the regulation of tight junction architecture is essential for the development of therapies (Bennett et al., 2010).

Kebir et al employed the EAE model to examine the effects of Th17 lymphocytes, which are known to have encephalitogenic potential, on BBB disruption, and found that significantly more Th17 lymphocytes migrated across the BBB *in vitro* than did either Th1 or *ex vivo* CD4+ lymphocytes. To confirm the ability of these lymphocytes to cross the BBB *in vitro*, cells were stained for IL-17 and IL-22, a cytokine product of Th17 cells, before and after migration. There was a significant increase in IL-17+ and IL-22+ lymphocytes after migration. Furthermore, it was found that both IL-17 and IL-22-producing lymphocytes expressed the cytolytic molecule granzyme B, enabling these cells to kill human fetal neuron-enriched cultures. Similar to the previously mentioned studies, the effect on tight junctions was also investigated. It was discovered that treating monolayers of human BBB-ECs with IL-17 produced an increase in the diffusion of fluorescently-labeled BSA, which coincided with a decrease in occludin and ZO-1 expression in EAE mice. Additionally, it was found that Th17 lymphocytes contribute to inflammation through the recruitment of CD4+ lymphocytes (Kebir et al., 2007).

The mechanisms of IL-17-induced BBB disruption were further investigated using the EAE model by Huppert et al. It was discovered that IL-17 treatment disrupted tight junction molecules by decreasing occludin levels and causing a reorganization of ZO-1, thus impairing BBB integrity. It was also found that IL-17 induced an increase in reactive oxygen species (ROS) formation, a mechanism known to be involved in BBB disruption. To link this observation to the effect on tight junctions, the involvement of ROS signaling was investigated, and DPI, an NAD(P)H oxidase inhibitor, was found to prevent the effect of IL-17 on occludin. Additionally, it has been demonstrated that phosphorylation of myosin light chain (MLC) in BECs is induced by IL-17, leading to BBB permeability. When EAE mice were treated with ML-7, a MLCK inhibitor, they developed significantly milder clinical signs and had a reduced number of infiltrating lymphocytes and macrophages when compared with vehicle-treated mice. This treatment also reduced the levels of IL-17 and IL-22, which are pathogenic cytokines associated with EAE. Furthermore, IL-17-deficient mice portrayed lower levels of oxidative stress and were protected from BBB disruption induced by EAE (Huppert et al., 2010). Taken together, these two studies portray a role for proinflammatory cytokines, particularly IL-17, on the integrity of the BBB. Targeting the mechanisms of these cytokines could bring about novel therapeutic strategies for inflammatory diseases such as ADEM and AHLE. The results from these studies can be incorporated into a model, which is shown in Figure 4.

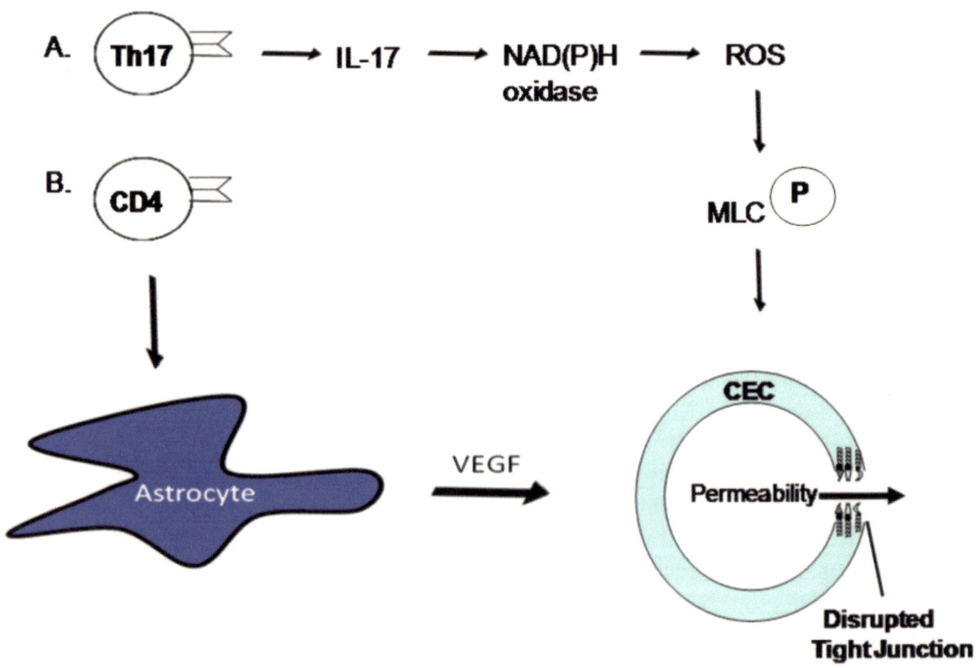

Fig. 4. Mechanisms of CD4 T cell initiated BBB disruption. (A) Th17 lymphocytes contribute to inflammation through IL-17, which induces NAD(P)H oxidase-dependent ROS formation, leading to phosphorylation of MLC, and subsequent BBB permeability. (B) Additionally, CD4 T cells induce astrocytes to release VEGF, causing down-regulation of the tight junction proteins claudin-5 and occludin, which promotes breakdown of the BBB.

7. Lipopolysaccharide (LPS) model

Injection of small amounts of lipopolysaccharide (LPS), a component of the cell wall of Gram-negative bacteria, can induce shock and systemic inflammation. The signaling pathway begins by LPS binding to LPS binding protein (LBP), with subsequent transfer of

LPS to CD14. In order for the proper targeting of TLR-4 to the surface and its ability to recognize LPS, MD-2 binds to TLR-4. This complex then interacts with CD14:LPS, sending a signal that activates the transcription factor NFkB, which activates genes that encode proteins that play a role in defense against infection.

Qin et al sought to understand the effects of systemic LPS on brain inflammation. Upon peripheral injection of LPS, there was a rapid increase in the cytotoxic factor TNFα, which remained elevated in the brain even 10 months after treatment. Injection of LPS also promoted the activation of brain microglia through TNFα receptors. Brain sections were immunostained with Iba1, an antibody specific for microglia. Increased cell size, irregular shape, and intensified Iba1 staining are apparent in LPS-treated mice when compared with controls. This activated microglia may lead to the production of more inflammatory factors, which could possibly lead to neuronal death. This reactive microgliosis may be the cause of progressive and chronic neuroinflammation (Crews et al., 2007).

Using a similar model, Brooks et al employed Complete Freund's adjuvant (CFA), which has also been known to stimulate the production of TNF. It was discovered that changes in certain transmembrane tight junction proteins alter the function of the BBB. For example, occludin was significantly decreased in CFA-injected rats, while claudin-3 and claudin-5 were both significantly increased when compared to saline-treated controls. The alteration of these tight junction protein levels coincided with BBB disruption (Brooks et al., 2005).

Matrix metalloproteinases (MMPs) mediate BBB disruption and trafficking of immune cells into the CNS and can be induced by LPS. It has previously been shown that expression of stromelysin-1 (MMP-3) occurs after intracerebral injection of LPS. To investigate the effect of MMP-3 on BBB disruption, MMP-3 knockout mice have been used. LPS injection increased CNS vascular permeability in wild-type mice but not in mice lacking MMP-3. Additionally, quantitative stereology showed that MMP-3 KO mice exhibited a significant reduction in neutrophil infiltration. Furthermore, when analyzing alterations in tight junction proteins, it was discovered that both claudin-5 and occludin were decreased after LPS injection in both WT and MMP-3 KO mice. However, there was less tight junction damage in the mice lacking MMP-3. Therefore, further investigating the mechanisms of MMP-3 activity may aid in the development of MMP inhibitors to be used in the treatment of neuroinflammatory diseases (Gurney et al., 2006). Importantly, this model system illustrates the potential of peripheral inflammation to induce microglia activation and subsequent BBB disruption in the CNS, the tentative model of which is put forward in Figure 5.

8. LCMV model of Vascular Permeability: Lymphocytic Choriomeningitis Virus (LCMV)

Lymphocytic choriomeningitis virus (LCMV) is a well-studied fatal model of CNS vascular permeability. CD8+ T cells are important mediators in the response to several viral infections. These immune cells are activated in secondary lymphoid organs, particularly the spleen, and then migrate to sites of infection, where they kill virus-infected cells and secrete pro-inflammatory cytokines such as IFN-γ and TNF-α. It has previously been shown that the immunopathology resulting from CNS infection with LCMV correlates with the cytotoxic activity of virus-specific CD8+ T cells and this process is perforin-dependent (Kagi et al., 1994). Storm et al sought to re-evaluate the role of perforin in this process. They discovered that perforin-deficient mice infected with LCMV still die from inflammation mediated by CD8+ T cells, although this death is delayed 2-5 days when compared to wild-type mice infected with LCMV. Nevertheless, death occurred despite the absence of perforin, impaired pro-inflammatory cytokine production, and a deficit in the cytotoxic ability of CD8+ T cells. However, it was also shown that CD8+ T cells were required for the lethality, because those that received CD8-depleting antibodies survived. The delay in fatality in the absence of perforin may be attributed to virus-specific T cells being prevented from entering the CNS. Additionally, these T cells may not be effectively recruited to the CNS within the first 6-7 days after infection. However, once they are able to enter the CNS, they have the ability to induce fatal CNS pathology (Storm et al., 2006).

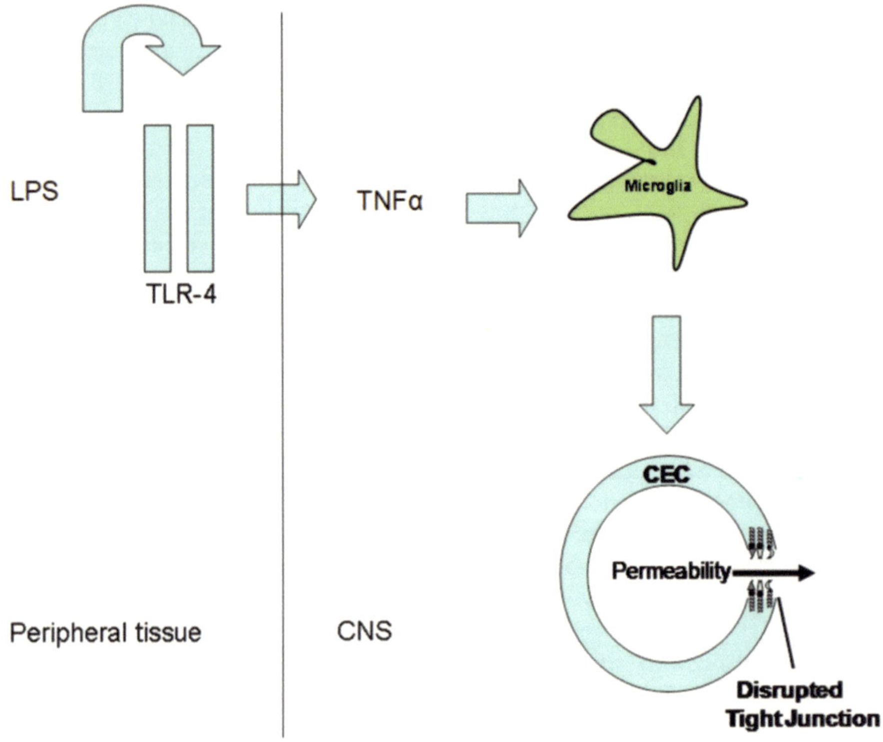

Fig. 5. Proposed model of LPS-induced systemic inflammation that results in BBB disruption. LPS binds to TLR-4, promoting shock and systemic inflammation that leads to BBB disruption. LPS causes an increase in TNFα, causing reactive microgliosis and chronic neuroinflammation. Additionally, tight junction proteins are altered, coinciding with BBB disruption.

Similarly, Kim et al, using the LCMV model, employed two-photon microscopy to visualize the dynamics of immune cells in the meninges. They observed motile CTL which expressed chemoattractants that recruited myelomonocytic cells, such as neutrophils. Therefore, it was inferred that a disorder that depends on CD8+ T cells may rely solely on CTL recruited myelomonocytic cells. Using mice with single mutations in all major CTL effector pathways, including perforin and TNF-α, it was found that mice still experienced convulsive seizures after LCMV infection. Therefore, no single deficiency had the ability to prevent disease. This group then questioned the potential role for monocytes and/or neutrophils in the seizure-induced death on day 6. To investigate this, they depleted both monocytes and neutrophils by administering high-dose anti-GR-1 to CCR2 knockout mice. This treatment extended survival by 3 days and preserved vascular integrity on day 6, as evidenced by leakage of Evans blue dye into the brain. Therefore, they concluded that CD8+ T cells may primarily serve to attract other effector populations. Potential therapies could involve reduction of myelomonocytic activation or targeting the CTL chemotactic mechanisms that recruit myelomonocytic cells (Kim et al., 2009).

Another study addressing LCMV-mediated death once again showed the importance of CD8+ T cells in generating the lethality of the disease. This study showed that CD8-deficient mice survived after i.c. injection of LCMV. Additionally, they showed that RAG knockout mice, which lack T and B cells, do not exhibit morbidity or mortality, thus providing evidence attributing these effects to immunopathology instead of viral damage. This group also addressed a possible connection between BBB disruption and LCMV pathogenesis through the use of Evans blue staining. While leakage of Evans blue dye was observed in C57BL/6 mice on day 5, before the onset of seizures, RAG knockout mice did not show signs of BBB disruption, indicating that BBB damage is induced by adaptive immunity. The role of perforin was also addressed in this study, with perforin knockout mice showing an intermediate phenotype after LCMV challenge and no clinical signs of the disease. However, surviving perforin knockout mice showed an increase in BBB disruption similar to C57BL/6 mice. Therefore, although BBB disruption occurs after LCMV infection, it may not be associated with mortality. This group proposed that other neuroanatomical changes, such as brain herniation, may be the most likely cause of mortality. Understanding the basis of LCMV neuropathogenesis may be helpful for designing therapies for viral hemorrhagic fevers in addition to ADEM and AHLE (Matullo et al., 2010).

9. Inducible model of severe vascular permeability: Peptide-Induced Fatal Syndrome (PIFS)

The Daniel's strain of Theiler's murine encephalomyelitis virus (TMEV) is a murine picornavirus that causes a transient early meningoencephalitis in all mouse strains, and persistent infection of the white matter with demyelination in susceptible strains (Njenga et al., 1997; Rodriguez & David, 1985; Rodriguez, 1986). During acute TMEV infection, mice of H-2^b haplotype mount an antiviral CD8 T cell response that is highly focused on an immunodominant TMEV peptide, $VP2_{121-130}$, presented in the context of the D^b class I molecule (Johnson et al., 1999; Johnson et al., 2001). It was demonstrated that intravenous injection of this $VP2_{121-130}$ peptide prior to TMEV infection inhibited VP2 peptide specific CD8 T cell expansion in the CNS and prevented IFN-γ receptor-/- mice from developing paralytic disease. However, injection of VP2 peptide during acute TMEV infection, after the expansion of D^b:$VP2_{121-130}$ epitope specific CD8 T cells in the CNS, resulted in death in 24 to 48 hours. It was determined that this fatal syndrome was antigen specific, because mice were asymptomatic when given the mock control D^b binding E7 peptide. In subsequent studies, our laboratory determined that CNS vascular permeability and hemorrhage are a major component of this condition. This peptide induced fatal syndrome (PIFS) is a readily reproducible means to investigate CD8 T cell-mediated CNS vascular permeability (Figure 6). The major advantage of this model system is that BBB disruption is inducible through administration of the antigenic VP2 peptide, enabling a kinetic analysis of early and late cellular and gene expression events. While BBB disruption is a common feature of numerous neurological conditions, the PIFS model with its high level of CNS vascular permeability, edema, rapid demyelination, and onset of multiple focal hemorrhages, most closely resembles AHLE (Figure 7).

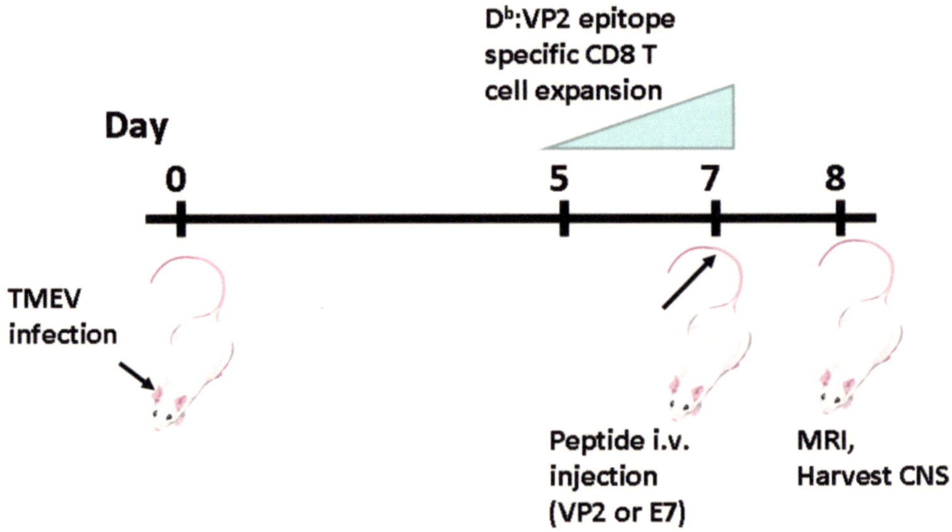

Fig. 6. Mouse model of CNS vascular permeability. CD8+ T cell-mediated vascular permeability is induced in C57BL/6 mice. Mice are intracranially infected with TMEV at day 0. During the peak of CD8 T cell expansion, mice are intravenously administered $VP2_{121\text{-}130}$ peptide to induce permeability or E7 control peptide. The CNS is harvested on the following day.

In addition to being mediated by antigen-specific CD8+ T cells, PIFS is influenced by perforin expression and genetic background. C57BL/6 perforin-deficient mice are resistant to this fatal syndrome. Another key determinant in the development of PIFS is the genetic background of the animal. While C57BL/6 mice are highly susceptible to PIFS, both FVB and 129 SvIm strains are significantly more resistant. Interestingly, this holds true despite these strains having a substantial population of antigen-specific CD8+ T cells (Johnson et al., 2005).

Another important aspect of the PIFS model is the observation that mice lacking major histocompatibility complex (MHC) class II, and thus CD4 T cells, IFN-γR, TNF-α, TNFR1, TNFR2, and TNFR1/TNFR2 still succumbed to the fatal syndrome. Inhibiting interleukin-1 and lymphotoxin-β did not serve to protect the mice from PIFS (Johnson et al., 2005). Therefore, it appears that the cytokines and CD4 T cell subsets heavily studied in other model systems of immune-mediated CNS vascular permeability do not play a role in the development of fatal blood brain barrier disruption in the PIFS model. However, removal of antigen-specific CD8+ T cells conferred protection, preventing mice from becoming moribund (Johnson et al., 2005). Suidan et al took this into consideration and investigated the contribution of the effector functions of CD8+ T cells, notably perforin and FasL, on disruption of the BBB and PIFS. It was first observed that the expansion of CNS infiltrating antigen-specific CD8+ T cells was not significantly different between C57BL/6 mice and C57BL/6 mice deficient in perforin or FasL. MRI analysis revealed that while C57BL/6 and C57BL/6 FasL deficient mice both exhibited extensive vascular permeability, mice lacking

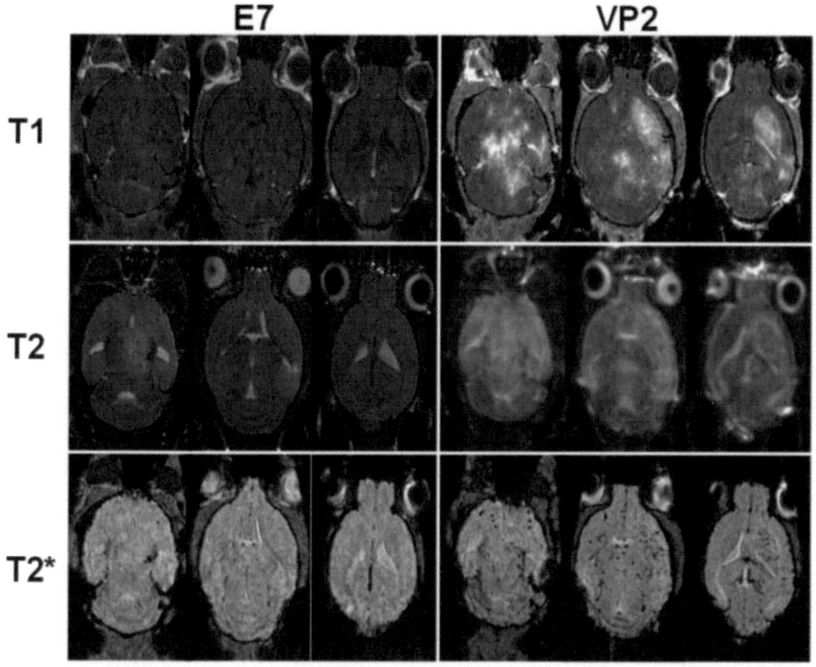

Fig. 7. In vivo MRI images of 8 day TMEV infected C57BL/6 mice, 24 hours after $VP2_{121-130}$ peptide injection (right panel) or irrelevant E7 peptide injection (left panel). Top row: axial images extracted from the gadolinium enhanced T1 weighted dataset demonstrate extensive contrast enhancement of confluent areas of the brain in the VP2 injected mouse, and very faint enhancement in the parahippocampal area in the E7 injected animal. Middle row: T2 weighted images demonstrate T2 hyperintensities, corresponding with areas of edema, inflammatory infiltrates, demyelination and tissue damage in the VP2 injected mouse; minimal hyperintense changes are also demonstrated in the parahippocampal areas of the E7 injected animal. Bottom row: T2* weighted images demonstrate punctuate T2 hypointensities, corresponding with areas of microhemorrhages in the VP2 injected mouse. (Reproduced with permission from Pirko, I., G. L. Suidan, et al. (2008). Acute hemorrhagic demyelination in a murine model of multiple sclerosis. *Journal of neuroinflammation* 5: 31).

perforin were protected. These same results were obtained when employing the FITC permeability assay, in which FITC-albumin is intravenously given to VP2 or E7 treated mice. Since albumin does not readily cross the BBB under normal conditions, this technique enables analysis of CNS vascular permeability with both microscopy and analysis of brain homogenate on an immunofluorescent plate reader. The combination of these two techniques, in addition to T1 gadolinium enhanced, T2 and T2* MRI, revealed that perforin, but not FasL, is essential for VP2 peptide induced CNS vascular permeability, edema and microhemorrhage formation, respectively. It was also found that astrocyte activation as measured by GFAP expression is dependent on perforin expression (Figure 8). High-resolution microscopy revealed the expression of GFAP co-localized with FITC-albumin leakage. This is important because astrocytes have been shown to be involved in regulation of BBB integrity (Suidan et al., 2008).

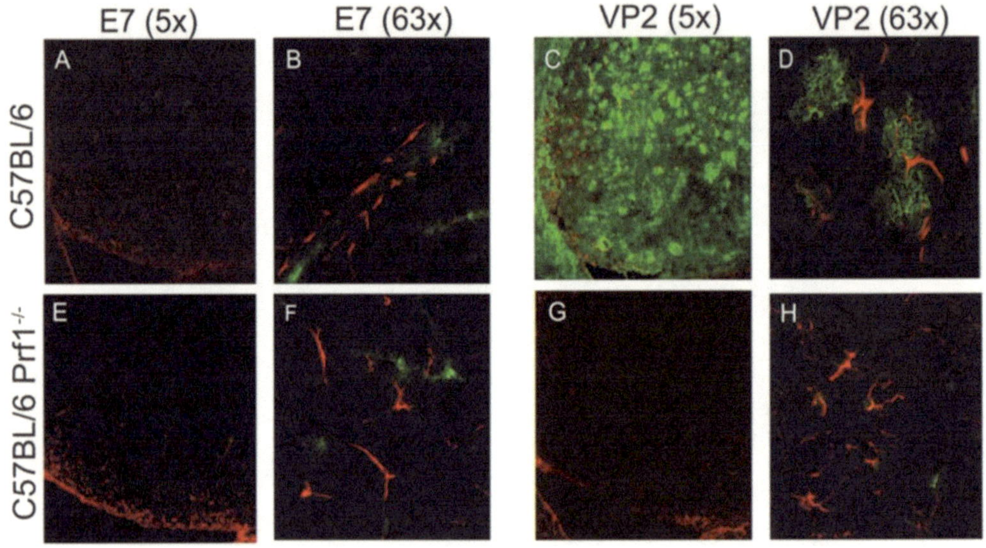

Fig. 8. Vascular permeability and astrocyte activation following administration of $VP2_{121-130}$ peptide is dependent on perforin expression. Tissue sections obtained from the brains of each animal were analyzed for astrocyte activation and vascular permeability as measured by leakage of FITC albumin into the CNS and expression of GFAP. Shown is GFAP expression and the extent of FITC-albumin leakage in the striatum of E7 control or $VP2_{121-130}$ peptide administered animals. Animals represented are (A) C57BL/6, E7 treatment, 5x, (B) C57BL/6, E7 treatment, 63x, (C) C57BL/6, $VP2_{121-130}$ treatment, 5x, (D) C57BL/6, $VP2_{121-130}$ treatment, 63x, (E) C57BL/6 Prf-/-, E7 treatment, 5x, (F) C57BL/6 Prf-/-, E7 treatment, 63x, (G) C57BL/6 Prf-/-, $VP2_{121-130}$ treatment, 5x, (H) C57BL/6 Prf-/-, $VP2_{121-130}$ treatment, 63x. (This figure was reproduced from Suidan, G. L., J. R. McDole, et al. (2008). Induction of blood brain barrier tight junction protein alterations by CD8 T cells. *PloS one* 3(8): e3037).

Time course experiments have been conducted in order to determine the sequence of events that occur in the development of PIFS. It was discovered that astrocyte activation and degradation of the tight junction protein occludin occur prior to peak levels of CNS vascular permeability and motor deficits. In accordance with the results from the LPS model employed by Brooks et al using the same microvessel isolation technique, it was found that expression of claudin-5 was significantly increased, while expression of occludin was significantly decreased. In both the LPS and the PIFS model, these alterations of tight junction protein levels coincide with BBB disruption. Furthermore, in the PIFS model, concurrent with a lack of vascular permeability, tight junction protein alterations were not observed in perforin-deficient mice. Additionally, to investigate the possibility that apoptosis is the cause of CNS vascular permeability, active caspase-3 protein levels were assessed. These levels did not increase until after peak levels of CNS vascular permeability, indicating that apoptosis does not initiate this permeability. In addition, the increase in claudin-5 levels serves as evidence that CECs were viable during peak permeability and not undergoing apoptosis (Suidan et al., 2008).

A putative mechanism of CD8+ T cell-mediated CNS vascular permeability is induction of vascular endothelial growth factor (VEGF) in the CNS. This cytokine has a highly vascular-permeating effect, and, along with its receptors, undergoes a change in expression following insult to the CNS (Deininger et al., 2003; Ferrara et al., 2003; Krum & Khaibullina, 2003; Krum et al., 2008; Lafuente et al., 2006; Proescholdt et al., 1999; Proescholdt, et al., 2002; Senger et al., 1983; Su et al., 2006; Srikiatkhachorn et al., 2007; Zhang et al., 2000). Because signal transduction through binding of VEGF to its receptor, fetal liver kinase-1 (flk-1), leads to vascular permeability, there may be an important role for this cytokine in disruption of the BBB during neuroinflammatory conditions (Ferrara et al., 2003). Through analysis of VEGF protein levels and FITC albumin-leakage into the brain, it was found that both VEGF protein and phosphorylation of flk-1 were significantly increased following administration of VP2 peptide. Coinciding with these increases was an increase in leakage of FITC-albumin, and thus CNS vascular permeability. During this permeability, in situ hybridization revealed that the major source of VEGF expression was neurons. Confocal microscopy further confirmed this by showing that immunostaining of the neuronal marker NeuN colocalizes VEGF cytokine (Suidan et al., 2010). However, since VEGF is not exclusively expressed by neurons clinically and in other model systems, alternative cell types, such as GR-1+ neutrophils, may also contribute to BBB disruption through a VEGF dependant mechanism.

Since it has been demonstrated that neuronal expression of VEGF occurred simultaneously with CD8 T cell-mediated CNS vascular permeability, VEGF had the potential to be a viable therapeutic target in neurological diseases such as AHLE. To investigate this possibility, Suidan et al administered the neuropilin-1 inhibitor, ATWLPPR, to 7-day TMEV-infected C57BL/6 mice given $VP2_{121-130}$ peptide or mock E7 peptide. Neuropilin-1 is a coreceptor for VEGF and has been shown to enhance processes mediated by the VEGF receptor flk-1 (Soker et al., 1998). Through analysis of FITC-albumin leakage into the brain, it was found that inhibition of neuropilin-1 with high doses of ATWLPPR VEGF inhibitor resulted in decreased CNS vascular permeability when compared to mice treated with PBS or scrambled RAPTLWP peptide. Furthermore, there was no significant difference between mice treated with VEGF inhibitor and mice treated with mock E7 peptide (Suidan et al., 2010). As previously reported using the PIFS model, degradation of the tight junction protein occludin occurs prior to CNS vascular permeability (Suidan et al., 2008). However, when mice were treated with ATWLPPR neuropilin-1 inhibitor, occludin protein levels were preserved, likely contributing to the maintenance of an impermeable BBB. Therefore, inhibition of VEGF-mediated pathways may serve as a strong therapeutic strategy for the treatment of neurological diseases characterized by BBB disruption.

The observation that high neuronal VEGF expression coincided with BBB disruption prompts the question of to what extent CNS-infiltrating CD8 T cells could actively engage Theiler's virus-infected neurons. This area of research has been controversial since neurons express little or no detectable levels of MHC class I (Corriveau et al., 1998; Horwitz et al., 1999; Joly et al., 1991; Neumann, et al., 1995; Rall et al., 1995). To address this controversy, GFP+ CD8+ cells were adoptively transferred to C57BL/6 mice, and it was found that these cells were highly specific for the D^b:$VP2_{121-130}$ epitope. The next major question is which cell types are potential targets for these cells. Confocal microscopy revealed that TMEV protein translation occurred in the hippocampus, striatum, hypothalamus, and cortex. Positive staining with the neuronal marker NeuN revealed that neurons were the main cell type translating virus protein. Furthermore, adoptively transferred GFP+ CD8+ cells were found in close proximity to TMEV infected neurons and their processes. (McDole et al., 2010). The finding that CD8 T cells engage neurons, as shown in Figure 9, also reveals a possible mechanism by which axonal and neuronal damage could take place in neuroinflammatory diseases such as AHLE and ADEM.

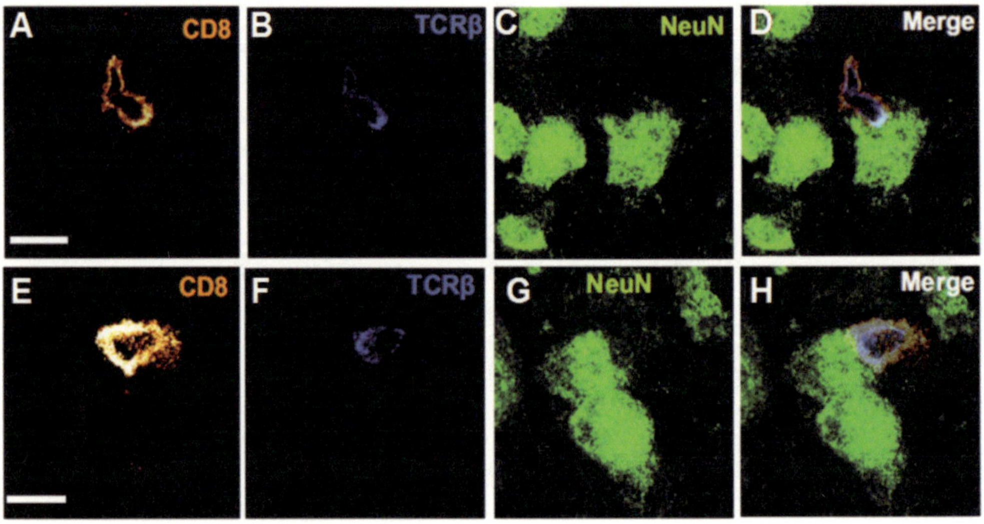

Fig. 9. CD8 T cells form immune synapses with target neurons. Both CD8 protein (**A** and **E**) and T cell receptor (**B** and **F**) polarized toward neurons (**C** and **G**) are highly indicative of an immune synapse. Merged images are shown (**D** and **H**). For **A–H**, results are representative of an analysis of eight mice. All microscopy was performed on hippocampus. Scale bars: 10 μm (This figure was reproduced from McDole, J.R., S.C. Danzer, et al. (2010). Rapid formation of extended processes and engagement of theiler's virus-infected neurons by CNS-infiltrating CD8 T cells. *The American Journal of Pathology* 177(4): 1823-1833. Permission was granted by Elsevier).

It is apparent that CD8 T cells and expression of VEGF contribute to BBB disruption in the PIFS model. However, it is possible that the NVU or other immune cell types, such as GR-1+ neutrophils, may also contribute to disruption of the BBB in accordance with previously published work with the LCMV models of BBB disruption highlighted above. These potential mechanisms of virus induced vascular permeability are illustrated in Figure 10. Traditional methods of neutrophil depletion, such as those used in the BBB studies of LCMV, employ the anti-GR-1 monoclonal antibody RB6-8C5. These studies conclude that neutrophils are the critical blood-derived cell type promoting BBB disruption (Kim et al., 2009). However, RB6-8C5 has been shown to bind to both Ly-6G on neutrophils and Ly-6C on lymphocytes and monocytes. Therefore, it is possible that GR-1-specific Ab depletion could also remove large numbers of activated CD8 T cells in addition to neutrophils. To address this controversy and determine whether CD8 T cells cause BBB disruption without the contribution of neutrophils, we have recently employed the TMEV model and used both the RB6-8C5 mAb and the Ly-6G-specific mAb 1A8 to deplete neutrophils *in vivo*. Ablation of epitope-specific CD8 T cells was seen in 7-day TMEV infected mice treated with RB6-8C5 but not those treated with 1A8 or normal rat serum. Therefore, the Ly-6G-specific mAb 1A8 is more selective for neutrophils in accordance with published results (Daley et al., 2008; Dunay et al., 2010). Additionally, anti-GR-1 depletion was shown to preserve motor function, as shown through assessment of the mice on a Rotamex Rotarod, and to reduce CNS vascular permeability as demonstrated by assaying FITC-albumin leakage into the CNS (data not shown). However, because 1A8 treatment somewhat reduced the levels of FITC-albumin leakage into the CNS, there may be a potential role for neutrophils in CD8 T cell initiated CNS vascular permeability, and this needs to be investigated further. Nevertheless, anti-GR-1 depletion strategies may hold promise as a potential therapeutic strategy for neurologic disorders characterized by altered permeability of the BBB.

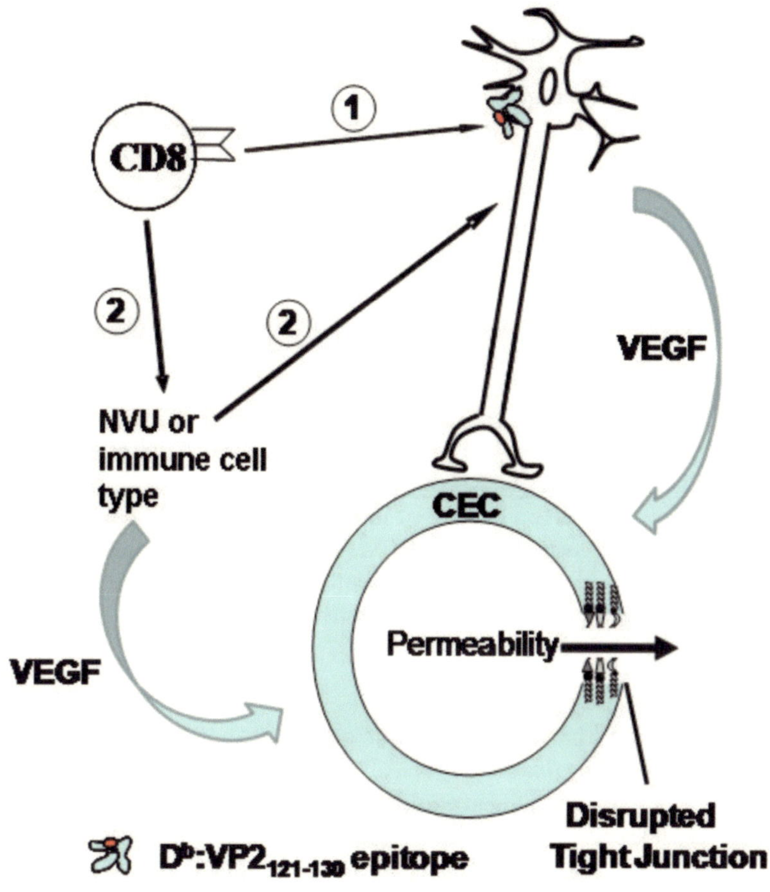

Fig. 10. BBB disruption in the PIFS model is induced through intravenous injection of VP2$_{121-130}$ peptide at 7 days post TMEV infection. At 7 days post TMEV infection, the CNS infiltrating D^b:VP2$_{121-130}$ specific CD8 T cell response peaks. Administration of VP2$_{121-130}$ peptide results in heightened activation of expanded CNS infiltrating D^b:VP2$_{121-130}$ specific CD8 T cells interacting with D^b class I expressing cells, which could include neurons, astrocytes, cerebral endothelial cells, pericytes and microglia. Our central hypothesis (1.) is that CD8 T cells engage neurons to promote upregulation of VEGF. Our alternative hypothesis (2.) is that CD8 T cells engage a different CNS cell type that results in BBB disruption and vascular permeability that is dependent or independent of neuronal VEGF.

10. Summary of the experimental model systems to illustrate the contribution of immune cells in BBB disruption

The EAE, LPS, and virus induced CNS vascular permeability model systems have enabled an understanding of how immune cells affect and alter CNS cell types of the neurovascular unit and ensuing BBB disruption. A defined role for CD4 T cells has been put forth through the EAE model, which also demonstrates that astrocyte-derived VEGF and IL-17 cause decreases in the tight junction proteins claudin-5 and occludin. The LPS model has portrayed a role for TNFα, activated microglia, and MMPs in BBB disruption. Similar to the EAE model, occludin has also been shown to be decreased in this model. However, claudin-3 and claudin-5 were found to be increased, and this coincided with BBB disruption. The virus induced models of vascular permeability have demonstrated a role for neutrophils, CD8 T cells, and VEGF. The LCMV model demonstrates an essential role for CD8 T cells in lethality, but puts emphasis on the fact that these cells may primarily serve to attract other effector populations, such as GR-1+ neutrophils. The PIFS model, which has the advantage of being inducible through the administration of an antigen peptide, also validates a role for CD8 T cells in contributing to CNS vascular permeability. Similar to the LPS model, the PIFS model also reveals a decrease in occludin and an increase in claudin-5, both of which are dependent on perforin expression. In accordance with the EAE model, VEGF is also shown to play a major role in BBB disruption. Furthermore, time course experiments using this model enabled the discovery of the order of events involved in BBB disruption, showing that astrocyte activation and degradation of occludin occur prior to CNS vascular permeability and motor deficits. Taken together, these models have put forward a defined role for neutrophils, CD4 and CD8 T cells, and VEGF in BBB disruption. This knowledge provides important information on the extent inflammatory immune cells contribute to CNS vascular permeability in diseases such as ADEM and AHLE. Therefore, continued efforts to control inflammation and dampen VEGF-mediated vascular permeability are important therapeutic approaches for treatment of these conditions.

11. Conclusion

Knowledge of the extent inflammatory immune cells contribute to disruption of the BBB is essential in order to develop treatments for ADEM and AHLE, two diseases that currently have no standard therapies and whose etiology is still not well understood. These potential therapies could also extend beyond ADEM and AHLE to other diseases characterized by increased BBB disruption, such as multiple sclerosis, viral hemorrhagic fevers, and cerebral malaria. The current experimental model systems available to address the contribution of inflammatory cells in BBB disruption open the door to several potential therapies. For example, it is apparent from both the EAE model and the PIFS model that targeting VEGF and inhibiting VEGF-mediated pathways may help ameliorate BBB disruption. In support of this therapeutic approach, we have determined that inhibition of neuropilin-1, a co-receptor for VEGF, decreased CNS vascular permeability (Suidan 2010). It is also evident through the EAE model that targeting the signaling pathways of occludin, the mechanisms of proinflammatory cytokines such as IL-17, and the tight junction architecture may provide avenues for potential therapeutic approaches. Results obtained from the LPS model demonstrate that directing research at MMP inhibitors and targeting microglia to potentially stop the production of inflammatory factors may also be valuable tools. The LCMV model portrays a need to investigate reducing myelomonocytic activation or targeting CTL chemotactic mechanisms that recruit myelomonocytic cells as a potential means of treatment. Finally, the PIFS model demonstrates that strategies that target CD8 T cells and VEGF cytokine may hold promise as potential therapies to ameliorate severe BBB disruption. Future research in these areas as well as in additional mechanisms by which immune cells cause BBB disruption will aid in the development of more specific therapies to address these devastating immune-mediated neurological disorders.

12. References

Abbott, N. J. (2002). Astrocyte-endothelial interactions and blood-brain barrier permeability. *Journal of Anatomy* 200(6): 629-638.

Abbott, N. J. (2005). Dynamics of CNS barriers: evolution, differentiation, and modulation. *Cellular and molecular neurobiology* 25(1): 5-23.

Abbott, N. J., L. Ronnback, et al. (2006). Astrocyte-endothelial interactions at the blood-brain barrier. *Nature Reviews Neuroscience* 7(1): 41-53.

Antonetti, D. A., A. J. Barber, et al. (1999). Vascular endothelial growth factor induces rapid phosphorylation of tight junction proteins occludin and zonula occluden 1 - A potential mechanism for vascular permeability in diabetic retinopathy and tumors. *Journal of Biological Chemistry* 274(33): 23463-23467.

Argaw, A. T., B. T. Gurfein, et al. (2009). VEGF-mediated disruption of endothelial CLN-5 promotes blood-brain barrier breakdown. *Proceedings of the National Academy of Sciences of the United States of America* 106(6): 1977-1982.

Ballabh, P., A. Braun, et al. (2004). The blood-brain barrier: an overview - Structure, regulation, and clinical implications. *Neurobiology of disease* 16(1): 1-13.

Befort, P., N. Gaillard, et al. (2010). Hemorrhagic leukoencephalitis linked to Epstein-Barr virus in an adult patient. *Clinical Neurology and Neurosurgery* 112: 829-831.

Begley, D. J. (2004). Delivery of therapeutic agents to the central nervous system: the problems and the possibilities. *Pharmacology & therapeutics* 104(1): 29-45.

Bennett, J., J. Basivireddy, et al. (2010). Blood-brain barrier disruption and enhanced vascular permeability in the multiple sclerosis model EAE. *Journal of Neuroimmunology* 229(1-2): 180-191.

Blamire, A. M., D. C. Anthony, et al. (2000). Interleukin-1beta -induced changes in blood-brain barrier permeability, apparent diffusion coefficient, and cerebral blood volume in the rat brain: a magnetic resonance study. *J Neurosci* 20(21): 8153-8159.

Brooks, T. A., B. T. Hawkins, et al. (2005). Chronic inflammatory pain leads to increased blood-brain barrier permeability and tight junction protein alterations. *American journal of physiology. Heart and circulatory physiology* 289(2): H738-743.

Burns, A. R., R. A. Bowden, et al. (2000). Analysis of tight junctions during neutrophil transendothelial migration. *Journal of Cell Science* 113(1): 45-57.

Callen, D. J. A., M. M. Shroff, et al. (2009). Role of MRI in the differentiation of ADEM from MS in children. *Neurology* 72(11): 968-973.

Carmeliet, P., V. Ferreira, et al. (1996). Abnormal blood vessel development and lethality in embryos lacking a single VEGF allele. *Nature* 380(6573): 435-439.

Carmeliet, P. and E. Storkebaum (2002). Vascular and neuronal effects of VEGF in the nervous system: implications for neurological disorders. *Seminars in cell & developmental biology* 13(1): 39-53.

Cauli, B., X. K. Tong, et al. (2004). Cortical GABA interneurons in neurovascular coupling: relays for subcortical vasoactive pathways. *The Journal of neuroscience : the official journal of the Society for Neuroscience* 24(41): 8940-8949.

Chen, L. and C. F. Brosnan (2006). Exacerbation of experimental autoimmune encephalomyelitis in P2X7R-/- mice: evidence for loss of apoptotic activity in lymphocytes. *Journal of immunology* 176(5): 3115-3126.

Chi, O. Z., C. Hunter, et al. (2005). Effects of VEGF and nitric oxide synthase inhibition on blood-brain barrier disruption in the ischemic and non-ischemic cerebral cortex. *Neurological research* 27(8): 864-868.

Corriveau, R. A., G. S. Huh, et al. (1998). Regulation of class I MHC gene expression in the developing and mature CNS by neural activity. *Neuron* 21(3): 505-520.

Crews, F. T., L. Y. Qin, et al. (2007). Systemic LPS causes chronic neuroinflammation and progressive neurodegeneration. *Glia* 55(5): 453-462.

Dale, R. C., C. de Sousa, et al. (2000). Acute disseminated encephalomyelitis, multiphasic disseminated encephalomyelitis and multiple sclerosis in children. *Brain : a journal of neurology* 123 Pt 12: 2407-2422.

Daley, J. M., A. A. Thomay, et al. (2008). Use of Ly6G-specific monoclonal antibody to deplete neutrophils in mice. *Journal of Leukocyte Biology* 83(1): 64-70.

Deininger, M. H., S. Winkler, et al. (2003). Angiogenic proteins in brains of patients who died with cerebral malaria. *Journal of Neuroimmunology* 142(1-2): 101-111.

Demeuse, P., A. Kerkhofs, et al. (2002). Compartmentalized coculture of rat brain endothelial cells and astrocytes: a syngenic model to study the blood-brain barrier. *Journal of neuroscience methods* 121(1): 21-31.

Didier, N., I. A. Romero, et al. (2003). Secretion of interleukin-1beta by astrocytes mediates endothelin-1 and tumour necrosis factor-alpha effects on human brain microvascular endothelial cell permeability. *Journal of neurochemistry* 86(1): 246-254.

Dohgu, S., F. Takata, et al. (2005). Brain pericytes contribute to the induction and up-regulation of blood-brain barrier functions through transforming growth factor-beta production. *Brain research* 1038(2): 208-215.

Dohgu, S., F. Takata, et al. (2005). Brain pericytes contribute to the induction and up-regulation of blood-brain barrier functions through transforming growth factor-beta production. *Brain Res* 1038(2): 208-215.

Dunay, I.R., A. Fuchs, et al. (2010). Inflammatory monocytes but not neutrophils are necessary to control infection with Toxoplasma gondii in mice. *Infection and Immunity* 78(4): 1564-1570.Esser, S., K. Wolburg, et al. (1998). Vascular endothelial growth factor induces endothelial fenestrations in vitro. *Journal of Cell Biology* 140(4): 947-959.

Fanning, A. S., L. L. Mitic, et al. (1999). Transmembrane proteins in the tight junction barrier. *Journal of the American Society of Nephrology : JASN* 10(6): 1337-1345.

Feng, D., J. A. Nagy, et al. (1999). Pathways of macromolecular extravasation across microvascular endothelium in response to VPF VEGF and other vasoactive mediators. *Microcirculation* 6(1): 23-44.

Ferrara, N., K. Carver-Moore, et al. (1996). Heterozygous embryonic lethality induced by targeted inactivation of the VEGF gene. *Nature* 380(6573): 439-442.

Ferrara, N., H. P. Gerber, et al. (2003). The biology of VEGF and its receptors. *Nature medicine* 9(6): 669-676.

Ferrari, C. C., A. M. Depino, et al. (2004). Reversible demyelination, blood-brain barrier breakdown, and pronounced neutrophil recruitment induced by chronic IL-1 expression in the brain. *American Journal of Pathology* 165(5): 1827-1837.

Fugate, J.E., E. Lam, et al. (2010). Acute hemorrhagic leukoencephalitis and hypoxic brain injury associated with H1N1 influenza. *Archives of Neurology* 67(6): 756-758.S

Geerts, Y., I. Dehaene, et al. (1991). Acute hemorrhagic leukoencephalitis. *Acta neurologica Belgica* 91(4): 201-211.

Gibbs, W. N., M. A. Kreidie, et al. (2005). Acute hemorrhagic leukoencephalitis - Neuroimaging features and neuropathologic diagnosis. *Journal of Computer Assisted Tomography* 29(5): 689-693.

Gurfein, B. T., Y. Zhang, et al. (2009). IL-11 regulates autoimmune demyelination. *Journal of immunology* 183(7): 4229-4240.

Gurney, K. J., E. Y. Estrada, et al. (2006). Blood-brain barrier disruption by stromelysin-1 facilitates neutrophil infiltration in neuroinflammation. *Neurobiology of disease* 23(1): 87-96.

Hamel, E. (2006). Perivascular nerves and the regulation of cerebrovascular tone. *Journal of Applied Physiology* 100(3): 1059-1064.

Hart, M. N. and K. M. Earle (1975). Haemorrhagic and perivenous encephalitis: a clinical-pathological review of 38 cases. *Journal of neurology, neurosurgery, and psychiatry* 38(6): 585-591.

Haseloff, R. F., I. E. Blasig, et al. (2005). In search of the astrocytic factor(s) modulating blood-brain barrier functions in brain capillary endothelial cells in vitro. *Cellular and molecular neurobiology* 25(1): 25-39.

Hawkins, B. T. and T. P. Davis (2005). The blood-brain barrier/neurovascular unit in health and disease. *Pharmacological reviews* 57(2): 173-185.

Hayashi, T., K. Abe, et al. (1997). Rapid induction of vascular endothelial growth factor gene expression after transient middle cerebral artery occlusion in rats. *Stroke; a journal of cerebral circulation* 28(10): 2039-2044.

Hayashi, Y., M. Nomura, et al. (1997). Induction of various blood-brain barrier properties in non-neural endothelial cells by close apposition to co-cultured astrocytes. *Glia* 19(1): 13-26.

Hellstrom, M., H. Gerhardt, et al. (2001). Lack of pericytes leads to endothelial hyperplasia and abnormal vascular morphogenesis. *The Journal of cell biology* 153(3): 543-553.

Horwitz, M. S., C. F. Evans, et al. (1999). Detailed in vivo analysis of interferon-gamma induced major histocompatibility complex expression in the the central nervous system: astrocytes fail to express major histocompatibility complex class I and II molecules. *Laboratory investigation; a journal of technical methods and pathology* 79(2): 235-242.

Huppert, J., D. Closhen, et al. (2010). Cellular mechanisms of IL-17-induced blood-brain barrier disruption. *Faseb Journal* 24(4): 1023-1034.

Ildiko R. Dunay, A. F., and L. David Sibley (2010). Inflammatory Monocytes but Not Neutrophils Are Necessary To Control Infection with Toxoplasma gondii in Mice. *Infection and Immunity* 78: 1564-1570.

Ingo Bechmann, I. G., V. Hugh Perry (2007). What is the blood–brain barrier (not)?. *Trends in Immunology* 28(1): 5-11.

Ishida, A., J. Murray, et al. (2001). Expression of vascular endothelial growth factor receptors in smooth muscle cells. *Journal of cellular physiology* 188(3): 359-368.

Issa, R., J. Krupinski, et al. (1999). Vascular endothelial growth factor and its receptor, KDR, in human brain tissue after ischemic stroke. *Laboratory investigation; a journal of technical methods and pathology* 79(4): 417-425.

Itoh, M., M. Furuse, et al. (1999). Direct binding of three tight junction-associated MAGUKs, ZO-1, ZO-2, and ZO-3, with the COOH termini of claudins. *The Journal of cell biology* 147(6): 1351-1363.

Janzer, R. C. and M. C. Raff (1987). Astrocytes induce blood-brain barrier properties in endothelial cells. *Nature* 325(6101): 253-257.

Johnson, A.J., M.K. Njenga, et al. (1999). Prevalent class I-restricted T-cell response to the Theiler's virus epitope D^b:$VP2_{121-130}$ in the absence of endogenous CD4 help, tumor necrosis factor alpha, gamma interferon, perforin, or costimulation through CD28. *Journal of Virology* 73(5): 3702-3708.

Johnson, A.J., J. Upshaw, et al. (2001). Preservation of motor function by inhibition of CD8+ virus peptide-specific T cells in Theiler's virus infection. *The FASEB Journal* 15(14): 2760-2762.

Johnson, A. J., Y. Mendez-Fernandez, et al. (2005). Antigen-specific CD8+ T cells mediate a peptide-induced fatal syndrome. *Journal of immunology* 174(11): 6854-6862.

Joly, E., L. Mucke, et al. (1991). "Viral persistence in neurons explained by lack of major histocompatibility class I expression. *Science* 253(5025): 1283-1285.

Kagi, D., B. Ledermann, et al. (1994). Cytotoxicity mediated by T cells and natural killer cells is greatly impaired in perforin-deficient mice. *Nature* 369(6475): 31-37.

Karamysheva, A. F. (2008). Mechanisms of angiogenesis. *Biochemistry. Biokhimiia* 73(7): 751-762.

Kebir, H., K. Kreymborg, et al. (2007). Human TH17 lymphocytes promote blood-brain barrier disruption and central nervous system inflammation. *Nature medicine* 13(10): 1173-1175.

Kim, J. V., S. S. Kang, et al. (2009). Myelomonocytic cell recruitment causes fatal CNS vascular injury during acute viral meningitis. *Nature* 457(7226): 191-195.

Koehler, R. C., D. Gebremedhin, et al. (2006). Role of astrocytes in cerebrovascular regulation. *Journal of Applied Physiology* 100(1): 307-317.

Krizanac-Bengez, L., M. Kapural, et al. (2003). Effects of transient loss of shear stress on blood-brain barrier endothelium: role of nitric oxide and IL-6. *Brain research* 977(2): 239-246.

Krum, J. M. and A. Khaibullina (2003). Inhibition of endogenous VEGF impedes revascularization and astroglial proliferation: roles for VEGF in brain repair. *Experimental neurology* 181(2): 241-257.

Krum, J. M., N. Mani, et al. (2008). Roles of the endogenous VEGF receptors flt-1 and flk-1 in astroglial and vascular remodeling after brain injury. *Experimental neurology* 212(1): 108-117.

Laflamme, N., S. Lacroix, and S. Rivest (1999). An essential role of interleukin-1beta in mediating NF-kappaB activity and COX-2 transcription in cells of the blood-brain barrier in response to a systemic and localized inflammation but not during endotoxemia. *J Neurosci* 19: 10923-10930.

Lafuente, J. V., E. G. Argandona, et al. (2006). VEGFR-2 expression in brain injury: its distribution related to brain-blood barrier markers. *Journal of Neural Transmission* 113(4): 487-496.

Lai, C. H., K. H. Kuo, et al. (2005). Critical role of actin in modulating BBB permeability. *Brain research. Brain research reviews* 50(1): 7-13.

Mack, C. L., C. L. Vanderlugt-Castaneda, et al. (2003). Microglia are activated to become competent antigen presenting and effector cells in the inflammatory environment of the Theiler's virus model of multiple sclerosis. *Journal of Neuroimmunology* 144(1-2): 68-79.

Marchi, N., Q. Fan, et al. (2009). Antagonism of peripheral inflammation reduces the severity of status epilepticus. *Neurobiology of disease* 33(2): 171-181.

Marti, H. H. and W. Risau (1998). Systemic hypoxia changes the organ-specific distribution of vascular endothelial growth factor and its receptors. *Proceedings of the National Academy of Sciences of the United States of America* 95(26): 15809-15814.

Marti, H. J., M. Bernaudin, et al. (2000). Hypoxia-induced vascular endothelial growth factor expression precedes neovascularization after cerebral ischemia. *The American journal of pathology* 156(3): 965-976.

Matullo, C. M., K. J. O'Regan, et al. (2010). Lymphocytic choriomeningitis virus-induced mortality in mice is triggered by edema and brain herniation. *Journal of virology* 84(1): 312-320.

Maxwell, K., J. A. Berliner, et al. (1987). Induction of gamma-glutamyl transpeptidase in cultured cerebral endothelial cells by a product released by astrocytes. *Brain research* 410(2): 309-314.

McDole, J.R., S.C. Danzer, et al. (2010). Rapid formation of extended processes and engagement of theiler's virus-infected neurons by CNS-infiltrating CD8 T cells. *The American Journal of Pathology* 177(4): 1823-1833.

Minagar, A. and J. S. Alexander (2003). Blood-brain barrier disruption in multiple sclerosis. *Multiple sclerosis* 9(6): 540-549.

Morgan, L., B. Shah, et al. (2007). Inflammation and dephosphorylation of the tight junction protein occludin in an experimental model of multiple sclerosis. *Neuroscience* 147(3): 664-673.

Neuhaus, J., W. Risau, et al. (1991). Induction of blood-brain barrier characteristics in bovine brain endothelial cells by rat astroglial cells in transfilter coculture. *Annals of the New York Academy of Sciences* 633: 578-580.

Neumann, H., A. Cavalie, et al. (1995). Induction of MHC class I genes in neurons. *Science* 269(5223): 549-552.

Njenga, M. K., K. Asakura, et al. (1997). The immune system preferentially clears Theiler's virus from the gray matter of the central nervous system. *Journal of virology* 71(11): 8592-8601.

Olsson, A. K., A. Dimberg, et al. (2006). VEGF receptor signalling - in control of vascular function. *Nature reviews. Molecular cell biology* 7(5): 359-371.

Paul, R., U. Koedel, et al. (2003). Lack of IL-6 augments inflammatory response but decreases vascular permeability in bacterial meningitis. *Brain : a journal of neurology* 126(Pt 8): 1873-1882.

Petty, M. A. and E. H. Lo (2002). Junctional complexes of the blood-brain barrier: permeability changes in neuroinflammation. *Progress in neurobiology* 68(5): 311-323.

Pinto, P.S., R. Taipa, et al. (2011). Acute hemorrhagic leukoencephalitis with severe brainstem and spinal cord involvement: MRI features with neuropathological confirmation. *Journal of Magnetic Resonance Imaging* 33: 957-961.

Pirko, I., G. L. Suidan, et al. (2008). Acute hemorrhagic demyelination in a murine model of multiple sclerosis. *Journal of neuroinflammation* 5: 31.

Plate, K. H., H. Beck, et al. (1999). Cell type specific upregulation of vascular endothelial growth factor in an MCA-occlusion model of cerebral infarct. *Journal of neuropathology and experimental neurology* 58(6): 654-666.

Posey, K., J. N. Alpert, et al. (1994). Acute hemorrhagic leukoencephalitis: a cause of acute brainstem dysfunction. *Southern medical journal* 87(8): 851-854.

Proescholdt, M. A., J. D. Heiss, et al. (1999). Vascular endothelial growth factor (VEGF) modulates vascular permeability and inflammation in rat brain. *Journal of neuropathology and experimental neurology* 58(6): 613-627.

Proescholdt, M. A., S. Jacobson, et al. (2002). Vascular endothelial growth factor is expressed in multiple sclerosis plaques and can induce inflammatory lesions in experimental allergic encephalomyelitis rats. *Journal of neuropathology and experimental neurology* 61(10): 914-925.

Rall, G. F., L. Mucke, et al. (1995). Consequences of cytotoxic T lymphocyte interaction with major histocompatibility complex class I-expressing neurons in vivo. *The Journal of experimental medicine* 182(5): 1201-1212.

Ramsauer, M., D. Krause, et al. (2002). Angiogenesis of the blood-brain barrier in vitro and the function of cerebral pericytes. *FASEB J* 16(10): 1274-1276.

Roberts, W. G. and G. E. Palade (1995). Increased Microvascular Permeability and Endothelial Fenestration Induced by Vascular Endothelial Growth-Factor. *Journal of Cell Science* 108: 2369-2379.

Rodriguez, M., and David, C.S. (1986). Immune-mediated injury of virus-infected oligodendrocytes. *Immunol. Today* 7: 9-363.

Rodriguez, M. and C. S. David (1985). Demyelination induced by Theiler's virus: influence of the H-2 haplotype. *Journal of immunology* 135(3): 2145-2148.

Rust, R. S. (2000). Multiple sclerosis, acute disseminated encephalomyelitis, and related conditions. *Seminars in pediatric neurology* 7(2): 66-90.

Schoch, H. J., S. Fischer, et al. (2002). Hypoxia-induced vascular endothelial growth factor expression causes vascular leakage in the brain. *Brain : a journal of neurology* 125: 2549-2557.

Schroeter, M. L., S. Muller, et al. (2001). Astrocytes induce manganese superoxide dismutase in brain capillary endothelial cells. *Neuroreport* 12(11): 2513-2517.

Senger, D. R., S. J. Galli, et al. (1983). Tumor cells secrete a vascular permeability factor that promotes accumulation of ascites fluid. *Science* 219(4587): 983-985.

Shulman, K., S. Rosen, et al. (1996). Expression of vascular permeability factor (VPF/VEGF) is altered in many glomerular diseases. *Journal of the American Society of Nephrology* 7(5): 661-666.

Siddharthan, V., Y. V. Kim, et al. (2007). Human astrocytes/astrocyte-conditioned medium and shear stress enhance the barrier properties of human brain microvascular endothelial cells. *Brain research* 1147: 39-50.

Smith (2007). Primary porcine brain microvascular endothelial cells: Biochemical and functional characterisation as a model for drug transport and targeting (vol 15, pg 253, 2007). *Journal of Drug Targeting* 15(6): 454-454.

Sobue, K., N. Yamamoto, et al. (1999). Induction of blood-brain barrier properties in immortalized bovine brain endothelial cells by astrocytic factors. *Neuroscience research* 35(2): 155-164.

Soker, S., S. Takashima, et al. (1998). Neuropilin-1 is expressed by endothelial and tumor cells as an isoform-specific receptor for vascular endothelial growth factor. *Cell* 92(6): 735-745.

Srikiatkhachorn, A., C. Ajariyakhajorn, et al. (2007). Virus-induced decline in soluble vascular endothelial growth receptor 2 is associated with plasma leakage in dengue hemorrhagic Fever. *Journal of virology* 81(4): 1592-1600.

Stoll, G., S. Jander, et al. (2000). Cytokines in CNS disorders: neurotoxicity versus neuroprotection. *Journal of neural transmission. Supplementum* 59: 81-89.

Storm, P., C. Bartholdy, et al. (2006). Perforin-deficient CD8+ T cells mediate fatal lymphocytic choriomeningitis despite impaired cytokine production. *Journal of virology* 80(3): 1222-1230.

Su, J. J., M. Osoegawa, et al. (2006). Upregulation of vascular growth factors in multiple sclerosis: Correlation with MRI findings. *Journal of the neurological sciences* 243(1-2): 21-30.

Suchowersky, O., V. P. Sweeney, et al. (1983). Acute hemorrhagic leukoencephalopathy. A clinical, pathological, and radiological correlation. *The Canadian journal of neurological sciences. Le journal canadien des sciences neurologiques* 10(1): 63-67.

Suidan, G. L., J. W. Dickerson, et al. (2010). CD8 T cell-initiated vascular endothelial growth factor expression promotes central nervous system vascular permeability under neuroinflammatory conditions. *Journal of immunology* 184(2): 1031-1040.

Suidan, G. L., J. R. McDole, et al. (2008). Induction of blood brain barrier tight junction protein alterations by CD8 T cells. *PloS one* 3(8): e3037.

Tenembaum, S., N. Chamoles, et al. (2002). Acute disseminated encephalomyelitis: a long-term follow-up study of 84 pediatric patients. *Neurology* 59(8): 1224-1231.

Tsukita, S., M. Furuse, et al. (1999). Structural and signalling molecules come together at tight junctions. *Current Opinion in Cell Biology* 11(5): 628-633.

Vidensky, S., Y. Zhang, et al. (2003). Neuronal overexpression of COX-2 results in dominant production of PGE2 and altered fever response. *Neuromolecular medicine* 3(1): 15-28.

Wang, G., W. Li, et al. (2010). Acute encephalopathy and encephalitis caused by influenza virus infection. *Current Opinion in Neurology*23: 305-311.

Weis, S. M. and D. A. Cheresh (2005). Pathophysiological consequences of VEGF-induced vascular permeability. *Nature* 437(7058): 497-504.

Wolburg, H. and A. Lippoldt (2002). Tight junctions of the blood-brain barrier: development, composition and regulation. *Vascular pharmacology* 38(6): 323-337.

Wolburg, H., K. Wolburg-Buchholz, et al. (2005). Diapedesis of mononuclear cells across cerebral venules during experimental autoimmune encephalomyelitis leaves tight junctions intact. *Acta Neuropathologica* 109(2): 181-190.

Wong, D., K. Dorovini-Zis, et al. (2004). Cytokines, nitric oxide, and cGMP modulate the permeability of an in vitro model of the human blood-brain barrier. *Experimental neurology* 190(2): 446-455.

Zhang, Z. G., L. Zhang, et al. (2000). VEGF enhances angiogenesis and promotes blood-brain barrier leakage in the ischemic brain. *Journal of Clinical Investigation* 106(7): 829-838.

Zhao, C., Z. Ling, et al. (2007). TNF-alpha knockout and minocycline treatment attenuates blood-brain barrier leakage in MPTP-treated mice. *Neurobiology of disease* 26(1): 36-46.

Zlokovic, B. V. (2008). The blood-brain barrier in health and chronic neurodegenerative disorders. *Neuron* 57(2): 178-201.

20

Development of Human and Macaque Antibodies Using Antibody Phage Display for the Detection of Equine Encephalitis Viruses

Philippe Thullier[1], Birgit Hülseweh[2], Thibaut Pelat[1], Torsten Rülker[3], Sebastian Miethe[3], Stefan Dübel[3] and Michael Hust[3,*]
[1]Groupe de biotechnologie des anticorps, Département de biologie des agents transmissibles, Centre de Recherche du Service de Santé des Armées
[2]Armed Forces Scientific Institute for Protection Technologies – NBC Protection (WIS)
[3]Technische Universität Braunschweig, Institut für Biochemie und Biotechnologie
[1]France
[2,3]Germany

1. Introduction

Antibody phage display is an *in vitro* technology to generate recombinant antibodies. In particular for pathogens or toxins, antibody phage display is an alternative to hybridoma technology, since it circumvents the limitations of the immune system. Furthermore, phage display allows generation of human antibodies when either immunised patients are not available or immunisation is not ethically feasible.

Equine encephalitis viruses, like VEEV, WEEV and EEEV, belong to the Alphavirus group. Several species and subspecies of this family are pathogenic for man and are recognized as potential agents of biological warfare and terrorism. In this review, we describe the generation of human antibodies from naive antibody gene libraries and macaque antibodies from immune antibody gene libraries. Furthermore, we give an overview about phage display derived recombinant antibodies against equine encephalitis viruses for diagnostics and therapy.

2. Short introduction to encephalitis viruses

Venezuelan equine encephalitis virus (VEEV), Western equine encephalitis virus (WEEV) and Eastern equine encephalitis virus (EEEV) were first isolated in the 1930s and belong to the Alphavirus genus within the *Togaviridae* family (Giltner and Shahan, 1933; King, 1939; Kubes and Ríos, 1939; Meyer et al., 1931; Powers et al., 2001; Weaver et al., 2004). Mosquitoes are the biological vectors of theses viruses and equine species and man are periodically infected

* Corresponding Author

(Strauss and Strauss, 1994). In the past epidemics caused by these viruses occured in North, Central and South America. These viruses can spread to the human central nervous system (CNS) causing symptoms ranging from mild febrile reactions to encephalitis, often resulting in fatal and permanent neurologic damages. The severity of the illness depends on virus strain, age of patients as well as dose and route of infection (Calisher, 1994; Deresiewicz et al., 1997; Feemster, 1938; Hoke, 2005; Leitenberg, 2001; Letson et al., 1993; Rivas et al., 1997; Rozdilsky et al., 1968; Sanchez et al., 1984; Sellers and Maarouf, 1993; Sudia et al., 1975; Weaver et al., 1996). Moreover, alphaviruses can be produced in large quantities, are moderately easy to disseminate and are highly infectious as aerosols (Phillpotts, 2006; Reed et al., 2005). Therefore, VEEV, WEEV and EEEV are potential biological weapons (Hawley and Eitzen, 2001). All three encephalitis virus species are classified as Bioterrorism Agent Category B by the Center of Disease Control (CDC) (http://www.bt.cdc.gov/agent/agentlist-category.asp).

For rapid detection, diagnosis and treatment of VEEV, WEEV and EEEV antibodies are indispensable tools and potential therapeutics.

3. Antibody phage display

Production of polyclonal antibodies by immunisation of animals is a method established for more than a century. The first antibody serum was produced in horses and directed against diphtheria (von Behring and Kitasato, 1890). Hybridoma technology was the next milestone, allowing the production of monoclonal antibodies (Köhler and Milstein, 1975). Hybridoma technology has drawbacks like limited number of candidates, possible instability of aneuploid cell lines (Pauza et al., 1993), inability to provide antibodies against highly conserved antigens and most of all its limited application to generate human antibodies (Winter and Milstein, 1991). Hybridoma technology thus essentially allows isolation of murine antibodies which have a broad detection range and can be applied for diagnostic or research uses. However, their therapeutic applications are limited because repeated administration of murine antibodies can cause human anti-mouse antibody reaction (HAMA), in turn leading to a diminution of the antibody half-life and to severe side effects including anaphylactic side effects (Courtenay-Luck et al., 1986; Tjandra et al., 1990). These difficulties might be alleviated by engineering these antibodies to reduce their fraction of murine origin. Chimerised antibodies have murine variable regions, retaining binding capacity of the original murine antibody, expressed in fusion with human constant regions. But, these variable murine regions are still large enough to be a cause for adverse reactions so that the smaller hypervariable regions, in direct contact with the antigen, might be preferred as the only murine part retained in the therapeutic molecule. The corresponding engineering process is known as humanisation, which is however more difficult to implement than chimerisation. Another possibility is to utilise transgenic mice whose loci coding antibodies have been replaced by their human counterparts. With these mice, human antibodies can be generated by hybridoma technology but these transgenic animals are available in a very limited number of laboratories only (Fishwild et al., 1996; Jakobovits, 1995; Lonberg and Huszar, 1995; Nelson et al., 2010). For the isolation of antibodies directed against toxins, animals are immunised by non-toxic subunits or even selected domains from these subunits (Pelat et al., 2009a; Pelat et al., 2007; Scotcher et al., 2010; Winterroth et al., 2010).

A technology which circumvents the limitations of the immune system is antibody phage display. This technology is completely independent from any immune system by an *in vitro* selection process. The display method most commonly used today is based on the work of

George P. Smith (Smith, 1985) on filamentous phage, which infect *E. coli*. By this technology, genotype and phenotype of a polypeptide e.g. an antibody are linked by fusing the antibody-encoding DNA to the coat protein III gene (gIII) of the filamentous bacteriophage M13. The resulting antibody::pIII fusion protein is displayed on the surface of phage particles, thus allowing affinity isolation of the antibody and consequently the purification of its coding DNA present within the phage (Breitling et al., 1991; Clackson et al., 1991; McCafferty et al., 1990).
In fact only antibody fragments like single chain fragment variable (scFv) or fragment antigen binding (Fab) are used routinely for phage display (Hoet et al., 2005; Hust et al., 2010), due to limitations of the *E. coli* protein folding machinery which can express full-sized IgGs only in rare cases (Mazor et al., 2007; Simmons et al., 2002). ScFv fragments consist of the variable domains of the heavy and light chain (Fv fragment) connected by a peptide linker (Bird et al., 1988; Huston et al., 1988). Other used formats for phage display are single chain Fabs (scFab), human VH domains (dAbs) and the variable domains of camel heavy chains (VHHs) (Holt et al., 2003; Hust et al., 2007b; Muyldermans, 2001; Muyldermans et al., 2009). Another interesting „antibody" format for phage display are immunoglobulins of sharks (IgNARs), which are very resistant to denaturation and well suitable for diagnostics. (Flajnik and Dooley, 2009; Nuttall et al., 2001; Nuttall et al., 2004).
The phage-displayed libraries are built from immunised or non-immunised lymphocyte donors or from synthetic repertoires. Libraries using the naïve IgM repertoire - the primary immune response - of a donor or synthetic antibody sequences are summarised as „single-pot" or universal libraries. These libraries are designed to isolate antibody fragments binding to every possible antigen, at least in theory (Dübel et al., 2010; Winter et al., 1994). Different types of universal libraries are available. Naïve libraries are constructed from rearranged V genes from B cells (IgM) of non-immunised donors. Examples for this library type are the naive human Fab library constructed by de Haard et al. (de Haard et al., 1999) and the HAL scFv libraries (Hust et al., 2011). Semi-synthetic libraries are constructed from unrearranged V genes from pre B germline cells (Griffiths et al., 1994) or from an antibody framework (Pini et al., 1998) in which one or several complementarity determining regions (CDR), including always the CDR H3, are randomised. For the FAB310 antibody gene library, a combination of naive and synthetic repertoire was used. Here, light chains from autoimmune patients were combined with a Fd fragment containing synthetic CDR1 and CDR2 in the human VH3-23 framework and naive CDR3 regions, derived from autoimmune patients (Hoet et al., 2005). Fully synthetic libraries are made of human frameworks with randomised CDR cassettes (Knappik et al., 2000; Rothe et al., 2008). Universal libraries have a repertoire of 10^8 - 10^{11} independent clones as molecular repertoire for phage display selection procedures. The difficulty of naïve libraries is that antibodies isolated thereof have lower affinities as hybridoma derived antibodies. Affinity and stability of the antibodies selected by phage display can be increased by additional *in vitro* affinity maturation steps (Finlay et al., 2009; Kobayashi et al., 2010; Thie et al., 2011; Thie et al., 2009).
To date, antibody phage display was used for the generation of antibodies against a large panel of human pathogenic viruses by using either recombinant viral proteins or complete virus particles for panning. Naïve antibody gene libraries were used to generate antibodies against Sin nombre virus (Velappan et al., 2007), Dengue virus (Cabezas et al., 2008; Moreland et al., 2010), Hepatitis C virus (Songsivilai and Dharakul, 1998), Influenza virus (Lim et al., 2008) or VEEV (Kirsch et al., 2008).
Opposite to these naive libraries are "immune libraries" which are constructed from antibody V-genes isolated from IgG secreting plasma cells from blood or bone marrow of

immunised donors. V genes of these libraries contain hypermutations and are affinity matured. From these immune libraries, human antibodies usable for therapeutic purposes against infectious pathogens (Clackson et al., 1991; Pelat et al., 2007; Schütte et al., 2009), including viruses (Duggan et al., 2001; Hunt et al., 2010; Kang et al., 2006; Sun et al., 2009; Throsby et al., 2008) have been isolated. Generally, immune libraries have a size of 10^6-10^8 independent clones, but can not be built for each antigen of interest, because man cannot be immunized with all antigens for ethical and practical reasons. An alternative are macaque immune libraries. The antibody genes of non-human primates (NHP) are closely related to human antibody genes (Pelat et al., 2009b) and might easily be humanised or germline humanised. In this latter case, the macaque amino acid sequence of the antibody is first compared with the corresponding human germline sequence. Differing macaque amino acid sequences are localised and are replaced by their human germline counterparts (Pelat et al., 2008; Pelat and Thullier, 2009) with respect to their affinity. Human germline sequences belong to the immunological self and are generally perfectly tolerated. However, this approach can even be used to reduce the potential immunogenicity of human antibodies.
The *in vitro* isolation of antibody fragments from libraries is performed independently from their immune or naïve origin. It relies on the binding activity of these antibody fragments and is called „panning" (Fig. 1), referring to the gold digger's tool (Parmley and Smith, 1988). For this panning, the antigen (a protein or a complete organism like a virus) is immobilised to a solid surface, mainly plastic surfaces like polystyrene tubes (Hust et al., 2002) or 96 well microtitre plates (Hust et al., 2011) and incubated with antibody phage of the antibody gene library. During this incubation step, chemical (e.g. pH), physical (e.g. temperature) or biological (e.g. competitor) parameters can be controlled to select antibodies which are able to bind the antigen. Antibody phage particles which bind weakly to the antigen and the vast excess of non-binding antibody phage are removed by strigent washing. Specifically binding antibody phage are eluted (e.g. by trypsin or pH shift) and reamplified by infection of *E. coli*. Subsequently, the phagemid bearing *E. coli* are infected with a helperphage, mainly M13K07, to produce new antibody phage which can be used for further panning rounds until a significant enrichment of antigen specific phage is achieved. Usually two or three panning rounds are necessary to select specifically binding antibody fragments. After panning, soluble individual monoclonal antibody fragments or antibody phage are produced and specific antigen binding is analysed by ELISA to identify individual binders. Afterwards, these individual binders can be sequenced and further biochemically characterised (Hust et al., 2007a; Winter et al., 1994). This panning process can also be performed in a high-throughput manner (Buckler et al., 2008; Hallborn and Carlsson, 2002; Hust et al., 2011; Konthur et al., 2005). Because the gene sequence of the binder is available, the antibody - depending on the desired application - can be converted into different antibody formats (e.g. scFv-Fc fusion or IgG) and produced in different production hosts (Hust et al., 2011; Schirrmann et al., 2008). In summary, recombinant antibody fragments derived from phage display can be adapted to the final assay requirements.

4. Antibodies for diagnostics and therapy of encephalitis viruses generated by phage display

In the beginning of 2011, 29 therapeutic monoclonal antibodies were approved in the USA or EU. For further antibodies approval is pending (http://www.landesbioscience.com /journals/mabs/about). The most admitted therapeutic antibodies are for cancer and

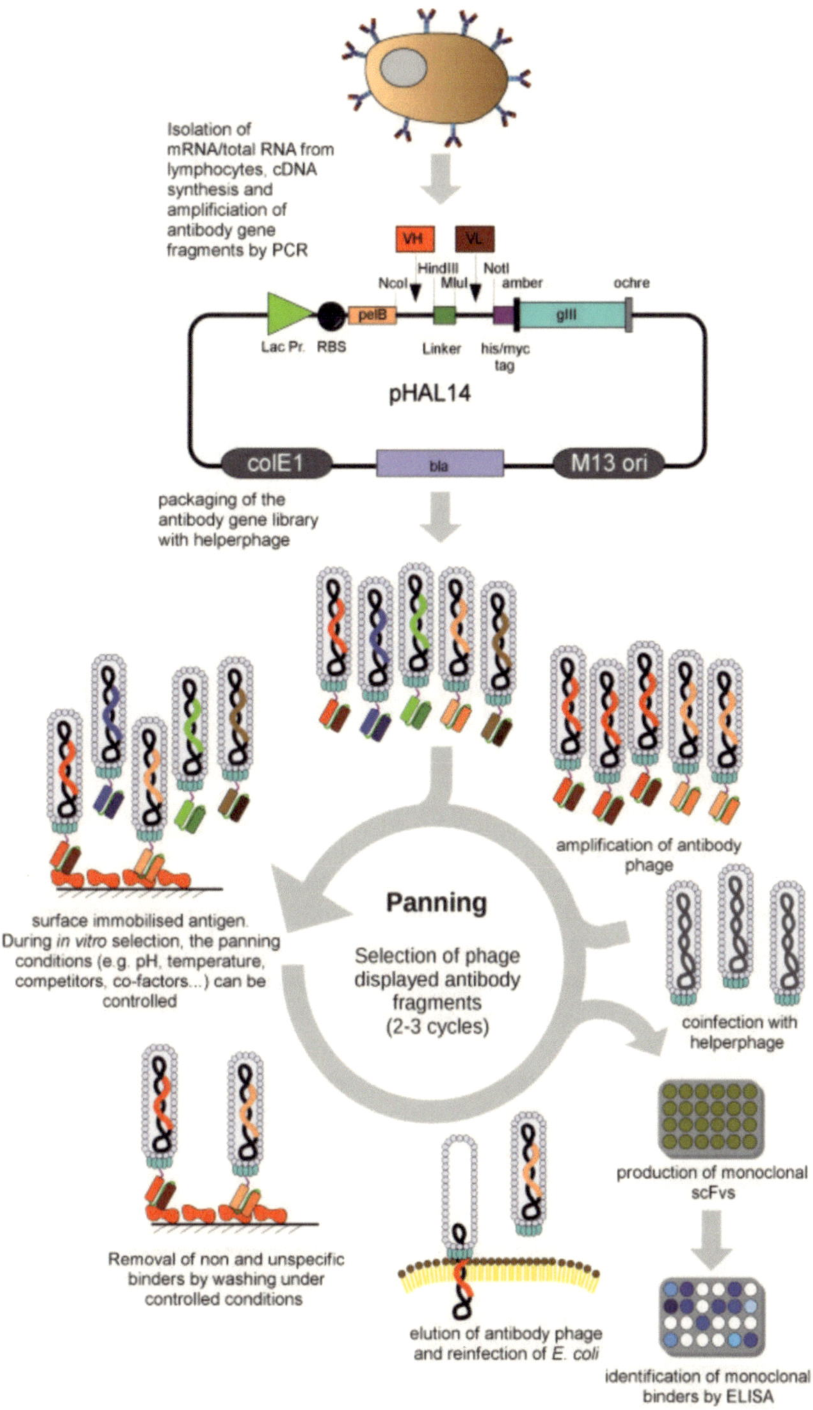

Fig. 1. Schematic overview about antibody gene library construction and the selection of binders (panning). This figure is a modified version of a former figure (Schirrmann and Hust, 2010).

autoimmune diseases (Dübel, 2007). Mechanisms of therapeutic antibodies are manifold and include neutralisation of substances e.g. toxins (Pelat et al., 2007) or cytokines like tumor necrosis factor (TNF) alpha (Alonso-Ruiz et al., 2008), blocking of receptors like epidermal growth factor receptor (EGFR) (Peeters et al., 2009), binding to cells and modulating the host immune system (Chatenoud and Bluestone, 2007), or combinations of these effects (Adams and Weiner, 2005). Interestingly, todate no recombinant antibodies are approved for the treatment of viral infections.

Rapid diagnosis of equine encephalitis is essential to allow an appropriate medical treatment, preventing viral replication. This may be allowed by point-of-care diagnosis tests based on antibodies or antibody fragments. After successful diagnosis, specific treatment might be considered and the use of recombinant (chimerized, humanized or human) neutralising antibodies is one choice. Also a prophylactic use of these recombinant antibodies might be considered for a time-limited protection, as human antibodies have a half-life of around 3 weeks in man (Eklund et al., 1982).

Since the administration of the original vaccine VEEV strain, TC83, developed in the sixties, had serious side effects to man (MCKINNEY et al., 1963), murine, macaque, humanised and human antibodies have been generated against VEEV by antibody phage display as an alternative in recent years. VEEV TC83 was used for example for the immunisation of mice from which the protective monoclonal antibody mAb 3B4C-4 was generated and later humanised (Hunt et al., 2006; Roehrig et al., 1982). The resulting antibody, mAb Hy4, turned out to be as protective as the original mouse antibody as demonstrated by virus challenge in Swiss Webster mice (Hunt et al., 2006). A further neutralising humanised antibody was developed by Hu et al (Hu et al., 2010).

The first anti-VEEV recombinant antibody fragments were derived from the murine IgG mAb 5B4D-6 by molecular cloning (Alvi et al., 1999). Murine scFvs aimed for diagnostic use were also isolated by phage display using immune libraries (Duggan et al., 2001), as phage display allows testing more candidates than hybridoma technology thus improving the search for selected specificities. Later, protective murine antibody fragments were generated using phage display. The broadly reacting scFv CUF37 was converted into the murine IgG2a format; this antibody was not neutralising *in vitro* but protective *in vivo* (O'Brien et al., 2009). The humanised version of this antibody (hu1A3B-7) protected mice in challenge experiments using the VEEV strain Trinidad Donkey (TrD) (Goodchild et al., 2011).

Regarding human antibody fragments, a panel of scFvs was selected for diagnostic assays from the naïve human libraries HAL4/7 using the antibody-displaying phage particles directly (Kirsch et al., 2008). Further human antibodies for therapeutic purposes were isolated using Fab (Fragment antigen binding) antibody phage display. The human immune library was constructed from sera of two VEEV strain TC-83 immunised US soldiers and two neutralising antibody fragments were identified. Hunt and coauthors suggested to use mAb F5 in combination with the earlier isolated humanised antibody mAb Hy4 for therapeutic purposes because they bind to different epitopes of the VEEV E2 glycoprotein (Hunt et al., 2010). The authors of the present review isolated a macaque scFv from an immune phage-displayed library directed against VEEV. Expressed as fusion with human constant regions, the resulting scFv-Fc protected mice against lethal challenge with Venezuelan equine encephalitis viruses (Rülker et al., in preparation).

To our knowledge no anti-WEEV antibody fragments derived from any kind of library is published. However, scFvs were generated from the murine IgGs 11D2 (Das et al., 2004; Xu

et al., 1999) and 10B5 E7E2 (Long et al., 2000) for diagnostic purposes. The authors of this review generated scFvs against WEEV by phage display using a macaque immune antibody gene library (Rülker et al. in preparation), both for diagnosis and therapeutic purposes.
Regarding EEEV, to our knowledge no recombinant human or murine antibodies have been published.
"At present there is no FDA-approved medical treatment for infection with these viruses." (Reichert et al., 2009). However, antibody phage display and other techniques have already delivered human or human-like antibodies as leads for the treatment or prophylaxis of equine encephalitis. Alternatively, the epitopes of these antibodies might also be candidate-vaccine.

5. References

Adams, G.P., Weiner, L.M. (2005). Monoclonal antibody therapy of cancer. *Nat Biotechnol* 23, 1147-1157.

Alonso-Ruiz, A., Pijoan, J.I., Ansuategui, E., Urkaregi, A., Calabozo, M., Quintana, A. (2008). Tumor necrosis factor alpha drugs in rheumatoid arthritis: systematic review and metaanalysis of efficacy and safety. *BMC Musculoskeletal Disorders* 9: 52.

Alvi, A.Z., Stadnyk, L.L., Nagata, L.P., Fulton, R.E., Bader, D.E., Roehrig, J.T., Suresh, M.R. (1999). Development of a functional monoclonal single-chain variable fragment antibody against Venezuelan equine encephalitis virus. *Hybridoma* 18, 413-421.

von Behring, E., Kitasato, S. (1890). Über das Zustandekommen der Diphtherie-Immunität und der Tetanus-Immunität bei Thieren. *Deutsche Medizinische Wochenzeitschrift* 16, 1113-1114.

Bird, R.E., Hardman, K.D., Jacobson, J.W., Johnson, S., Kaufman, B.M., Lee, S.M., Lee, T., Pope, S.H., Riordan, G.S., Whitlow, M. (1988). Single-chain antigen-binding proteins. *Science* 242, 423-426.

Breitling, F., Dübel, S., Seehaus, T., Klewinghaus, I., Little, M. (1991). A surface expression vector for antibody screening. *Gene* 104, 147-153.

Buckler, D.R., Park, A., Viswanathan, M., Hoet, R.M., Ladner, R.C. (2008). Screening isolates from antibody phage-display libraries. *Drug Discov Today* 13, 318-324.

Cabezas, S., Rojas, G., Pavon, A., Alvarez, M., Pupo, M., Guillen, G., Guzman, M.G. (2008). Selection of phage-displayed human antibody fragments on Dengue virus particles captured by a monoclonal antibody: application to the four serotypes. *J Virol Methods* 147, 235-243.

Calisher, C.H. (1994). Medically important arboviruses of the United States and Canada. *Clin Microbiol Rev* 7, 89-116.

Chatenoud, L., Bluestone, J.A. (2007). CD3-specific antibodies: a portal to the treatment of autoimmunity. *Nat Rev Immunol* 7, 622-632.

Clackson, T., Hoogenboom, H.R., Griffiths, A.D., Winter, G. (1991). Making antibody fragments using phage display libraries. *Nature* 352, 624-628.

Courtenay-Luck, N.S., Epenetos, A.A., Moore, R., Larche, M., Pectasides, D., Dhokia, B., Ritter, M.A. (1986). Development of primary and secondary immune responses to mouse monoclonal antibodies used in the diagnosis and therapy of malignant neoplasms. *Cancer Res* 46, 6489-6493.

Das, D., Kriangkum, J., Nagata, L.P., Fulton, R.E., Suresh, M.R. (2004). Development of a biotin mimic tagged ScFv antibody against western equine encephalitis virus: bacterial expression and refolding. *J Virol Methods* 117, 169-177.

Deresiewicz, R.L., Thaler, S.J., Hsu, L., Zamani, A.A. (1997). Clinical and neuroradiographic manifestations of eastern equine encephalitis. *N Engl J Med* 336, 1867-1874.

Dübel, S. (2007). Recombinant therapeutic antibodies. *Appl Microbiol Biotechnol* 74, 723 -729.

Dübel, S., Stoevesandt, O., Taussig, M.J., Hust, M. (2010). Generating recombinant antibodies to the complete human proteome. *Trends Biotechnol* 28, 333-339.

Duggan, J.M., Coates, D.M., Ulaeto, D.O. (2001). Isolation of single-chain antibody fragments against Venezuelan equine encephalomyelitis virus from two different immune sources. *Viral Immunol* 14, 263-273.

Eklund, J., Hermann, M., Kjellman, H., Pohja, P. (1982). Turnover rate of anti-D IgG injected during pregnancy. *Br Med J (Clin Res Ed)* 284, 854-855.

Feemster, R.F. (1938). Outbreak of Encephalitis in Man Due to the Eastern Virus of Equine Encephalomyelitis. *Am J Public Health Nations Health* 28, 1403-1410.

Finlay, W.J., Cunningham, O., Lambert, M.A., Darmanin-Sheehan, A., Liu, X., Fennell, B.J., Mahon, C.M., Cummins, E., Wade, J.M., O'Sullivan, C.M., Tan, X.Y., Piche, N., Pittman, D.D., Paulsen, J., Tchistiakova, L., Kodangattil, S., Gill, D., Hufton, S.E. (2009). Affinity maturation of a humanized rat antibody for anti-RAGE therapy: comprehensive mutagenesis reveals a high level of mutational plasticity both inside and outside the complementarity-determining regions. *J Mol Biol* 388, 541-558.

Fishwild, D.M., O'Donnell, S.L., Bengoechea, T., Hudson, D.V., Harding, F., Bernhard, S.L., Jones, D., Kay, R.M., Higgins, K.M., Schramm, S.R., Lonberg, N. (1996). High-avidity human IgG kappa monoclonal antibodies from a novel strain of minilocus transgenic mice. *Nat Biotechnol* 14, 845-851.

Flajnik, M.F., Dooley, H. (2009). The generation and selection of single-domain, v region libraries from nurse sharks. *Methods Mol Biol* 562, 71-82.

Giltner, L.T., Shahan, M.S. (1933). The immunological relationship of eastern and western strains of equine encephalomyelitis virus. *Science* 78, 587-588.

Goodchild, S.A., O'Brien, L.M., Steven, J., Muller, M.R., Lanning, O.J., Logue, C.H., D'Elia, R.V., Phillpotts, R.J., Perkins, S.D. (2011). A humanised murine monoclonal antibody with broad serogroup specificity protects mice from challenge with Venezuelan equine encephalitis virus. *Antiviral Res* 90, 1-8.

Griffiths, A.D., Williams, S.C., Hartley, O., Tomlinson, I.M., Waterhouse, P., Crosby, W.L., Kontermann, R.E., Jones, P.T., Low, N.M., Allison, T.J. (1994). Isolation of high affinity human antibodies directly from large synthetic repertoires. *EMBO* J 13, 3245-3260.

de Haard, H.J., van Neer, N., Reurs, A., Hufton, S.E., Roovers, R.C., Henderikx, P., de Bruïne, A.P., Arends, J.W., Hoogenboom, H.R. (1999). A large non-immunized human Fab fragment phage library that permits rapid isolation and kinetic analysis of high affinity antibodies. *J Biol Chem* 274, 18218-18230.

Hallborn, J., Carlsson, R. (2002). Automated screening procedure for high-throughput generation of antibody fragments. *Biotechniques Suppl*, 30-7.

Hawley, R.J., Eitzen, E.M. (2001). Biological weapons--a primer for microbiologists. *Annu Rev Microbiol* 55, 235-253.

Hoet, R.M., Cohen, E.H., Kent, R.B., Rookey, K., Schoonbroodt, S., Hogan, S., Rem, L., Frans, N., Daukandt, M., Pieters, H., van Hegelsom, R., Neer, N.C.-van, Nastri, H.G., Rondon, I.J., Leeds, J.A., Hufton, S.E., Huang, L., Kashin, I., Devlin, M., Kuang, G., Steukers, M., Viswanathan, M., Nixon, A.E., Sexton, D.J., Hoogenboom, H.R., Ladner, R.C. (2005). Generation of high-affinity human antibodies by combining donor-derived and synthetic complementarity-determining-region diversity. *Nat Biotechnol* 23, 344-348.

Hoke, C.H. (2005). History of U.S. military contributions to the study of viral encephalitis. *Mil Med* 170, 92-105.

Holt, L.J., Herring, C., Jespers, L.S., Woolven, B.P., Tomlinson, I.M. (2003). Domain antibodies: proteins for therapy. *Trends Biotechnol* 21, 484-490.

Hunt, A.R., Frederickson, S., Hinkel, C., Bowdish, K.S., Roehrig, J.T. (2006). A humanized murine monoclonal antibody protects mice either before or after challenge with virulent Venezuelan equine encephalomyelitis virus. *J Gen Virol* 87, 2467-2476.

Hunt, A.R., Frederickson, S., Maruyama, T., Roehrig, J.T., Blair, C.D. (2010). The first human epitope map of the alphaviral E1 and E2 proteins reveals a new E2 epitope with significant virus neutralizing activity. *PLoS Negl Trop Dis* 4, e739.

Hust, M., Dübel, S., Schirrmann, T. (2007a). Selection of recombinant antibodies from antibody gene libraries. *Methods Mol Biol* 408, 243-255.

Hust, M., Jostock, T., Menzel, C., Voedisch, B., Mohr, A., Brenneis, M., Kirsch, M.I., Meier, D., Dübel, S. (2007b). Single chain Fab (scFab) fragment. *BMC Biotechnol* 7: 14.

Hust, M., Maiss, E., Jacobsen, H.-J., Reinard, T. (2002). The production of a genus-specific recombinant antibody (scFv) using a recombinant potyvirus protease. *J Virol Methods* 106, 225-233.

Hust, M., Meyer, T., Voedisch, B., Rülker, T., Thie, H., El-Ghezal, A., Kirsch, M.I., Schütte, M., Helmsing, S., Meier, D., Schirrmann, T., Dübel, S. (2011). A human scFv antibody generation pipeline for proteome research. *J Biotechnol* 152, 159-170.

Huston, J.S., Levinson, D., Mudgett-Hunter, M., Tai, M.S., Novotný, J., Margolies, M.N., Ridge, R.J., Bruccoleri, R.E., Haber, E., Crea, R. (1988). Protein engineering of antibody binding sites: recovery of specific activity in an anti-digoxin single-chain Fv analogue produced in Escherichia coli. *Proc Natl Acad Sci USA* 85, 5879-5883.

Hu, W.-G., Phelps, A.L., Jager, S., Chau, D., Hu, C.C., O'Brien, L.M., Perkins, S.D., Gates, A.J., Phillpotts, R.J., Nagata, L.P. (2010). A recombinant humanized monoclonal antibody completely protects mice against lethal challenge with Venezuelan equine encephalitis virus. *Vaccine* 28, 5558-5564.

Jakobovits, A. (1995). Production of fully human antibodies by transgenic mice. *Curr Opin Biotechnol* 6, 561-566.

Kang, X., Yang, B.-A., Hu, Y., Zhao, H., Xiong, W., Yang, Y., Si, B., Zhu, Q. (2006). Human neutralizing Fab molecules against severe acute respiratory syndrome coronavirus generated by phage display. *Clin Vaccine Immunol* 13, 953-957.

King, L.S. (1939). Studies on eastern equine encephalomyelitis : III. intraocular infection with fixed virus in the guinea pig. *J Exp Med* 69, 691-704.

Kirsch, M., Hülseweh, B., Nacke, C., Rülker, T., Schirrmann, T., Marschall, H.-J., Hust, M., Dübel, S. (2008). Development of human antibody fragments using antibody phage display for the detection and diagnosis of Venezuelan equine encephalitis virus (VEEV). *BMC Biotechnol* 8:66.

Knappik, A., Ge, L., Honegger, A., Pack, P., Fischer, M., Wellnhofer, G., Hoess, A., Wölle, J., Plückthun, A., Virnekäs, B. (2000). Fully synthetic human combinatorial antibody libraries (HuCAL) based on modular consensus frameworks and CDRs randomized with trinucleotides. *J Mol Biol* 296, 57-86.

Kobayashi, N., Oyama, H., Kato, Y., Goto, J., Söderlind, E., Borrebaeck, C.A.K. (2010). Two-step in vitro antibody affinity maturation enables estradiol-17beta assays with more than 10-fold higher sensitivity. *Anal Chem* 82, 1027-1038.

Köhler, G., Milstein, C. (1975). Continuous cultures of fused cells secreting antibody of predefined specificity. *Nature* 256, 495-497.

Konthur, Z., Hust, M., Dübel, S. (2005). Perspectives for systematic in vitro antibody generation. *Gene* 364, 19-29.

Kubes, V., Ríos, F.A. (1939). The causative agent of infectious equine encephalomyelitis in venezuela. *Science* 90, 20-21.

Leitenberg, M. (2001). Biological weapons in the twentieth century: a review and analysis. *Crit Rev Microbiol* 27, 267-320.

Letson, G.W., Bailey, R.E., Pearson, J., Tsai, T.F. (1993). Eastern equine encephalitis (EEE): a description of the 1989 outbreak, recent epidemiologic trends, and the association of rainfall with EEE occurrence. *Am J Trop Med Hyg* 49, 677-685.

Lim, A.P.C., Chan, C.E.Z., Wong, S.K.K., Chan, A.H.Y., Ooi, E.E., Hanson, B.J. (2008). Neutralizing human monoclonal antibody against H5N1 influenza HA selected from a Fab-phage display library. *Virol J* 5: 130.

Lonberg, N., Huszar, D. (1995). Human antibodies from transgenic mice. *Int Rev Immunol* 13, 65-93.

Long, M.C., Jager, S., Mah, D.C., Jebailey, L., Mah, M.A., Masri, S.A., Nagata, L.P. (2000). Construction and characterization of a novel recombinant single-chain variable fragment antibody against Western equine encephalitis virus. *Hybridoma* 19, 1-13.

Mazor, Y., Van Blarcom, T., Mabry, R., Iverson, B.L., Georgiou, G. (2007). Isolation of engineered, full-length antibodies from libraries expressed in Escherichia coli. *Nat Biotechnol* 25, 563-565.

McCafferty, J., Griffiths, A.D., Winter, G., Chiswell, D.J. (1990). Phage antibodies: filamentous phage displaying antibody variable domains. *Nature* 348, 552-554.

Mckinney, R.W., Berge, T.O., Sawyer, W.D., Tigertt, W.D., Crozier, D. (1963). Use of an attenuated strain of venezuelan equine encephalomyelitis virus for immunization in man. *Am J Trop Med Hyg* 12, 597-603.

Meyer, K.F., Haring, C.M., Howitt, B. (1931). The etiology of epizootic encephalomyelitis of horses in the san joaquin valley, 1930. *Science* 74, 227-228.

Moreland, N.J., Tay, M.Y.F., Lim, E., Paradkar, P.N., Doan, D.N.P., Yau, Y.H., Geifman Shochat, S., Vasudevan, S.G., 2010. High affinity human antibody fragments to dengue virus non-structural protein 3. PLoS Negl Trop Dis 4: e881.

Muyldermans, S. (2001). Single domain camel antibodies: current status. *J Biotechnol* 74, 277-302.

Muyldermans, S., Baral, T.N., Retamozzo, V.C., De Baetselier, P., De Genst, E., Kinne, J., Leonhardt, H., Magez, S., Nguyen, V.K., Revets, H., Rothbauer, U., Stijlemans, B., Tillib, S., Wernery, U., Wyns, L., Hassanzadeh-Ghassabeh, G., Saerens, D. (2009). Camelid immunoglobulins and nanobody technology. *Vet Immunol Immunopathol* 128, 178-183.

Nelson, A.L., Dhimolea, E., Reichert, J.M. (2010). Development trends for human monoclonal antibody therapeutics. *Nat Rev Drug Discov* 9, 767-774.

Nuttall, S.D., Krishnan, U.V., Hattarki, M., De Gori, R., Irving, R.A., Hudson, P.J. (2001). Isolation of the new antigen receptor from wobbegong sharks, and use as a scaffold for the display of protein loop libraries. *Mol Immunol* 38, 313-326.

Nuttall, S.D., Humberstone, K.S., Krishnan, U.V., Carmichael, J.A., Doughty, L., Hattarki, M., Coley, A.M., Casey, J.L., Anders, R.F., Foley, M., Irving, R.A., Hudson, P.J. (2004). Selection and affinity maturation of IgNAR variable domains targeting Plasmodium falciparum AMA1. *Proteins* 55, 187-197.

O'Brien, L.M., Underwood-Fowler, C.D., Goodchild, S.A., Phelps, A.L., Phillpotts, R.J. (2009). Development of a novel monoclonal antibody with reactivity to a wide range of Venezuelan equine encephalitis virus strains. *Virol J* 6: 206.

Parmley, S.F., Smith, G.P. (1988). Antibody-selectable filamentous fd phage vectors: affinity purification of target genes. *Gene* 73, 305-318.

Pauza, M.E., Rehmann, J.A., LeBien, T.W. (1993). Unusual patterns of immunoglobulin gene rearrangement and expression during human B cell ontogeny: human B cells can simultaneously express cell surface kappa and lambda light chains. *J Exp Med* 178, 139-149.

Peeters, M., Price, T., Van Laethem, J.-L. (2009). Anti-epidermal growth factor receptor monotherapy in the treatment of metastatic colorectal cancer: where are we today? *Oncologist* 14, 29-39.

Pelat, T., Bedouelle, H., Rees, A.R., Crennell, S.J., Lefranc, M.-P., Thullier, P. (2008). Germline humanization of a non-human primate antibody that neutralizes the anthrax toxin, by in vitro and in silico engineering. *J Mol Biol* 384, 1400-1407.

Pelat, T., Hust, M., Hale, M., Lefranc, M.-P., Dübel, S., Thullier, P. (2009a). Isolation of a human-like antibody fragment (scFv) that neutralizes ricin biological activity. *BMC Biotechnol* 9: 60.

Pelat, T., Hust, M., Laffly, E., Condemine, F., Bottex, C., Vidal, D., Lefranc, M.-P., Dübel, S., Thullier, P. (2007). High-affinity, human antibody-like antibody fragment (single-chain variable fragment) neutralizing the lethal factor (LF) of Bacillus anthracis by inhibiting protective antigen-LF complex formation. *Antimicrob Agents Chemother* 51, 2758-2764.

Pelat, T., Hust, M., Thullier, P. (2009b). Obtention and engineering of non-human primate (NHP) antibodies for therapeutics. *Mini Rev Med Chem* 9, 1633-1638.

Pelat, T., Thullier, P. (2009). Non-human primate immune libraries combined with germline humanization: an (almost) new, and powerful approach for the isolation of therapeutic antibodies. *MAbs* 1, 377-381.

Phillpotts, R.J. (2006). Venezuelan equine encephalitis virus complex-specific monoclonal antibody provides broad protection, in murine models, against airborne challenge with viruses from serogroups I, II and III. *Virus Res* 120, 107-112.

Pini, A., Viti, F., Santucci, A., Carnemolla, B., Zardi, L., Neri, P., Neri, D. (1998). Design and use of a phage display library. Human antibodies with subnanomolar affinity against a marker of angiogenesis eluted from a two-dimensional gel. *J Biol Chem* 273, 21769-21776.

Powers, A.M., Brault, A.C., Shirako, Y., Strauss, E.G., Kang, W., Strauss, J.H., Weaver, S.C. (2001). Evolutionary relationships and systematics of the alphaviruses. *J Virol* 75, 10118-10131.

Reed, D.S., Larsen, T., Sullivan, L.J., Lind, C.M., Lackemeyer, M.G., Pratt, W.D., Parker, M.D. (2005). Aerosol exposure to western equine encephalitis virus causes fever and encephalitis in cynomolgus macaques. *J Infect Dis* 192, 1173-1182.

Reichert, E., Clase, A., Bacetty, A., Larsen, J. (2009). Alphavirus antiviral drug development: scientific gap analysis and prospective research areas. *Biosecur Bioterror* 7, 413-427.

Rivas, F., Diaz, L.A., Cardenas, V.M., Daza, E., Bruzon, L., Alcala, A., De la Hoz, O., Caceres, F.M., Aristizabal, G., Martinez, J.W., Revelo, D., De la Hoz, F., Boshell, J., Camacho, T., Calderon, L., Olano, V.A., Villarreal, L.I., Roselli, D., Alvarez, G., Ludwig, G., Tsai, T. (1997). Epidemic Venezuelan equine encephalitis in La Guajira, Colombia, 1995. *J Infect Dis* 175, 828-832.

Roehrig, J.T., Day, J.W., Kinney, R.M. (1982). Antigenic analysis of the surface glycoproteins of a Venezuelan equine encephalomyelitis virus (TC-83) using monoclonal antibodies. *Virology* 118, 269-278.

Rothe, C., Urlinger, S., Löhning, C., Prassler, J., Stark, Y., Jäger, U., Hubner, B., Bardroff, M., Pradel, I., Boss, M., Bittlingmaier, R., Bataa, T., Frisch, C., Brocks, B., Honegger, A., Urban, M. (2008). The human combinatorial antibody library HuCAL GOLD combines diversification of all six CDRs according to the natural immune system with a novel display method for efficient selection of high-affinity antibodies. *J Mol Biol* 376, 1182-1200.

Rozdilsky, B., Robertson, H.E., Chorney, J. (1968). Western encephalitis: report of eight fatal cases. Saskatchewan epidemic, 1965. *Can Med Assoc* J 98, 79-86.

Sanchez, J.L., Takafuji, E.T., Lednar, W.M., LeDuc, J.W., Macasaet, F.F., Mangiafico, J.A., Rosato, R.R., Driggers, D.P., Haecker, J.C. (1984). Venezuelan equine encephalomyelitis: report of an outbreak associated with jungle exposure. *Mil Med* 149, 618-621.

Schirrmann, T., Al-Halabi, L., Dübel, S., Hust, M. (2008). Production systems for recombinant antibodies. *Front Biosci* 13, 4576-4594.

Schirrmann, T., Hust, M. (2010). Construction of human antibody gene libraries and selection of antibodies by phage display. *Methods Mol Biol* 651, 177-209.

Schütte, M., Thullier, P., Pelat, T., Wezler, X., Rosenstock, P., Hinz, D., Kirsch, M.I., Hasenberg, M., Frank, R., Schirrmann, T., Gunzer, M., Hust, M., Dübel, S. (2009). Identification of a putative Crf splice variant and generation of recombinant antibodies for the specific detection of Aspergillus fumigatus. *PLoS ONE* 4: e6625.

Scotcher, M.C., Cheng, L.W., Stanker, L.H. (2010). Detection of botulinum neurotoxin serotype B at sub mouse LD(50) levels by a sandwich immunoassay and its application to toxin detection in milk. *PLoS ONE* 5: e11047.

Sellers, R.F., Maarouf, A.R. (1993). Weather factors in the prediction of western equine encephalitis epidemics in Manitoba. Epidemiol. *Infect* 111, 373-390.

Simmons, L.C., Reilly, D., Klimowski, L., Raju, T.S., Meng, G., Sims, P., Hong, K., Shields, R.L., Damico, L.A., Rancatore, P., Yansura, D.G. (2002). Expression of full-length immunoglobulins in Escherichia coli: rapid and efficient production of aglycosylated antibodies. *J Immunol Methods* 263, 133-147.

Smith, G.P. (1985). Filamentous fusion phage: novel expression vectors that display cloned antigens on the virion surface. *Science* 228, 1315-1317.

Songsivilai, S., Dharakul, T. (1998). Genetically engineered single-chain Fvs of human immunoglobulin against hepatitis C virus nucleocapsid protein derived from universal phage display library. *Asian Pac J Allergy Immunol* 16, 31-41.

Strauss, J.H., Strauss, E.G. (1994). The alphaviruses: gene expression, replication, and evolution. *Microbiol Rev* 58, 491-562.

Sudia, W.D., McLean, R.G., Newhouse, V.F., Johnston, J.G., Miller, D.L., Trevino, H., Bowen, G.S., Sather, G. (1975). Epidemic Venezuelan equine encephalitis in North America in 1971: vertebrate field studies. *Am J Epidemiol* 101, 36-50.

Sun, L., Lu, X., Li, C., Wang, M., Liu, Q., Li, Z., Hu, X., Li, J., Liu, F., Li, Q., Belser, J.A., Hancock, K., Shu, Y., Katz, J.M., Liang, M., Li, D. (2009). Generation, characterization and epitope mapping of two neutralizing and protective human recombinant antibodies against influenza A H5N1 viruses. *PLoS ONE* 4:e5476.

Thie, H., Toleikis, L., Li, J., von Wasielewski, R., Bastert, G., Schirrmann, T., Esteves, I.T., Behrens, C.K., Fournes, B., Fournier, N., de Romeuf, C., Hust, M., Dübel, S. (2011). Rise and fall of an anti-MUC1 specific antibody. *PLoS ONE* 6:e15921.

Thie, H., Voedisch, B., Dübel, S., Hust, M., Schirrmann, T. (2009). Affinity maturation by phage display. *Methods Mol Biol* 525, 309-322.

Throsby, M., van den Brink, E., Jongeneelen, M., Poon, L.L.M., Alard, P., Cornelissen, L., Bakker, A., Cox, F., van Deventer, E., Guan, Y., Cinatl, J., ter Meulen, J., Lasters, I., Carsetti, R., Peiris, M., de Kruif, J., Goudsmit, J. (2008). Heterosubtypic neutralizing monoclonal antibodies cross-protective against H5N1 and H1N1 recovered from human IgM+ memory B cells. *PLoS ONE* 3:e3942.

Tjandra, J.J., Ramadi, L., McKenzie, I.F. (1990). Development of human anti-murine antibody (HAMA) response in patients. Immunol. *Cell Biol* 68, 367-376.

Velappan, N., Martinez, J.S., Valero, R., Chasteen, L., Ponce, L., Bondu-Hawkins, V., Kelly, C., Pavlik, P., Hjelle, B., Bradbury, A.R.M. (2007). Selection and characterization of scFv antibodies against the Sin Nombre hantavirus nucleocapsid protein. *J Immunol Methods* 321, 60-69.

Weaver, S.C., Ferro, C., Barrera, R., Boshell, J., Navarro, J.-C. (2004). Venezuelan equine encephalitis. *Annu Rev Entomol* 49, 141-174.

Weaver, S.C., Salas, R., Rico-Hesse, R., Ludwig, G.V., Oberste, M.S., Boshell, J., Tesh, R.B. (1996). Re-emergence of epidemic Venezuelan equine encephalomyelitis in South America. VEE Study Group. *Lancet* 348, 436-440.

Winter, G., Griffiths, A.D., Hawkins, R.E., Hoogenboom, H.R. (1994). Making antibodies by phage display technology. *Annu Rev Immunol* 12, 433-455.

Winter, G., Milstein, C. (1991). Man-made antibodies. *Nature* 349, 293-299.

Winterroth, L., Rivera, J., Nakouzi, A.S., Dadachova, E., Casadevall, A. (2010). Neutralizing monoclonal antibody to edema toxin and its effect on murine anthrax. *Infect Immun* 78, 2890-2898.

Xu, B., Kriangkum, J., Nagata, L.P., Fulton, R.E., Suresh, M.R. (1999). A single chain Fv specific against Western equine encephalitis virus. *Hybridoma* 18, 315-323.

21

Modelling of Autoimmune Encephalomyelitis in a Non-Human Primate

S. Anwar Jagessar, Nicole Heijmans, Nikki van Driel,
Bert A. 't Hart and Yolanda S. Kap
Biomedical Primate Research Centre
The Netherlands

1. Introduction

Multiple sclerosis (MS) is a chronic disabling disease characterized by inflammation, demyelination, and axonal damage in the central nervous system (CNS), affecting both white and grey matter. Commonly observed symptoms are visual and balance disturbances, spasticity, bladder dysfunction, pain, and fatigue. At a later disease stage, paralysis may occur (Compston& Coles 2008; Sospedra& Martin 2005).
For both exploratory and applied research into MS the use of a valid animal model is indispensable. The most widely used animal model for MS is experimental autoimmune encephalomyelitis (EAE), which is induced by active immunization with myelin derivatives formulated in adjuvant. EAE has been induced in a wide variety of species, including rabbits, guinea pigs, rats, mice, and non-human primates (Brok et al 2000; Genain et al 1995; Gold et al 2006; Massacesi et al 1995; Wekerle 2006).
The EAE model in the common marmoset (*Callithrix jacchus*), a small-sized New World monkey, is exquisitely suitable for translational research into pathogenic mechanisms and therapy development for MS. A feature that distinguishes the model from classical rodent EAE models is that marmosets are exposed to the same environmental cues as humans, including those associated with MS susceptibility, i.e. viral pathogens. In this chapter, we will summarize our investigations into the core pathogenic autoimmune mechanisms underlying the development of pathology and clinical symptoms. In addition, we will discuss the separate and combined role of B cells and T cells, in this model. Finally, we will briefly discuss how the model can be used for testing new therapies.

1.1 Immunology and genetics of the common marmoset

The marmoset is immunologically, anatomically, and neurologically more closely related to humans than rodents. In contrast to laboratory rodent strains, the marmoset is an outbred species, and the clinical and pathologically heterogeneity of the EAE model resembles the heterogeneous situation in MS.
A particularly interesting aspect of marmosets is the stable bone marrow chimerism between twin siblings that is caused by the sharing of the placental blood stream. Consequently, the immune systems of twins are educated in the same thymic environment, making fraternal siblings immunologically more similar than siblings from different births

(Niblack et al 1977). This principle can be used in therapy trials where one twin sibling is treated with an experimental agent and the other sibling with placebo.
The strongest genetic influence on MS susceptibility in the human population is exerted by the major histocompatibility complex (MHC). The MHC is a highly polymorphic genetic region that encodes for antigen presentation molecules, which according to international consensus nomenclature are indicated with the acronym Caja, being derived from *Callithrix jacchus*. MHC class II molecules are constitutively expressed on B cells and antigen presenting cells (APC) and are involved in the activation of $CD4^+$ T cell responses. MHC class I molecules are expressed on all nucleated cells and are involved in the activation of $CD8^+$ T cells. In the marmoset, MHC class I diversity is more limited than in humans. The classical *A*, *B*, and *C* molecules could not be identified in marmosets, but non-classical E (oligomorphic) and G genes (polymorphic) have been described (Cadavid et al 1997; Knapp et al 1998). The marmoset MHC class II region contains *DQA1*, *DQB1*, and *DQB2* genes, but *DQA2* and *DP* genes could not be identified. Marmosets contain one *DRB* region configuration, containing the three lineages *DRB1*03*, *DRB*W12*, and *DRB*W16*. *Caja-DRB1*03* and *-DRB*W16* are polymorphic with 13 and 20 alleles, respectively. *Caja-DRB*W12* appears to be monomorphic with two alleles, which differ only at two codons. All marmosets express *DRB*W1201* or DRB**W1202* (Antunes et al 1998; Doxiadis et al 2006; Prasad et al 2006; Wu et al 2000).
Despite the limited polymorphism of the MHC, marmosets contain a diverse and evolutionary stable T cell receptor α- and β-chain repertoire (Fujii et al 2010; Uccelli et al 1997).

1.2 Myelin oligodendrocyte glycoprotein

Demyelination is the pathological hallmark of MS and is caused by a combined cellular and humoral autoimmune attack on myelin. The myelin sheath is produced by oligodendrocytes and is wrapped around axons to ensure fast saltatory pulse conduction. Myelin is composed of 80% lipids and 20% proteins, such as myelin basic protein (MBP), proteolipid protein (PLP), and myelin oligodendrocyte glycoprotein (MOG).
MOG is a type I membrane glycoprotein and a member of the Ig superfamily produced by oligodendrocytes. MOG is located on the outer myelin sheath with the N-terminal amino acids 1 to 125 exposed to the extracellular environment where it is accessible for immune cells (Kroepfl et al 1996; Ohler et al 2004). MOG probably forms homodimers (Clements et al 2003) and is highly conserved among species (Delarasse et al 2006; Mesleh et al 2002).
The function of MOG in the CNS is unknown, as MOG-deficient mice do not present clinical or histological abnormalities (Delarasse et al 2003). However, MOG is an important target of the autoimmune attack in EAE. Autoimmunity against MOG is crucial for the progression of EAE in Biozzi ABH mice (Smith et al 2005) and marmosets (Jagessar et al 2008). Immunization with recombinant human MOG (rhMOG) protein or MOG peptides induces pathogenic antibody and T cell responses (Iglesias et al 2001; von Büdingen et al 2001). Antibodies against MOG facilitate demyelination and phagocytosis *in vitro* (Kerlero de Rosbo et al 1990; Van der Goes et al 1999) and enhance demyelination *in vivo* in mice (Morris-Downes et al 2002), rats (Linington et al 1988; Schluesener et al 1987), and marmosets (Genain et al 1995; McFarland et al 1999). T cell responses against MOG are found in EAE models in mice (Mendel et al 1995), rats (Stefferl et al 2000), marmosets (Brok et al 2000), and rhesus macaques (Kerlero de Rosbo et al 2000).

2. Modelling of MS in the common marmoset

The marmoset EAE model was first developed by Genain and co-workers (Massacesi et al 1995). Since then, the model has been continuously refined to improve the similarity with MS ('t Hart et al 2009). All EAE models that have been developed in the past years vary in their clinical and pathological features, see Table 1.

The first documented EAE model in the marmoset was induced with human myelin emulsified in complete Freund's adjuvant (CFA) supplemented with *Bordetella pertussis* particles. The disease was very acute and gave an acute disseminated encephalomyelitis (ADEM) like disease (Massacesi et al 1995). Several large seriously destructive lesions in the white matter of the brain and spinal cord were detected in this model.

EAE induction with human or mouse myelin in CFA, but without *Bordetella pertussis*, gave essentially the same pathology but had a slower disease progression. We observed in these models high T and B cell responses against various myelin proteins, i.e. MOG, MBP and PLP; we chose to study the role of MOG in more detail. To confirm the pathogenic significance of MOG, one sibling of a marmoset twin was sensitized against myelin derived from wild type C57BL/6 mice and the other sibling with myelin derived from MOG deficient mice of the same strain (Jagessar et al 2008). Animals immunized with MOG deficient myelin showed only mild clinical EAE symptoms, inflammation and small demyelinated areas in the white matter. We assume that these are caused by autoimmune reactions against other myelin proteins, such as MBP and PLP.

The addition of a physiological dose of recombinant MOG to mice immunized with MOG-deficient myelin restored the induction of chronic relapsing EAE in Biozzi ABH mice (Smith et al 2005). This observation emphasizes the immunodominance of MOG, which was investigated in further detail in marmosets immunized with recombinant human MOG (rhMOG) in CFA. This formulation induced a more chronic disease and a typical MS like pathology, characterized by active lesions in the CNS with macrophages containing myelin degraded products (Kap et al 2008). Moreover antibody formation against the whole MOG protein and specific MOG peptides were observed, such as $MOG_{14\text{-}36}$, $MOG_{34\text{-}56}$ and $MOG_{54\text{-}76}$. Interestingly, animals that developed clinical EAE signs showed specific T cell proliferation against $MOG_{34\text{-}56}$ and $MOG_{74\text{-}96}$.

To test the immunogenicity of the peptides, marmosets were immunized with some of the peptides separately in CFA. It was observed that $MOG_{14\text{-}36}$ is only moderately encephalitogenic inducing only small-sized inflammatory lesions (Brok et al 2000). $MOG_{74\text{-}96}$ was not encephalitogenic, whereas marmosets immunized with $MOG_{34\text{-}56}$ displayed essentially similar pathology and disease course as the EAE model with rhMOG in CFA (Kap et al 2008). Antibodies against rhMOG, $MOG_{34\text{-}56}$ and the overlapping peptide $MOG_{24\text{-}46}$ were formed in the $MOG_{34\text{-}56}$/CFA EAE model.

The absence of antibodies binding MOG protein directs the attention to the $MOG_{34\text{-}56}$ specific cytotoxic T cells as a cause of the widespread demyelination that was observed in the $MOG_{34\text{-}56}$/CFA model. T cell lines raised against $MOG_{34\text{-}56}$ were phenotypically characterized as $CD4^+$, $CD8^+$ or CD4/8 double positive, expressing also $CD56^+$ but not CD16 (Kap et al 2008). Interestingly, T cells with a similar phenotype have been associated with demyelination in MS (Vergelli et al 1996; Antel et al 1998). Further phenotypical characterization in humans showed that the T cells were $CD45RO^-$, $CD27^+CD28^-CCR7^-$, being a phenotype reminiscent to the NK-CTL effector memory subpopulation (Mazzarino et al 2005).

CFA is a major cause of the serious discomfort experienced by animals engaged in the EAE model. This prompted us to test if EAE could be induced without usage of CFA. Hence, animals were subjected to a challenge-boost protocol with MOG_{34-56} in incomplete Freund's adjuvant (IFA) (Jagessar et al 2010). It is of note that the inoculum lacked microbial antigens for innate immune activation. Nevertheless, all animals developed clinically evident EAE, which was characterized by marked inflammation and demyelination in the grey and white matter of the brain and spinal cord. Freshly isolated T cells also showed the NK-CTL phenotype, with cytolytic capacities and a Th17 cytokine profile as immunological hallmark. The replacement of CFA by IFA makes this model more useful for the study of subtle regulatory networks that keep T and B cells in check and maintain homeostasis within the CNS.

Antigen	Adjuvant	Disease type	Demyelination		T cells	IgG to rhMOG
			Grey matter	White matter		
Human myelin	CFA+ *B. pertussis*	Acute	N/A	+	N/A	N/A
Human myelin	CFA	Acute	N/A	+	N/A	N/A
Mouse myelin	CFA	Acute	N/A	+	N/A	N/A
MBP	CFA	Mild	N/A	+/-	N/A	N/A
$MOG^{-/-}$ mouse myelin	CFA	Mild	N/A	+/-	N/A	-
rhMOG	CFA	Chronic	+	+	Th1/Th17	+
MOG_{14-36}	CFA	Chronic	N/A	+	N/A	+
MOG_{34-56}	CFA	Chronic	+	+	Th1/Th17	+
MOG_{34-56}	IFA	Chronic	+	+	Th17	-

CFA, complete Freund's adjuvant; IFA, incomplete Freund's adjuvant; MOG, myelin oligodendrocyte glycoprotein; N/A, not available

Table 1. All marmosets EAE models with their characteristics.

3. Role of B cells in the marmoset EAE models

We observed no relation between the diversity of the antibody response and the rate of EAE progression in marmosets (Kap et al 2008). In addition, EAE can be induced in the absence of anti-rhMOG antibodies (Jagessar et al 2010). This was not entirely unexpected. Although a role of anti-MOG antibodies in the induction of CNS demyelination has been proven (Genain et al 1995; Genain et al 1999), the main pathogenic antibody reactivity is thought to be mainly directed against non-linear/conformational epitopes (von Büdingen et al 2004).

Recently, treatment with Rituximab, an anti-CD20 antibody, in MS patients showed clear beneficial effect. The amount of lesions and relapses reduced significantly in the anti-CD20 treated group compared to the placebo group, although antibody levels did not reduce significantly (Hauser et al 2008; Bar-Or et al 2008). These data suggest that Rituximab does not deplete plasma cells, which lack CD20 expression, and that the antigen presentation or a regulatory role by B cells may play a key role in disease development.

A similar study in marmoset monkeys was performed to understand the role of B cells in further detail (Kap et al 2010b). This study showed a profound effect of anti-CD20 treatment in animals with EAE, see also section 6.4. In addition to the study in MS patients, impaired activation of autoreactive T cells in lymphoid organs was observed and reduced mRNA levels of IL-7 and pro-inflammatory cytokines, e.g. IL-6, IFNγ and TNFα. Also less inflammation and demyelination was detected in the white as well as the grey matter.
It is assumed that there is a relation between MS and EBV infected B cells, see section 5.2. To investigate the role of EBV transformed B cells, we are creating an *in vivo* model for EBV infection in marmosets. Marmoset monkeys will be infused with autologous B lymphoblastoid cell (B-LCL) induced with the marmoset EBV B95-8 virus. By *ex vivo* pulsing of the B-LCL with the dominant MOG peptide 34 to 56, and injecting them back, the B-LCL will acquire the capacity to activate encephalitogenic T cells. As control, the sibling will be infused with B-LCL, but these cells will not be pulsed with the MOG peptide.

4. Role of T cells in the marmoset EAE models

T cells reactive against MOG are present in the natural T cell repertoire of healthy human individuals (Diaz-Villoslada et al 1999; Koehler et al 2002) as well as in healthy marmosets (Villoslada et al 2001). These autoreactive T cells are not depleted during development of the immune system because MOG is absent outside the CNS (Bruno et al 2002) and is likely expressed within the CNS relatively late during fetal development (Allamargot & Gardinier 2007). A significant increase in the number of MOG-specific T cells was reported in blood and cerebrospinal fluid (CSF) of MS patients (Kerlero de Rosbo et al 1993; Sun et al 1991).
T cells play a central role in the marmoset EAE model, as EAE can be induced by the activity of MOG-specific T cells without support of autoantibodies. Below, the specificity, phenotype, and function of the T cells that are activated in the EAE model will be discussed.

4.1 Specificity

Immunization of marmosets with rhMOG in CFA leads to a 100% disease incidence that maps to the MHC class II allele *Caja-DRB*W1201*, which is ubiquitously expressed in marmosets (Antunes et al 1998; Brok et al 2000; Doxiadis et al 2006). In marmosets immunized with rhMOG, *Caja-DRB*W1201* presentation of MOG_{24-36} leads to the activation of MOG_{24-36} specific Th1-cells in all animals (Brok et al 2000). However, T cells against this peptide alone are not sufficient to induce the full aspect of the disease as shown by immunization (Brok et al 2000) or adoptive transfer (Villoslada et al 2001). This suggests an important pathogenic role of T cells directed against other MOG epitopes.
In a meta-analysis of T cell response profiles from about 30 rhMOG-immunized marmosets, we observed that T cells from monkeys developing clinically evident EAE early after immunization (fast progressors) proliferate against a wider range of MOG peptides than T cells from monkeys developing overt disease at a later time point (slow progressors) (Kap et al 2008). T cell responses against the peptide MOG_{34-56} were confined to fast progressor monkeys. As discussed above, immunization with MOG_{34-56} in either CFA or IFA leads to EAE (Jagessar et al 2010; Kap et al 2008). This shows that MOG_{34-56} contains crucial T cell epitopes for the activation of T cells that can induce neurological disease.
The T cell response in marmosets against MOG is similar to MS, being mainly directed against three domains in the extracellular part of MOG, i.e. 1-22, 34-56, and 64-96 (Bielekova & Martin 2004; Kerlero de Rosbo et al 1997; Van der Aa et al 2003).

4.2 Phenotype and function

It has long been thought that $CD4^+$/Th1 cells were the main pathogenic T cells in MS, but more recent literature highlights an important pathogenic contribution of Th17 cells and $CD8^+$ T cells as well (Brucklacher-Waldert et al 2009; Ifergan et al 2008; Kebir et al 2007; Serafini et al 2007; Tzartos et al 2008). We have investigated the role of the different T cells subsets in more detail in the marmoset EAE model.

Immunization of marmosets with rhMOG or MOG_{34-56} leads to the proliferation of $CD4^+CD8^-$, $CD4^-CD8^+$, and $CD4^+CD8^+$ MOG_{34-56}-specific T cells. In addition, a large population of these T cells expresses CD56, which is a marker for natural killer-cytotoxic T lymphocytes (NK-CTL).

MOG_{34-56}-specific T cells have also other characteristics of NK-CTLs, as they are able to lyse MOG_{34-56} pulsed cells (Jagessar et al 2010; Kap et al 2008). This is similar to MS patients, in which cytotoxic MOG-specific T cells have also been observed (Koehler et al 2002; Van der Aa et al 2003). This suggests that MOG_{34-56} specific T cells can induce cytolysis of oligodendrocytes leading to demyelination.

The contribution of IFN-γ producing Th1 and IL-17A producing Th17 cells is an ongoing debate in MS, but also in the EAE models (Haak et al 2009; Komiyama et al 2006; Kroenke et al 2008; Langrish et al 2005; O'Connor et al 2008). Immunization of marmosets with rhMOG in CFA leads to the activation of both Th1 and Th17 cells (Kap et al 2010a). Inhibition of IL-17A in this model has only a marginal effect on the disease course, suggesting that Th1 cells or the cytotoxicity of these T cells are more crucial than the single cytokine (Kap et al 2010a). Immunization of marmosets with MOG_{34-56} in IFA leads to the production of IL-17A, but not to IFN-γ, suggesting that Th17 and cytotoxic T cells dominate in this model.

5. Role of viruses

It is believed that the origin of autoimmune diseases, i.e. MS, has multiplex backgrounds. The role of genetic predisposition and environmental factors are much less defined, although viral infections have long been associated with MS development. Viral infections are known as the most critical environmental factors. Herpesviruses, such as human herpesvirus type 6 (HHV-6) (Fotheringham & Jacobson 2005; Lunemann et al 2007), Epstein-Barr virus (EBV) and to a lesser extent cytomegalovirus (CMV) (Kanzaki & Yabuki 1994) are suspects.

5.1 CMV

CMV is a beta herpes virus and a leading cause of opportunistic infection in the human population. CMV infection is estimated at a range from 50% to 80% in humans, and remains asymptomatic in the vast majority of infected individuals (Staras et al 2006). The prevalence is quite variable as it varies in different geographic areas, different social economic population and ethnic origin. CMV has been associated with several autoimmune diseases, i.e. Systemic Lupus Erythematosus (Sekigawa et al 2002), diabetes mellitus type 1 and 2 (Filippi & von Herrath 2005; Roberts& Cech 2005) and with the Guillain-Barré Syndrome, a demyelinating disorder of peripheral nervous system (Yuki et al 2001), but there is no obvious association with MS. However, the virus has been involved in acute CNS inflammatory disorders, causing meningo-encephalitis in immunocompromised and immunocompetent individuals (Devetag & Boscariolo 2000). Moreover, recently it was observed that MS patients sufficient for Vitamin D were associated with an increased CMV antibody level, while such an association was absent or in the opposite direction in controls (Mowry et al 2010). Furthermore, $CD8^+$ T cells specific against CMV could be isolated from brain lesions of MS patients (Scotet et al 1999). In support of a role of CMV in MS is the observation that $CD8^+$ T cells from rhesus EAE monkeys immunized with $MOG_{34\text{-}56}$ in CFA display high proliferation against a 9-mer peptide derived from the immunodominant UL86 antigen of human CMV, encoding the major capsid protein (Sylwester et al 2005). Interestingly, the amino acid sequence 986 to 993 (WLRSPFSR) of the major capsid protein showed striking similarity with the MOG sequence 39 to 46 (WYRPPFSR). T cells from rhesus monkeys sensitized against the mimicry motif proliferated against $MOG_{34\text{-}56}$, whereas $CD3^+$ T cells infiltrates were detected within the CNS white matter and meninges (Brok et al 2007). This data suggests that anti-CMV memory T cells can be activated by APC that present $MOG_{34\text{-}56}$. We hypothesise that CMV does not provoke MS, but those individuals that are predisposed with CMV generate a repertoire of memory T cells. These memory T cells might exacerbate CNS inflammation and demyelination upon activation with $MOG_{34\text{-}56}$ presenting APC as in the marmoset EAE model (Kap et al 2008).

5.2 EBV

EBV is a gamma herpes virus, which causes lymphoproliferative diseases, such as Hodgkins lymphoma, nasopharyngeal carcinoma and acute infectious mononucleosis (Levin et al 2003). The prevalence of EBV infection in Western countries is very high; in adulthood more than 90% of the population are infected with EBV. Half of this population becomes EBV positive after the age of ten. Individuals (30-50%) who experience a primary EBV infection in adolescence will develop infectious mononucleosis. A $CD8^+$ T cell response develops against an impressive expansion of EBV infected B cells, where 10 to 30% of the B cells carry the virus (Cohen et al 2000).

In developing countries most of the children become in contact with EBV, before the age of ten; all children are EBV infected and mostly without symptoms. This indicates an age-related association between a primary EBV infection and infectious mononucleosis.

Over the years many studies have found an association between EBV infection and the development of MS. MS patients showed a significant increase of anti-EBV antibody levels, i.e. anti-EBNA-1, compared to controls (Sumaya et al 1980). It was also found that the antibody levels increased before the onset of MS (Levin et al 2005). Meta-analysis of thirteen studies has found an odd ratio of 0.06 for the risk to develop MS, when EBV seronegative individuals were compared with seropositive individuals. Of all MS patients, 99.5% were seropositive for EBV related to 94% of the controls. In children with MS 99% were positive for EBV, while 72% of the age-matched controls were negative (Ascherio& Munger 2007; Pohl et al 2006). In MS patients also increased $CD4^+$ T cell responses to EBNA-1 were observed compared to controls (Lunemann et al 2006; Lunemann et al 2008).

6. Immunotherapies tested in the marmoset EAE model

The immunological proximity to humans and the clinico-pathological similarity with MS makes the EAE model in marmosets an exquisite test system for the preclinical evaluation of novel immunotherapies. This is especially the case for biological agents, which due to high species-specificity are inactive in lower species. A particularly attractive aspect of the marmoset model is the possibility to visualize the large-sized lesions in the brain with clinically relevant magnetic resonance techniques (Blezer et al 2007; 't Hart & van Kooyk

2004). This has enabled determination of the direct effect of new immunotherapies on lesions independent of the effects on neurological signs ('t Hart & Heije 2005).
In the past years a variety of biological agents was tested mainly aiming at modulating APC-T cell interactions.

6.1 Anti-human CD40 mAb

CD40 is a costimulatory molecule that is constitutively expressed on B cells and induced on myeloid antigen presenting cells, e.g. dendritic cells and macrophages. The interaction of CD40 with its ligand CD154 induced on activated T cells plays an important role in the activation of T and B cells as well as of myeloid antigen presenting cells and macrophage effector functions. The pleiotropic effects of CD40-CD154 interaction on immune functions create an attractive target of immunotherapy in autoimmune diseases, such as MS. Indeed, it was found that a chimeric antagonist anti-CD40 antibody administered during the onset of EAE in marmosets had a strong inhibitory effect on the disease (Boon et al 2001).

6.2 Anti-human IL-12p40 mAb

One of the factors produced by activated APC of the myeloid lineage is IL-12, which is a critical cytokine in the induction of Th1 responses. The notion that Th1 cells have a key pathogenic role in relapsing-remitting MS warranted efficacy evaluation of ustekinumab, a novel human-anti-human IL-12p40 antibody, in the marmoset EAE model. A prophylactic study-design in marmoset EAE induced with human myelin in CFA, showed complete protection against EAE (Brok et al 2002). Next, the same antibody was tested in a therapeutic setting, i.e. starting treatment when brain white matter lesions could be detected on T2-weighted MR images. This experiment showed complete suppression of the inflammatory activity in lesions as well as of lesion enlargement, but only delayed the onset of neurological deficit ('t Hart et al 2005).

6.3 Anti-human IL17A mAb

Many of the immunopathogenic mechanisms driving EAE that were previously assigned to the IL-12-Th1 pathway are actually mediated via the IL-23-induced activation of Th17 cells (Cua et al 2003; Langrish et al 2005), which exerts its pro-inflammatory effects via IL-17A/F, IL-6 and TNF-α. Therefore, we tested the effect of a neutralizing human antibody against human IL-17A in the rhMOG/CFA-induced EAE model. It was observed that the antibody did not protect against EAE, but caused only a moderate delayed onset of neurological signs (Kap et al 2010a). Our interpretation of this experiment is that it supports a role of IL-17A in late stage disease, rather than in the disease onset. This is in agreement with the observation that the MOG_{34-56} specific T cells that are associated with onset of neurological signs display IL-17A production as immunological hallmark.

6.4 Anti-human CD20 mAb

MS has for a long time been regarded as a T cell-driven disease, with a less important contribution of B cells, i.e. only the amplification of demyelination via the secretion of anti-myelin antibodies that elicit complement- (CDC) or macrophage-dependent (ADCC) cytotoxicity reactions. In this light it was rather unexpected that antibody-mediated depletion of $CD20^{+}$ B cells with rituximab had an almost immediate and longlasting beneficial effect on relapsing-remitting MS (Hauser et al 2008). As serum antibody levels remained essentially unaltered the mechanism underlying this remarkable clinical effect is poorly understood. Recent work in rheumatoid arthritis shows a reduction of Th17 responses in patients treated with rituximab, an effect that could be highly relevant for MS as well.

We have tested another human-anti-human CD20 antibody related to ofatumumab in the rhMOG/CFA induced marmoset EAE model. It was observed that weekly administration of the $CD20^+$ B cell depleting antibody, which was started at day 21 post-immunization, had a similar profound clinical effect as rituximab in relapsing-remitting MS (Kap et al 2010b). Remarkably, at the pathological level we observed the complete absence of lesions in the white as well as the grey matter. Mechanistically, suppressed autoantibody levels and profoundly altered cytokine profiles, especially of IL-7 and IL-17A, were detected.

7. Conclusion

The data discussed above clearly demonstrated that the outcome of a preclinical efficacy test with a new candidate therapeutic is strongly influenced by the chosen animal model. It is not surprising that reagents targeting Th1 cells are effective in EAE models induced with CFA, as CFA skews cellular immune reactions into the direction of Th1, with a less prominent pathogenic role of Th17 cells. By contrast, our data show that the marmoset EAE model induced with antigen in IFA is more dominated by Th17 cells; thus would thus be the elected model for testing reagents targeting Th17 cells. Obviously, the most important question is which model is the best representation of MS. Much could be learned from mechanistic analysis of successful and failed trials in MS. There is a marked discrepancy between the positive effect of the anti-human IL-12p40 antibody, ustekinumab, in the rhMOG/CFA-induced marmoset EAE model (Brok et al 2002; 't Hart et al 2005) and the inefficacy in relapsing-remitting MS. This may suggest that Th1 cells have a less prominent role in relapsing MS than in the EAE model, being consistent with the notion that Th17 cells may be pathogenetically more relevant in MS (Langrish et al 2005). On the other hand, depletion of $CD20^+$ B cells has a similar beneficial effect in the rhMOG/CFA-induced marmoset EAE model and relapsing MS (Hauser et al 2008; Kap et al 2010b). Intriguingly, the depletion of B cells also diminishes IL-7 mRNA levels in the lymphoid organs (Kap et al 2010b), which could impair the activation of Th17 effector memory cells (Liu et al 2011). The MOG_{34-56}/IFA EAE model shows that the T cells that mediate CNS inflammation and demyelination in marmosets can be *in vivo* activated without the need of APC activating innate receptor ligands, suggesting that they may be effector memory cells (Jagessar et al 2010). Data obtained from MS patients suggests that this may also be the case in MS (Bielekova et al 2004).

As discussed, the marmoset EAE model resembles MS closely and is a valid model for exploratory and applied research. Future work should make clear which model resembles MS most and should be used for preclinical testing.

8. References

Allamargot, C, Gardinier, MV. (2007). Alternative isoforms of myelin/oligodendrocyte glycoprotein with variable cytoplasmic domains are expressed in human brain. *J Neurochem*, 101, 2, (Apr), 298-312, 0022-3042 (Print)

Antel, JP, McCrea, E, Ladiwala, U, Qin, YF, Becher, B. (1998). Non-MHC-restricted cell-mediated lysis of human oligodendrocytes in vitro: relation with CD56 expression. *J Immunol*, 160, 4, (Feb 15), 1606-11, 0022-1767 (Print)

Antunes, SG, de Groot, NG, Brok, H, Doxiadis, G, Menezes, AA, Otting, N, Bontrop, RE. (1998). The common marmoset: a new world primate species with limited Mhc class II variability. *Proc Natl Acad Sci U S A*, 95, 20, (Sep 29), 11745-50, 0027-8424 (Print)

Ascherio, A, Munger, KL. (2007). Environmental risk factors for multiple sclerosis. Part I: the role of infection. *Ann Neurol*, 61, 4, (Apr), 288-99, 0364-5134 (Print)

Bar-Or, A, Calabresi, PA, Arnold, D, Markowitz, C, Shafer, S, Kasper, LH, Waubant, E, Gazda, S, Fox, RJ, Panzara, M, Sarkar, N, Agarwal, S, Smith, CH. (2008). Rituximab in relapsing-remitting multiple sclerosis: a 72-week, open-label, phase I trial. *Ann Neurol*, 63, 3, (Mar), 395-400, 1531-8249 (Electronic)

Bielekova, B, Martin, R. (2004). Development of biomarkers in multiple sclerosis. *Brain*, 127, Pt 7, (Jul), 1463-78, 0006-8950 (Print)

Bielekova, B, Sung, MH, Kadom, N, Simon, R, McFarland, H, Martin, R. (2004). Expansion and functional relevance of high-avidity myelin-specific CD4+ T cells in multiple sclerosis. *J Immunol*, 172, 6, (Mar 15), 3893-904, 0022-1767 (Print)

Blezer, EL, Bauer, J, Brok, HP, Nicolay, K, 't Hart, BA. (2007). Quantitative MRI-pathology correlations of brain white matter lesions developing in a non-human primate model of multiple sclerosis. *NMR Biomed*, 20, 2, (Apr), 90-103, 0952-3480 (Print)

Boon, L, Brok, HP, Bauer, J, Ortiz-Buijsse, A, Schellekens, MM, Ramdien-Murli, S, Blezer, E, van Meurs, M, Ceuppens, J, de Boer, M, 't Hart, BA, Laman, JD. (2001). Prevention of experimental autoimmune encephalomyelitis in the common marmoset (Callithrix jacchus) using a chimeric antagonist monoclonal antibody against human CD40 is associated with altered B cell responses. *J Immunol*, 167, 5, (Sep 1),

Brok, HP, Boven, L, van Meurs, M, Kerlero de Rosbo, N, Celebi-Paul, L, Kap, YS, Jagessar, A, Hintzen, RQ, Keir, G, Bajramovic, J, Ben-Nun, A, Bauer, J, Laman, JD, Amor, S, 't Hart, BA. (2007). The human CMV-UL86 peptide 981-1003 shares a crossreactive T-cell epitope with the encephalitogenic MOG peptide 34-56, but lacks the capacity to induce EAE in rhesus monkeys. *J Neuroimmunol*, 182, 1-2, (Jan), 135-52, 0165-5728 (Print)

Brok, HP, Uccelli, A, Kerlero De Rosbo, N, Bontrop, RE, Roccatagliata, L, de Groot, NG, Capello, E, Laman, JD, Nicolay, K, Mancardi, GL, Ben-Nun, A, 't Hart, BA. (2000). Myelin/oligodendrocyte glycoprotein-induced autoimmune encephalomyelitis in common marmosets: the encephalitogenic T cell epitope pMOG24-36 is presented by a monomorphic MHC class II molecule. *J Immunol*, 165, 2, (Jul 15), 1093-101, 0022-1767 (Print)

Brok, HP, van Meurs, M, Blezer, E, Schantz, A, Peritt, D, Treacy, G, Laman, JD, Bauer, J, 't Hart, BA. (2002). Prevention of experimental autoimmune encephalomyelitis in common marmosets using an anti-IL-12p40 monoclonal antibody. *J Immunol*, 169, 11, (Dec 1), 6554-63, 0022-1767 (Print)

Brucklacher-Waldert, V, Stuerner, K, Kolster, M, Wolthausen, J, Tolosa, E. (2009). Phenotypical and functional characterization of T helper 17 cells in multiple sclerosis. *Brain*, 132, Pt 12, (Dec), 3329-41, 1460-2156 (Electronic)

Bruno, R, Sabater, L, Sospedra, M, Ferrer-Francesch, X, Escudero, D, Martinez-Caceres, E, Pujol-Borrell, R. (2002). Multiple sclerosis candidate autoantigens except myelin oligodendrocyte glycoprotein are transcribed in human thymus. *Eur J Immunol*, 32, 10, (Oct), 2737-47, 0014-2980 (Print)

Cadavid, LF, Shufflebotham, C, Ruiz, FJ, Yeager, M, Hughes, AL, Watkins, DI. (1997). Evolutionary instability of the major histocompatibility complex class I loci in New World primates. *Proc Natl Acad Sci U S A*, 94, 26, (Dec 23), 14536-41, 0027-8424 (Print)

Clements, CS, Reid, HH, Beddoe, T, Tynan, FE, Perugini, MA, Johns, TG, Bernard, CC, Rossjohn, J. (2003). The crystal structure of myelin oligodendrocyte glycoprotein, a key autoantigen in multiple sclerosis. *Proc Natl Acad Sci U S A*, 100, 19, (Sep 16), 11059-64, 0027-8424 (Print)

Cohen, PA, Peng, L, Plautz, GE, Kim, JA, Weng, DE, Shu, S. (2000). CD4+ T cells in adoptive immunotherapy and the indirect mechanism of tumor rejection. *Crit Rev Immunol*, 20, 1, 17-56, 1040-8401 (Print)

Compston, A, Coles, A. (2008). Multiple sclerosis. *Lancet*, 372, 9648, (Oct 25), 1502-17, 1474-547X (Electronic)

Cua, DJ, Sherlock, J, Chen, Y, Murphy, CA, Joyce, B, Seymour, B, Lucian, L, To, W, Kwan, S, Churakova, T, Zurawski, S, Wiekowski, M, Lira, SA, Gorman, D, Kastelein, RA, Sedgwick, JD. (2003). Interleukin-23 rather than interleukin-12 is the critical cytokine for autoimmune inflammation of the brain. *Nature*, 421, 6924, (Feb 13), 744-8, 0028-0836 (Print)

Delarasse, C, Daubas, P, Mars, LT, Vizler, C, Litzenburger, T, Iglesias, A, Bauer, J, Della Gaspera, B, Schubart, A, Decker, L, Dimitri, D, Roussel, G, Dierich, A, Amor, S, Dautigny, A, Liblau, R, Pham-Dinh, D. (2003). Myelin/oligodendrocyte glycoprotein-deficient (MOG-deficient) mice reveal lack of immune tolerance to MOG in wild-type mice. *J Clin Invest*, 112, 4, (Aug), 544-53, 0021-9738 (Print)

Delarasse, C, Della Gaspera, B, Lu, CW, Lachapelle, F, Gelot, A, Rodriguez, D, Dautigny, A, Genain, C, Pham-Dinh, D. (2006). Complex alternative splicing of the myelin oligodendrocyte glycoprotein gene is unique to human and non-human primates. *J Neurochem*, 98, 6, (Sep), 1707-17, 0022-3042 (Print)

Devetag, FC, Boscariolo, L. (2000). Cytomegalovirus meningoencephalitis with paroxysmal course in immunocompetent adults: a new nosographical entity. Clinical, diagnostic and therapeutic correlations, and pathogenetic hypothesis. *Eur Neurol*, 44, 4, 242-7, 0014-3022 (Print)

Diaz-Villoslada, P, Shih, A, Shao, L, Genain, CP, Hauser, SL. (1999). Autoreactivity to myelin antigens: myelin/oligodendrocyte glycoprotein is a prevalent autoantigen. *J Neuroimmunol*, 99, 1, (Sep 1), 36-43, 0165-5728 (Print)

Doxiadis, GG, van der Wiel, MK, Brok, HP, de Groot, NG, Otting, N, 't Hart, BA, van Rood, JJ, Bontrop, RE. (2006). Reactivation by exon shuffling of a conserved HLA-DR3-

like pseudogene segment in a New World primate species. *Proc Natl Acad Sci U S A*, 103, 15, (Apr 11), 5864-8, 0027-8424 (Print)

Filippi, C, von Herrath, M. (2005). How viral infections affect the autoimmune process leading to type 1 diabetes. *Cell Immunol*, 233, 2, (Feb), 125-32, 0008-8749 (Print)

Fotheringham, J, Jacobson, S. (2005). Human herpesvirus 6 and multiple sclerosis: potential mechanisms for virus-induced disease. *Herpes*, 12, 1, (Jun), 4-9, 0969-7667 (Print)

Fujii, Y, Matsutani, T, Kitaura, K, Suzuki, S, Itoh, T, Takasaki, T, Suzuki, R, Kurane, I. (2010). Comprehensive analysis and characterization of the TCR alpha chain sequences in the common marmoset. *Immunogenetics*, 62, 6, (Jun), 383-95, 1432-1211 (Electronic)

Genain, CP, Cannella, B, Hauser, SL, Raine, CS. (1999). Identification of autoantibodies associated with myelin damage in multiple sclerosis. *Nat Med*, 5, 2, (Feb), 170-5, 1078-8956 (Print)

Genain, CP, Nguyen, MH, Letvin, NL, Pearl, R, Davis, RL, Adelman, M, Lees, MB, Linington, C, Hauser, SL. (1995). Antibody facilitation of multiple sclerosis-like lesions in a nonhuman primate. *J Clin Invest*, 96, 6, (Dec), 2966-74, 0021-9738 (Print)

Gold, R, Linington, C, Lassmann, H. (2006). Understanding pathogenesis and therapy of multiple sclerosis via animal models: 70 years of merits and culprits in experimental autoimmune encephalomyelitis research. *Brain*, 129, Pt 8, (Aug), 1953-71, 1460-2156 (Electronic)

Haak, S, Croxford, AL, Kreymborg, K, Heppner, FL, Pouly, S, Becher, B, Waisman, A. (2009). IL-17A and IL-17F do not contribute vitally to autoimmune neuro-inflammation in mice. *J Clin Invest*, 119, 1, (Jan), 61-9, 0021-9738 (Print)

Hauser, SL, Waubant, E, Arnold, DL, Vollmer, T, Antel, J, Fox, RJ, Bar-Or, A, Panzara, M, Sarkar, N, Agarwal, S, Langer-Gould, A, Smith, CH. (2008). B-cell depletion with rituximab in relapsing-remitting multiple sclerosis. *N Engl J Med*, 358, 7, (Feb 14), 676-88, 1533-4406 (Electronic)

Ifergan, I, Kebir, H, Bernard, M, Wosik, K, Dodelet-Devillers, A, Cayrol, R, Arbour, N, Prat, A. (2008). The blood-brain barrier induces differentiation of migrating monocytes into Th17-polarizing dendritic cells. *Brain*, 131, Pt 3, (Mar), 785-99, 1460-2156 (Electronic)

Iglesias, A, Bauer, J, Litzenburger, T, Schubart, A, Linington, C. (2001). T- and B-cell responses to myelin oligodendrocyte glycoprotein in experimental autoimmune encephalomyelitis and multiple sclerosis. *Glia*, 36, 2, (Nov), 220-34, 0894-1491 (Print)

Jagessar, SA, Kap, YS, Heijmans, N, van Driel, N, van Straalen, L, Bajramovic, JJ, Brok, HP, Blezer, EL, Bauer, J, Laman, JD, 't Hart, BA. (2010). Induction of progressive demyelinating autoimmune encephalomyelitis in common marmoset monkeys using MOG34-56 peptide in incomplete freund adjuvant. *J Neuropathol Exp Neurol*, 69, 4, (Apr), 372-85, 0022-3069 (Print)

Jagessar, SA, Smith, PA, Blezer, E, Delarasse, C, Pham-Dinh, D, Laman, JD, Bauer, J, Amor, S, 't Hart, B. (2008). Autoimmunity against myelin oligodendrocyte glycoprotein is dispensable for the initiation although essential for the progression of chronic encephalomyelitis in common marmosets. *J Neuropathol Exp Neurol*, 67, 4, (Apr), 326-40, 0022-3069 (Print)

Kanzaki, A, Yabuki, S. (1994). [Acute disseminated encephalomyelitis (ADEM) associated with cytomegalovirus infection--a case report]. *Rinsho Shinkeigaku*, 34, 5, (May), 511-3, 0009-918X (Print)

Kap, YS, Jagessar, SA, van Driel, N, Blezer, E, Bauer, J, van Meurs, M, Smith, P, Laman, JD, 't Hart, BA. (2010a). Effects of Early IL-17A Neutralization on Disease Induction in a Primate Model of Experimental Autoimmune Encephalomyelitis. *J Neuroimmune Pharmacol*, (Aug 12), 1557-1904 (Electronic)

Kap, YS, Smith, P, Jagessar, SA, Remarque, E, Blezer, E, Strijkers, GJ, Laman, JD, Hintzen, RQ, Bauer, J, Brok, HP, 't Hart, BA. (2008). Fast progression of recombinant human myelin/oligodendrocyte glycoprotein (MOG)-induced experimental autoimmune encephalomyelitis in marmosets is associated with the activation of MOG34-56-specific cytotoxic T cells. *J Immunol*, 180, 3, (Feb 1), 1326-37, 0022-1767 (Print)

Kap, YS, van Driel, N, Blezer, E, Parren, PW, Bleeker, WK, Laman, JD, Craigen, JL, 't Hart, BA. (2010b). Late B cell depletion with a human anti-human CD20 IgG1kappa monoclonal antibody halts the development of experimental autoimmune encephalomyelitis in marmosets. *J Immunol*, 185, 7, (Oct 1), 3990-4003, 1550-6606 (Electronic)

Kebir, H, Kreymborg, K, Ifergan, I, Dodelet-Devillers, A, Cayrol, R, Bernard, M, Giuliani, F, Arbour, N, Becher, B, Prat, A. (2007). Human TH17 lymphocytes promote blood-brain barrier disruption and central nervous system inflammation. *Nat Med*, 13, 10, (Oct), 1173-5, 1078-8956 (Print)

Kerlero de Rosbo, N, Brok, HP, Bauer, J, Kaye, JF, 't Hart, BA, Ben-Nun, A. (2000). Rhesus monkeys are highly susceptible to experimental autoimmune encephalomyelitis induced by myelin oligodendrocyte glycoprotein: characterisation of immunodominant T- and B-cell epitopes. *J Neuroimmunol*, 110, 1-2, (Oct 2), 83-96, 0165-5728 (Print)

Kerlero de Rosbo, N, Hoffman, M, Mendel, I, Yust, I, Kaye, J, Bakimer, R, Flechter, S, Abramsky, O, Milo, R, Karni, A, Ben-Nun, A. (1997). Predominance of the autoimmune response to myelin oligodendrocyte glycoprotein (MOG) in multiple sclerosis: reactivity to the extracellular domain of MOG is directed against three main regions. *Eur J Immunol*, 27, 11, (Nov), 3059-69, 0014-2980 (Print)

Kerlero de Rosbo, N, Honegger, P, Lassmann, H, Matthieu, JM. (1990). Demyelination induced in aggregating brain cell cultures by a monoclonal antibody against myelin/oligodendrocyte glycoprotein. *J Neurochem*, 55, 2, (Aug), 583-7, 0022-3042 (Print)

Kerlero de Rosbo, N, Milo, R, Lees, MB, Burger, D, Bernard, CC, Ben-Nun, A. (1993). Reactivity to myelin antigens in multiple sclerosis. Peripheral blood lymphocytes respond predominantly to myelin oligodendrocyte glycoprotein. *J Clin Invest*, 92, 6, (Dec), 2602-8, 0021-9738 (Print)

Knapp, LA, Cadavid, LF, Watkins, DI. (1998). The MHC-E locus is the most well conserved of all known primate class I histocompatibility genes. *J Immunol*, 160, 1, (Jan 1), 189-96, 0022-1767 (Print)

Koehler, NK, Genain, CP, Giesser, B, Hauser, SL. (2002). The human T cell response to myelin oligodendrocyte glycoprotein: a multiple sclerosis family-based study. *J Immunol*, 168, 11, (Jun 1), 5920-7, 0022-1767 (Print)

Komiyama, Y, Nakae, S, Matsuki, T, Nambu, A, Ishigame, H, Kakuta, S, Sudo, K, Iwakura, Y. (2006). IL-17 plays an important role in the development of experimental autoimmune encephalomyelitis. *J Immunol*, 177, 1, (Jul 1), 566-73, 0022-1767 (Print)

Kroenke, MA, Carlson, TJ, Andjelkovic, AV, Segal, BM. (2008). IL-12- and IL-23-modulated T cells induce distinct types of EAE based on histology, CNS chemokine profile, and response to cytokine inhibition. *J Exp Med*, 205, 7, (Jul 7), 1535-41, 1540-9538 (Electronic)

Kroepfl, JF, Viise, LR, Charron, AJ, Linington, C, Gardinier, MV. (1996). Investigation of myelin/oligodendrocyte glycoprotein membrane topology. *J Neurochem*, 67, 5, (Nov), 2219-22, 0022-3042 (Print)

Langrish, CL, Chen, Y, Blumenschein, WM, Mattson, J, Basham, B, Sedgwick, JD, McClanahan, T, Kastelein, RA, Cua, DJ. (2005). IL-23 drives a pathogenic T cell population that induces autoimmune inflammation. *J Exp Med*, 201, 2, (Jan 17), 233-40, 0022-1007 (Print)

Levin, LI, Munger, KL, Rubertone, MV, Peck, CA, Lennette, ET, Spiegelman, D, Ascherio, A. (2003). Multiple sclerosis and Epstein-Barr virus. *JAMA*, 289, 12, (Mar 26), 1533-6, 0098-7484 (Print)

Levin, LI, Munger, KL, Rubertone, MV, Peck, CA, Lennette, ET, Spiegelman, D, Ascherio, A. (2005). Temporal relationship between elevation of epstein-barr virus antibody titers and initial onset of neurological symptoms in multiple sclerosis. *JAMA*, 293, 20, (May 25), 2496-500, 1538-3598 (Electronic)

Linington, C, Bradl, M, Lassmann, H, Brunner, C, Vass, K. (1988). Augmentation of demyelination in rat acute allergic encephalomyelitis by circulating mouse monoclonal antibodies directed against a myelin/oligodendrocyte glycoprotein. *Am J Pathol*, 130, 3, (Mar), 443-54, 0002-9440 (Print)

Liu, YS, Wu, L, Tong, XH, Wu, LM, He, GP, Zhou, GX, Luo, LH, Luan, HB. (2011). Study on the relationship between th17 cells and unexplained recurrent spontaneous abortion. *Am J Reprod Immunol*, 65, 5, (May), 503-11, 1600-0897 (Electronic)

Lunemann, JD, Edwards, N, Muraro, PA, Hayashi, S, Cohen, JI, Munz, C, Martin, R. (2006). Increased frequency and broadened specificity of latent EBV nuclear antigen-1-specific T cells in multiple sclerosis. *Brain*, 129, Pt 6, (Jun), 1493-506, 1460-2156 (Electronic)

Lunemann, JD, Gelderblom, H, Sospedra, M, Quandt, JA, Pinilla, C, Marques, A, Martin, R. (2007). Cerebrospinal fluid-infiltrating CD4+ T cells recognize Borrelia burgdorferi lysine-enriched protein domains and central nervous system autoantigens in early lyme encephalitis. *Infect Immun*, 75, 1, (Jan), 243-51, 0019-9567 (Print)

Lunemann, JD, Jelcic, I, Roberts, S, Lutterotti, A, Tackenberg, B, Martin, R, Munz, C. (2008). EBNA1-specific T cells from patients with multiple sclerosis cross react with myelin antigens and co-produce IFN-gamma and IL-2. *J Exp Med*, 205, 8, (Aug 4), 1763-73, 1540-9538 (Electronic)

Massacesi, L, Genain, CP, Lee-Parritz, D, Letvin, NL, Canfield, D, Hauser, SL. (1995). Active and passively induced experimental autoimmune encephalomyelitis in common marmosets: a new model for multiple sclerosis. *Ann Neurol*, 37, 4, (Apr), 519-30, 0364-5134 (Print)

Mazzarino, P, Pietra, G, Vacca, P, Falco, M, Colau, D, Coulie, P, Moretta, L, Mingari, MC. (2005). Identification of effector-memory CMV-specific T lymphocytes that kill CMV-infected target cells in an HLA-E-restricted fashion. *Eur J Immunol*, 35, 11, (Nov), 3240-7, 0014-2980 (Print)

McFarland, HI, Lobito, AA, Johnson, MM, Nyswaner, JT, Frank, JA, Palardy, GR, Tresser, N, Genain, CP, Mueller, JP, Matis, LA, Lenardo, MJ. (1999). Determinant spreading associated with demyelination in a nonhuman primate model of multiple sclerosis. *J Immunol*, 162, 4, (Feb 15), 2384-90, 0022-1767 (Print)

Mendel, I, Kerlero de Rosbo, N, Ben-Nun, A. (1995). A myelin oligodendrocyte glycoprotein peptide induces typical chronic experimental autoimmune encephalomyelitis in H-2b mice: fine specificity and T cell receptor V beta expression of encephalitogenic T cells. *Eur J Immunol*, 25, 7, (Jul), 1951-9, 0014-2980 (Print)

Mesleh, MF, Belmar, N, Lu, CW, Krishnan, VV, Maxwell, RS, Genain, CP, Cosman, M. (2002). Marmoset fine B cell and T cell epitope specificities mapped onto a homology model of the extracellular domain of human myelin oligodendrocyte glycoprotein. *Neurobiol Dis*, 9, 2, (Mar), 160-72, 0969-9961 (Print)

Morris-Downes, MM, Smith, PA, Rundle, JL, Piddlesden, SJ, Baker, D, Pham-Dinh, D, Heijmans, N, Amor, S. (2002). Pathological and regulatory effects of anti-myelin antibodies in experimental allergic encephalomyelitis in mice. *J Neuroimmunol*, 125, 1-2, (Apr), 114-24, 0165-5728 (Print)

Mowry, EM, Krupp, LB, Milazzo, M, Chabas, D, Strober, JB, Belman, AL, McDonald, JC, Oksenberg, JR, Bacchetti, P, Waubant, E. (2010). Vitamin D status is associated with relapse rate in pediatric-onset multiple sclerosis. *Ann Neurol*, 67, 5, (May), 618-24, 1531-8249 (Electronic)

Niblack, GD, Kateley, JR, Gengozian, N. (1977). T-and B-lymphocyte chimerism in the marmoset. *Immunology*, 32, 2, (Feb), 257-63, 0019-2805 (Print)

O'Connor, RA, Prendergast, CT, Sabatos, CA, Lau, CW, Leech, MD, Wraith, DC, Anderton, SM. (2008). Cutting edge: Th1 cells facilitate the entry of Th17 cells to the central nervous system during experimental autoimmune encephalomyelitis. *J Immunol*, 181, 6, (Sep 15), 3750-4, 1550-6606 (Electronic)

Ohler, B, Graf, K, Bragg, R, Lemons, T, Coe, R, Genain, C, Israelachvili, J, Husted, C. (2004). Role of lipid interactions in autoimmune demyelination. *Biochim Biophys Acta*, 1688, 1, (Jan 20), 10-7, 0006-3002 (Print)

Pohl, D, Krone, B, Rostasy, K, Kahler, E, Brunner, E, Lehnert, M, Wagner, HJ, Gartner, J, Hanefeld, F. (2006). High seroprevalence of Epstein-Barr virus in children with multiple sclerosis. *Neurology*, 67, 11, (Dec 12), 2063-5, 1526-632X (Electronic)

Prasad, S, Humphreys, I, Kireta, S, Gilchrist, RB, Bardy, P, Russ, GR, Coates, PT. (2006). MHC Class II DRB genotyping is highly predictive of in-vitro alloreactivity in the common marmoset. *J Immunol Methods*, 314, 1-2, (Jul 31), 153-63, 0022-1759 (Print)

Roberts, BW, Cech, I. (2005). Association of type 2 diabetes mellitus and seroprevalence for cytomegalovirus. *South Med J*, 98, 7, (Jul), 686-92, 0038-4348 (Print)

Schluesener, HJ, Sobel, RA, Linington, C, Weiner, HL. (1987). A monoclonal antibody against a myelin oligodendrocyte glycoprotein induces relapses and demyelination in central nervous system autoimmune disease. *J Immunol*, 139, 12, (Dec 15), 4016-21, 0022-1767 (Print)

Scotet, E, Peyrat, MA, Saulquin, X, Retiere, C, Couedel, C, Davodeau, F, Dulphy, N, Toubert, A, Bignon, JD, Lim, A, Vie, H, Hallet, MM, Liblau, R, Weber, M, Berthelot, JM, Houssaint, E, Bonneville, M. (1999). Frequent enrichment for CD8 T cells reactive against common herpes viruses in chronic inflammatory lesions: towards a reassessment of the physiopathological significance of T cell clonal expansions found in autoimmune inflammatory processes. *Eur J Immunol*, 29, 3, (Mar), 973-85, 0014-2980 (Print)

Sekigawa, I, Nawata, M, Seta, N, Yamada, M, Iida, N, Hashimoto, H. (2002). Cytomegalovirus infection in patients with systemic lupus erythematosus. *Clin Exp Rheumatol*, 20, 4, (Jul-Aug), 559-64, 0392-856X (Print)

Serafini, B, Rosicarelli, B, Franciotta, D, Magliozzi, R, Reynolds, R, Cinque, P, Andreoni, L, Trivedi, P, Salvetti, M, Faggioni, A, Aloisi, F. (2007). Dysregulated Epstein-Barr virus infection in the multiple sclerosis brain. *J Exp Med*, (Nov 5),

Smith, PA, Heijmans, N, Ouwerling, B, Breij, EC, Evans, N, van Noort, JM, Plomp, AC, Delarasse, C, 't Hart, B, Pham-Dinh, D, Amor, S. (2005). Native myelin oligodendrocyte glycoprotein promotes severe chronic neurological disease and demyelination in Biozzi ABH mice. *Eur J Immunol*, 35, 4, (Apr), 1311-9, 0014-2980 (Print)

Sospedra, M, Martin, R. (2005). Immunology of multiple sclerosis. *Annu Rev Immunol*, 23, 683-747, 0732-0582 (Print)

Staras, SA, Dollard, SC, Radford, KW, Flanders, WD, Pass, RF, Cannon, MJ. (2006). Seroprevalence of cytomegalovirus infection in the United States, 1988-1994. *Clin Infect Dis*, 43, 9, (Nov 1), 1143-51, 1537-6591 (Electronic)

Stefferl, A, Brehm, U, Linington, C. (2000). The myelin oligodendrocyte glycoprotein (MOG): a model for antibody-mediated demyelination in experimental autoimmune encephalomyelitis and multiple sclerosis. *J Neural Transm Suppl*, 58, 123-33, 0303-6995 (Print)

Sumaya, CV, Myers, LW, Ellison, GW. (1980). Epstein-Barr virus antibodies in multiple sclerosis. *Arch Neurol*, 37, 2, (Feb), 94-6, 0003-9942 (Print)

Sun, J, Link, H, Olsson, T, Xiao, BG, Andersson, G, Ekre, HP, Linington, C, Diener, P. (1991). T and B cell responses to myelin-oligodendrocyte glycoprotein in multiple sclerosis. *J Immunol*, 146, 5, (Mar 1), 1490-5, 0022-1767 (Print)

Sylwester, AW, Mitchell, BL, Edgar, JB, Taormina, C, Pelte, C, Ruchti, F, Sleath, PR, Grabstein, KH, Hosken, NA, Kern, F, Nelson, JA, Picker, LJ. (2005). Broadly targeted human cytomegalovirus-specific CD4+ and CD8+ T cells dominate the memory compartments of exposed subjects. *J Exp Med*, 202, 5, (Sep 5), 673-85, 0022-1007 (Print) 't Hart, BA, Brok, HP, Remarque, E, Benson, J, Treacy, G, Amor, S, Hintzen, RQ, Laman, JD, Bauer, J, Blezer, EL. (2005). Suppression of ongoing disease in a nonhuman primate model of multiple sclerosis by a human-anti-human IL-12p40 antibody. *J Immunol*, 175, 7, (Oct 1), 4761-8, 0022-1767 (Print)

't Hart, BA, Heije, K. (2005). Broad spectrum immune monitoring in immune-mediated inflammatory disorders. *Drug Discov Today*, 10, 20, (Oct 15), 1348-51, 1359-6446 (Print)

't Hart, BA, Hintzen, RQ, Laman, JD. (2009). Multiple sclerosis - a response-to-damage model. *Trends Mol Med*, 15, 6, (Jun), 235-44, 1471-499X (Electronic)

't Hart, BA, van Kooyk, Y. (2004). Yin-Yang regulation of autoimmunity by DCs. *Trends Immunol*, 25, 7, (Jul), 353-9,

Tzartos, JS, Friese, MA, Craner, MJ, Palace, J, Newcombe, J, Esiri, MM, Fugger, L. (2008). Interleukin-17 production in central nervous system-infiltrating T cells and glial cells is associated with active disease in multiple sclerosis. *Am J Pathol*, 172, 1, (Jan), 146-55, 0002-9440 (Print)

Uccelli, A, Oksenberg, JR, Jeong, MC, Genain, CP, Rombos, T, Jaeger, EE, Giunti, D, Lanchbury, JS, Hauser, SL. (1997). Characterization of the TCRB chain repertoire in the New World monkey Callithrix jacchus. *J Immunol*, 158, 3, (Feb 1), 1201-7, 0022-1767 (Print)

Van der Aa, A, Hellings, N, Bernard, CC, Raus, J, Stinissen, P. (2003). Functional properties of myelin oligodendrocyte glycoprotein-reactive T cells in multiple sclerosis patients and controls. *J Neuroimmunol*, 137, 1-2, (Apr), 164-76, 0165-5728 (Print)

Van der Goes, A, Kortekaas, M, Hoekstra, K, Dijkstra, CD, Amor, S. (1999). The role of anti-myelin (auto)-antibodies in the phagocytosis of myelin by macrophages. *J Neuroimmunol*, 101, 1, (Nov 1), 61-7, 0165-5728 (Print)

Vergelli, M, Le, H, van Noort, JM, Dhib-Jalbut, S, McFarland, H, Martin, R. (1996). A novel population of CD4+CD56+ myelin-reactive T cells lyses target cells expressing CD56/neural cell adhesion molecule. *J Immunol*, 157, 2, (Jul 15), 679-88, 0022-1767 (Print)

Villoslada, P, Abel, K, Heald, N, Goertsches, R, Hauser, SL, Genain, CP. (2001). Frequency, heterogeneity and encephalitogenicity of T cells specific for myelin oligodendrocyte glycoprotein in naive outbred primates. *Eur J Immunol*, 31, 10, (Oct), 2942-50, 0014-2980 (Print)

von Büdingen, HC, Hauser, SL, Ouallet, JC, Tanuma, N, Menge, T, Genain, CP. (2004). Frontline: Epitope recognition on the myelin/oligodendrocyte glycoprotein differentially influences disease phenotype and antibody effector functions in autoimmune demyelination. *Eur J Immunol*, 34, 8, (Aug), 2072-83, 0014-2980 (Print)

von Büdingen, HC, Tanuma, N, Villoslada, P, Ouallet, JC, Hauser, SL, Genain, CP. (2001). Immune responses against the myelin/oligodendrocyte glycoprotein in experimental autoimmune demyelination. *J Clin Immunol*, 21, 3, (May), 155-70, 0271-9142 (Print)

Wekerle H, KF. (2006). Animal models of multiple sclerosis. *Drug Discovery Today: Disease models*, 3, 4, 359-367,

Wu, MS, Tani, K, Sugiyama, H, Hibino, H, Izawa, K, Tanabe, T, Nakazaki, Y, Ishii, H, Ohashi, J, Hohjoh, H, Iseki, T, Tojo, A, Nakamura, Y, Tanioka, Y, Tokunaga, K, Asano, S. (2000). MHC (major histocompatibility complex)-DRB genes and polymorphisms in common marmoset. *J Mol Evol*, 51, 3, (Sep), 214-22, 0022-2844 (Print)

Yuki, N, Susuki, K, Odaka, M, Hirata, K. (2001). Overlapping Guillain-Barre syndrome and Bickerstaff's brainstem encephalitis associated with anti-GQ1b IgG antibody after herpes simplex virus infection. *Acta Neurol Scand*, 104, 1, (Jul), 57-60, 0001-6314 (Print)

22

Alternative Medicines for Encephalitis

Kenji Sorimachi and Takaaki Nakamoto
Dokkyo Medical University
Japan

1. Introduction

Encephalitis can be caused by several viruses, including western equine encephalitis (WEE) virus, Japanese encephalitis virus, herpes simplex virus (HSV), human immunodeficiency virus (HIV), influenza viruses and the measles virus. Bacteria such as *Neisseria meningitidis* and *Treponema pallidum* have also been shown to be causative agents of encephalitis. There are no medications currently available that selectively target virus-infected cells, although some nucleotide derivatives, and oseltamivir, are exceptionally effective against herpes simplex and influenza viruses, respectively.

Vaccination is one way to prevent infection; however, vaccines have not been developed for every viral disease. Western medicines based on herbal extracts, and alternative Eastern medicines have been used for treatment and as preventative measures in instances of viral infection. In particular, the latter has been developed based on daily life from ancient times when molecular biological knowledge was lacking. An example of this is the bark of *Cinchona succirubra,* which contains quinine and has been used as a remedy for malaria.

Following infection, certain viruses cause cytopathic effects (CPE) in cells that grow as monolayers *in vitro*. This phenomenon is a useful tool in virology to determine whether a material is applicable for treatment of viral diseases. Viral infection is usually controlled by species specificity, and inhibited by interferons produced by infected cells. Not every cell line exhibits a CPE following infection. African Green Monkey (Vero) cells (Yasumura & Kawakita, 1963) are defective in the production of interferons, and are highly susceptible to arboviruses and many other pathogenic viruses (Simizu & Terasima,). The Vero cell line is used for basic virus research in laboratories, diagnostics in hospitals, epidemiological surveys and bacterial toxin assays. Additionally, the potential of Vero cells for vaccine production has been examined. The cell line has been distributed to scientists globally by services such as the American Type Culture Collection.

It has been shown that *Agaricus blazei* Murille water extracts, prepared as an alternative medicine, inhibit the formation of CPE in Vero cell cultures caused by the WEE virus. Vero cells were continuously cultured in a modified Eagle's minimal essential medium without serum, protein and lipids (Yasumura et al., 1978). The cells were grown on 24-well plastic culture plates in a chemically defined medium for viral assay experiments, cells infected after they reached confluency. Before virus infection, the cells were washed with the phosphate-buffered saline (PBS, pH 7.4) without Mg^{2+} and Ca^{2+}. A virus-containing solution (0.2 ml) with a 50% tissue culture infective dose ($TCID_{50}$) of 100 was added to each well and allowed to adsorb for 90 min at room temperature. The virus solution was then removed from the wells, and fresh culture medium with and without *Agaricus* extracts added (Sorimachi et al., 2001).

2. Effect of alternative medicine on viruses

2.1 Effect of Agaricus blazei water extracts on virus-infected VERO cells

When Vero cells were infected with WEE virus, CPE was observed as shown in Figure 1-D and Table 1. The original water extract from *Agaricus blazei* mycelia (A-0) and other fractions (A-1, A-2 and A-3) showed a significant inhibitory effect on CPE formation by WEE virus after 1 week in culture, but this effect was no longer observable after 2 weeks in culture (Table 1) (Sorimachi et al., 2001). Fractions A-4 and A-5 showed a small inhibitory effect on the occurrence of CPE induced by HSV (Table 1). However, neither the original water extracts of *Agaricus blazei* fruiting bodies nor their fractions obtained by ethanol precipitation demonstrated significant inhibitory effects on CPE due to WEE virus or HSV.

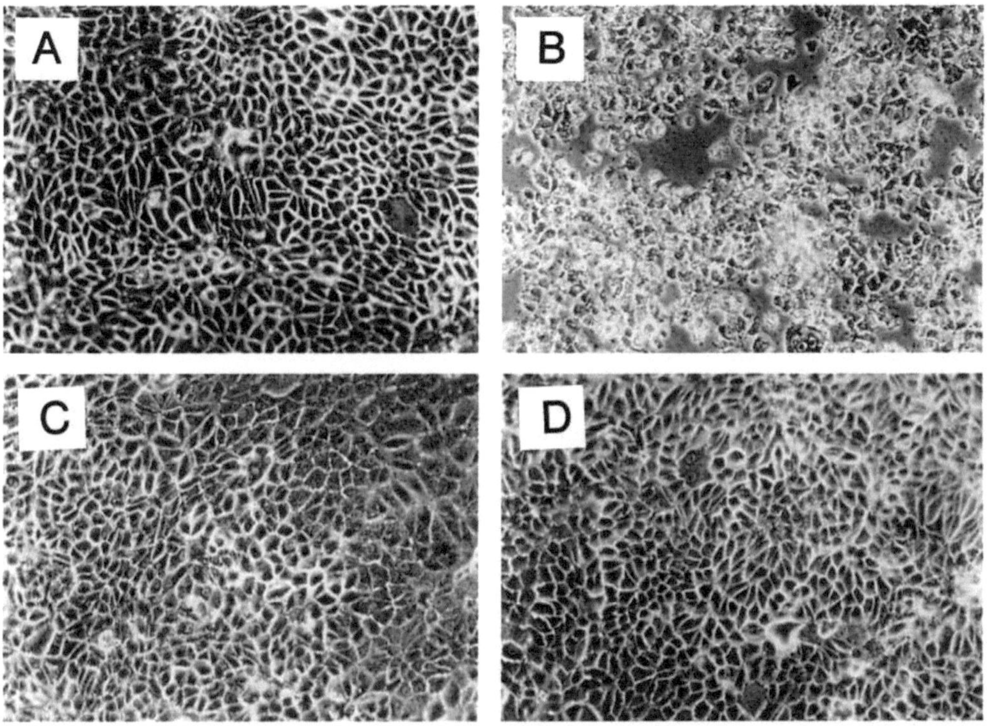

Fig. 1. Inhibitory effect of *Agaricus blazei* fractions on the CPE of Vero cells induced with western equine encephalitis (WEE) virus. Cells were infected with WEE virus and cultured for 1 week. (A) Control, uninfected Vero cells; (B) cells infected with WEE virus; (C) cells treated with fraction A-4; and (D) cells infected with WEE virus and cultured with fraction A-4. The concentration of *Agaricus* fraction A-4 was 100 μg/ml. This figure is reproduced from *Bioscience, Biotechnology and Biochemistry*, 65 (7); 1645–1647, 2001, and has been used with permission from Japan Society for Bioscience, Biotechnology, and Agrochemistry.

Fraction	Ethanol (%)	WEE	HSV
A-0	0	(++)	-
A-1	17	(+)	-
A-2	29	(++)	-
A-3	38	(++)	-
A-4	44	+++	(++)
A-5	50	+++	(+)
A-6	50 Sup	-	-

Table 1. Inhibitory effect of *Agaricus blazei* mycelia fractions on CPE induced by western equine encephalitis (WEE) virus and herpes simplex virus (HSV).
Cells were cultured for 2 weeks following virus inoculation.
(+), small inhibitory effect observed after 1 week in culture, but absent after 2 weeks in culture. (++), significant inhibitory effect observed after 1 week in culture, but no longer observable after 2 weeks in culture. +++, complete inhibition was observed after 2 weeks in culture. -, no significant inhibition was observed. The 50% tissue culture infective dose was 100. The concentration of *Agaricus* fractions was 100 μg/ml.

2.2 Effect of lignin derivatives on virus-infected VERO cells

Lignin derivatives, such as EP3, extracted from the culture medium of the edible Japanese mushroom, *Lentinus edodes*, inhibit the formation of CPE usually caused by HSV and WEE virus (Table 2) (Sorimachi et al., 1990). Other lignin derivatives, such as lignosulfonate (LS), obtained from the waste liquor of acid sulfite pulping processes, demonstrate similar anti-viral activity as EP3. Both EP3 and LS partially inhibit the formation of CPE caused by other viruses including polio, mumps and measles viruses. It is well known that a small proportion of measles cases can cause subacute sclerosing panencephalitis many years after the initial infection.

Virus	EP3	LS
Vaccinia	(+)	(+)
Herpes simplex		
(Yasumura, type 1)	+++	+++
(UR-3, type 1)	+++	+++
(UW, type 2)	+++	+++
(MS, type 2)	+++	+++
WEE	+++	+++
Polio	+	++
Mumps	+	+
Measles (Sugiyama)	+	+

Table 2. Inhibitory effects of EP3 and LS on CPE induced by various viruses.
+++, complete inhibition; ++, a few cytopathogenic effects were observed; +, a small effect was observed; and (+), a small drug effect was observed after 4 days in culture.

2.3 Effect of alternative medicines on HIV

Encephalitis caused by HIV is another serious problem that needs to be considered. HIV has been well characterized at a molecular biological level and clinically, but with a complete remedy yet to be established. Reasons for this include antigenic variation of HIV surface proteins and a lack of adequate medications. The compound agaritine, which is a carcinogen and is contained in *Agaricus bisuporus* and *Agaricus blazei* Murrile, inhibits HIV protease activity (Gao et al., 2007). Although agaritine is found within alternative medicines and is toxic to healthy people, it is useful in treating HIV-positive patients. Additionally, the method to specifically remove agaritine from *Agaricus blazei* water extracts has been recently established in our laboratory (Koge et al., 2011). Thus, we can now select *Agaricus* water extracts with or without agaritine products depending on their end purpose. EP3 (Suzuki et al., 1989a) and LS (Suzuki et al., 1989b) showed anti-viral activity against HIV *in vitro*, and the oral administration of LEM, which contains EP3, improved the hepatic functions of hepatitis B patients *in vivo* without serious side effects. Therefore, *Agaricus blazei* extracts and lignin derivatives, which are used as alternative medicines, may be promising antiviral compounds, even though we do not understand the inhibitory mechanisms of these drugs on certain viruses *in vitro* or *in vivo*.

3. References

Gao, W.-N., Wei, D.-Q., Li, Y., Gao, H., Xu, W. -R., Li, A.-X., et al. (2007). Agaritine and its derivatives are potential inhibitors against HIV proteases. *Medicinal Chemistry*, Vol. 3, pp. 221-226

Koge, T., Komatsu, W. & Sorimachi, K. (2011). Heat Stability of agartitine in water extracts from Agaricus blazei and other edible fungi, and removal of agaritine by ethanol fractionation. Food Chemistry, Vol. 126, No. 3, pp. 1172-1177.

Simizu, B. & Terasima, T. (Eds.). (1987). *VERO CELLS - Origin, Properties and Biological Applications*. Department of Microbiology, School of Medicine, Chiba University, Soft Science Publications, Tokyo, Japan

Sorimachi, K., Niwa, A., Yamazaki, S., Toda, S. & Yasumura, Y. (1990). Anti-viral activity of water-solubilized lignin derivatives in vitro. *Agricultural and Biological Chemistry*, Vol. 54, No. 5, pp. 1337-1339.

Sorimachi, K., Ikehara, Y., Maezato, G., Okubo, A., Yamazaki, S., Akimoto, K. & Niwa, A. (2001). Inhibition by *Agaricus blazei* Murill fractions of cytophathic effect induced by western equine encephalitis (WEE) virus on VERO cells in vitro. *Bioscence, Biotechnology and Biochemistry*, Vol. 65, No. 7, pp. 1645-1647.

Suzuki, H., Okubo, A., Yamazaki, S., Suzuki, K., Mitsuya, H. & Toda, S. (1989a). Inhibition of the infectivity and cytophathic effect of human immunodeficiency virus by water-soluble lignin in an extract of the culture medium of *Lentinus edodes* mycelia (LEM). *Biochemical and Biophysical Research Communications*, Vol. 160, No. 1, pp. 3369-3372.

Suzuki, H., Tochikura, T.S., Iiyama, K., Yamazaki, S., Yamamoto, N. & Toda, S. (1989b). Lignosulfonate, a water-solubilized lignin from the waste liquor of pulping process, inhibits the infectivity and cytophatic effect of human immunodeficiency virus in vitro. *Agricultural and Biological Chemistry*, Vol. 53, No. 12, pp. 1201-1215.

Yasumura, Y. & Kawakita, Y. (1963). Studies on SV40 in tissue culture – Preliminary step for cancer research in vitro. *Nihon Rinsho* (in Japanese), Vol. 21, No. 6, pp. 1201-1215

Yasumura, Y., Niwa, A. & Yamamoto, K. (1978). Phenotypic requirement for glutamine of kidney cells and for glutamine and arginine of liver cells in culture. In: *Nutritional Requirements of Culture Cells*, H. Katsuta (Ed.), Japan Sci. Soc. Press, Tokyo and University Park Press, Baltimore, pp. 223-255